From Hunger to Malnutrition

The Political Economy of Scientific Knowledge in Europe, 1918-1960

AF793843

P.I.E. Peter Lang

Bruxelles • Bern • Berlin • Frankfurt am Main • New York • Oxford • Wien

Josep L. Barona

From Hunger to Malnutrition

The Political Economy of Scientific Knowledge in Europe, 1918-1960

European Food Issues
n° 3

This book is sponsored by the Spanish Ministry of Science and Technology [Sanidad Internacional y transferencia de conocimiento científico. Europa 1900-1975, MICINN, HAR2011-23233]

Cover Picture : "Sanidad y Asistencia Social", Vicente Ballester Marco, Universitat de València

No part of this book may be reproduced in any form, by print, photocopy, microfilm or any other means, without prior written permission from the publisher. All rights reserved.

© P.I.E. PETER LANG S.A.
Éditions scientifiques internationales
Brussels, 2012
1 avenue Maurice, B-1050 Brussels, Belgique
www.peterlang.com ; info@peterlang.com

ISSN 2033-7892
ISBN 978-90-5201-856-0

D/2012/5678/51

Library of Congress Cataloging-in-Publication Data
Barona Vilar, Josep Lluis.
From hunger to malnutrition : the political economy of scientific knowledge in Europe, 1818-1960 / Josep L. Barona.
p. cm. — (European food issues, 2033-7892 ; no.3)
Includes bibliographical references and index.
ISBN 978-90-5201-856-0 (alk. paper)
1. Food supply—Europe—History. 2. Diet—Europe—History. 3. Nutrition—Europe—History. I. Title.
HD9015.A2B37 2012 363.8094'09041—dc23 2012020322

Bibliographic information published by "Die Deutsche Nationalbibliothek"
"Die Deutsche Nationalbibliothek" lists this publication in the "Deutsche National-bibliografie"; detailed bibliographic data is available on the Internet at <http://dnb.d-nb.de>.

*This book is devoted to the memory of the two most generous people
I ever met, José Barona Alcalá and Carmen Vilar Sanchis.
They were child survivors of wartime nutrition.*

Contents

Acknowledgements

This book is a result of research on the historical relations between hunger and health in contemporary Europe. It has benefited in the past from the support of the Spanish Ministry of Science and Innovation[1] and is part of a research project on *International Health and the Transfer of Scientific Knowledge in Europe (1900-1975)*. I have had the opportunity to discuss particular aspects of the book, such as the role of international agencies and the rural perspective, thanks to the Bergen Workshops on Health and Medicine. The author is most grateful to B. Pejovic, former archivist of the League of Nations Archives (Geneva), Laura Rinovatti, a librarian at the David Lubin Memorial Library FAO (Rome), as well as Fabio Ciccarello and Giuliano Fregoli, archivists at the Records and Archives Department of the FAO.

I am grateful to Rengenier Rittersma, the editor of the journal *Food and History*, for the discussion about particular aspects regarding experimental research on the physiology of nutrition. With Peter Scholliers (Institute for Food Studies, Free University, Brussels) I had the opportunity to address the historiographical aspects and new trends in historical research on food and diets. With Steve Sturdy (Science, Technology and Innovation Studies, University of Edinburgh), Astri Andresen and Tore Grønlie (History of Health and Medicine research group, University of Bergen), I discussed the historiography and methodological aspects of the transfer of scientific knowledge in health and medicine. Bartolomé Yun-Casalilla (Department of History and Civilisation, European University Institute, Florence) lent me his support in the final writing of the book, including long conversations on historiographical issues. Mark Harrison (Wellcome Unit for the History of Medicine, Oxford) accompanied me to the facilities at Oxford and to the patient discussions in master seminars, while Josep Bernabeu (Universitat d'Alacant) and Ximo Guillem (Universitat de València) also provided constant support, sharing valuable comments and encouragement. Some particular aspects benefited from discussions at

1 Research projects, *La lucha contra la desnutrición en la España contemporánea y el contexto internacional, 1874-1975*, Ministerio de Ciencia e Innovación (HAR2009-13504-C02-01); *La sanidad española en el contexto internacional: conferencias sanitarias, sociedad de naciones y organismos internacionales (1851-1975).* Ministerio de Educación y Ciencia (HUM200606098/HIST).

the Wellcome Unit for the History of Medicine, Oxford and at the Department of Anthropology, History, Cultural Sciences and Religion, University of Bergen, Norway. I want to thank Elisa Cuenca for her support with the linguistic review. This book is sponsored by the Spanish Ministry of Science and Technology [*Sanidad Internacional y transferencia de conocimiento científico. Europa 1900-1975*, MICINN, HAR2011-23233].

The most important question today is whether man has attained the wisdom to adjust the old systems to suit the new powers of science and to realize that we are now one world in which all nations will ultimately share the same fate.

Lord John Boyd Orr, *As I Recall*.
London, MacGibbon & Kee, 1966, p. 288.

CHAPTER 1

Hunger in Europe

Hunger and Health: a Discussion

Hunger and nutrition are essential components of individual and public health, as well as main factors for the economy, social peace and people's wellbeing. Nowadays the availability of foodstuffs represents one of the main challenges for the United Nations, as serious shortages affect wide regions in the world, with famine and malnutrition still a terrible plight. In Europe and other parts of the world, after decades of economic growth and globalisation of the food market, a portion of humankind has achieved good nutritional standards, according to clinical and scientific patterns, as well as satisfactory levels of individual and social wellbeing. Although this statement is permanently threatened by the evolution of the chronic crisis that started in 2008, and the future of the welfare state is debatable, one can accept that the European model is still at work and that access to food constitutes a legally accepted human right. Conversely, poverty and malnutrition still pose tremendous problems for millions of human beings on most continents. At present, Europe is the most tangible exception.

A quick overview of the global situation shows that at the beginning of the 21st century about 30% of children under the age of five still suffer from severe malnutrition.[1] Ever since the inter-war period, international agencies have warned about the extension of hunger and the risk associated with chronic deficient nutrition for public health and international stability. The latest reports by the *Standing Committee on Nutrition* of the United Nations raise an alert about the consequences of persisting malnutrition[2] and call for globalised nutritional health to be the starting point of the implementation of human rights and the extension of democracy. Access to food is therefore a responsibility for the international community and national governments. Hunger has now

1 On the prevalence of malnutrition affecting child populations and present global tendencies, see De Onís, M., Blössner, M., "The World Health Organization Global Database on Child Growth and Malnutrition: methodology and applications", *International Journal of Epidemiology*, No. 32, 2003, pp. 518-526.

2 http://www.unscn.org/

become an intolerable load for poor and developing countries;[3] it is one of the main obstacles to progress and wellbeing and the largest hindrance to social, cultural and economic growth in many countries in Africa, Asia and Latin America.

It is generally admitted that the fight against hunger by European governments and other Western institutions started in the 19th century. Although the traditional demographic crisis caused by famine decreased from the central decades of the 19th century, health problems associated with hunger, famine and malnutrition persisted up until the second half of the 20th century due to international conflicts, political and economic crises, as well as the effects of war and post-war depression. Factors that caused hunger and the food supply to remain big issues during the first half of the 20th century included political tensions, financial and economic crises, unemployment, trade protectionist barriers, as well as national, regional and international wars.[4]

In an earlier context, famine and starvation hit most European territories between 1846 and 1848. The great famine that shook the Irish between 1845 and 1849[5] must also be noted. The destruction of the Global Food Market, which had been built during the second half of the 19th century, was one of the outcomes of international conflicts in the first decades of the 20th century. Its negative consequences affected the most vulnerable sectors of the population, such as children, women and the elderly. These groups, together with the unemployed, those living in the country and other citizens, fell prey to marginality. They became the victims of alimentary deficiencies, starvation, chronic malnutrition and several health problems caused by the international blockade, difficulties in the food supply and extended conflicts. War was a fundamental and usual cause of famine and malnutrition in the first half of the 20th century, and the examples of Russia (1919), Ukraine (1932-33), Greece (1941-42) and The Netherlands (1944-45) illustrate the reach of the problem. Although the political, social and economic

---

3 Svedberg, P., *Poverty and undernutrition. Theory, measurement, and policy. With a foreword by Amartya Sen*, Oxford, Oxford University Press, 2000; Bhargava A., *Food, economics, and health*, Oxford, Oxford University Press, 2008.

4 Bengtsson, T., Saito, O. (eds.), *Population and economy. From hunger to modern economic growth*, Oxford, Oxford University Press, 2000. About famine and starvation, a global perspective could be found in Ó Gráda, C., *Famine: A Short History*, Princeton, Princeton University Press, 2009.

5 Mokyr, J., Ó Gráda, C., "What do people die of during famines: the Great Irish Famine in comparative perspective", *European Review of Economic History*, No. 6, 2002, pp. 339-363; Lindeboom, F., Portrait, F., Van den Berg, G.J., "Long-run effects on longevity of a nutritional shock early in life: the Dutch Potato Famine of 1846-1847", *International Journal of Epidemiology*, No. 29, 2010, pp. 617-629.

consequences of war were possibly the most important causes behind famine and malnutrition in Europe during the middle decades of the 20th century, the wrong agricultural policies, isolation and totalitarianism also contributed to reinforcing the problem.[6]

From Demographic to Nutritional Transition

Historical research on hunger and nutrition has taken on different historiographical orientations. Economic history and historical demography have been traditional approaches when carrying out research on hunger and nutrition, and are considered to be factors that influence the productivity, disease and mortality that condition the demographic evolution, growth and decrease of a population.[7] The concept of *nutritional transition* has been recently introduced by economy historians to express the importance of nutrition and diet as a meaningful factor in the changes in living standards during the social development of Western societies in the 20th century. The idea of a *nutritional transition* has added a new perspective to the process of modernisation experienced by Western societies in the 19th and 20th centuries. Prior to that, the concept of *demographic transition* had been proposed and generally introduced into historiography as a useful historiographical tool since the middle decades of the last century. The process of *demographic transition* helped to explain the changes identified in the internal structure of the populations during the modernisation period, as a consequence of changes in mortality, fertility and life expectancy.

Later, the idea of an *epidemiologic transition* underlying demographic changes pointed to specific transformations in the patterns of dominant diseases, morbidity and mortality rates. The notion of *epidemiologic transition* paved the way for a more general *health transition* accompanied by a *transition of risks* resulting from the spread of medical technologies, the urban/rural divide, agricultural/industrial societies, labour structure, health care organisation, sanitary campaigns, life expectancy and other social transformations affecting the levels of health and the way in which disease, as a social reality, appears at a specific time and place.

With the aim of explaining the transition followed by industrialised societies, economy and demography historians suggested in the 1990s

---

6 Sen, A., *Poverty and Famines: An Essay on Entitlements and Deprivation*, Oxford, Clarendon Press, 1982.

7 Livi-Bacci, M., *Population and Nutrition: An Essay on European Demographic History*, Cambridge, Cambridge University Press, 1991.

the idea of a *nutritional transition*, which would have taken place simultaneously to the demographic and epidemiologic transitions, directly related to the availability of foodstuffs and the changes experienced in the composition of diets among the different social groups. Obviously, the idea of a transition to modernisation from any other form of traditional society, as defined by historiography, implies the acceptance of a common pattern in the process of evolution of any society regarding the changes experienced by the structure of the population, the standards of health and the dietary habits. All countries, since the end of the 18th century, would have followed the same evolution at different speeds, something that could be accepted for the greater picture but which had to be discussed for each particular factor and context. To a great extent, those models of transition were proposed not only to explain past and present issues, but also to foresee and successfully face future challenges. The picture they showed aimed to draft economic, social and health policies in order to reduce deficiencies and inequalities in the standards of living of the Western population after World War II, especially in poor regions.[8]

Since transitional patterns include a prospective target as a practical tool to analyse future tendencies and shape new political strategies to improve nutritional and living standards, the definition of factors influencing social development – apart from the level of income and economic growth – has become increasingly essential. Demographic and health problems after World War II in countries with slow economic growth pointed out the necessity of taking into consideration any variable factor influencing the health status of the population, with the evolution of the income level proving insufficient to explain the transitional processes. Housing, environmental conditions, access to foodstuffs, the amount and composition of the diet, medical technologies, hygiene, levels of education and cultural habits appeared as complementary factors. This was confirmed by the inability of more simple indicators such as the levels of income and economic growth to explain the evolution of health improvements.[9] A wider approach that

8 Nicolau Nos, R., Pujol Andreu, J., "Los factores condicionantes de la transición nutricional en la Europa Occidental: Barcelona, 1890-1936", *Scripta Nova: Revista Electrónica de Geografía y Ciencias Sociales*, No. 12, 2008, pp. 256-265; Nicolau, R., Pujol-Andreu, J. "Aspectos políticos y científicos del Modelo de la Transición Nutricional: evaluación crítica y nuevas perspectivas", in Bernabeu-Mestre, J., Barona, J.L. (eds.), *Nutrición, Salud y Sociedad. España y Europa en los siglos XIX-XX*, Valencia, SEC/PUV, 2011, pp. 19-58.

9 Bernabeu-Mestre, J., Perdiguero, E., Barona, J.L., "Determinanti della mortalità infantile e transizione sanitaria. Una riflessiones a partire dall'esperienza spagnola",

included not only simple economic factors was required and at least three groups of factors were considered as influencing the evolution of health: environmental and cultural conditions; the health care service/system and social assistance organisation; and techno-scientific improvements, not only in medical therapy and prevention technologies but also in food production, agricultural modernisation, industrialisation of food production, distribution channels, global access and dietary habits.

Considering the fact that all these factors have changed over time and that they vary across countries, different patterns of transition have been accepted, which means that the idea of a *nutritional transition* that includes all such factors appears to be more complex nowadays than the previous approach based on demographic, epidemiologic and sanitary features. However, demographic, epidemiologic, sanitary, risk and nutritional transitions were proposed in different contexts according to the availability of records on the evolution of mortality and birth rates, causes of death and disease, access to foodstuffs and composition of the diet. Usually, such records were reported for a very specific group of developed countries and forecasts were made about the future evolution of the population, health and diet in other countries with more deficient statistics and also in poor countries that lack reliable records. Is this type of projection a solid instrument to analyse and foresee what is going on in those countries?

It is worth highlighting the political dimension of the transitional patterns proposed by recent historiography as a reference for political strategies aimed at reducing tensions, managing demographic pressure and facing foodstuff crises during the inter-war years and the period after World War II. Those models served as a reference for programmes of stabilisation during the Cold War, a period characterised by demographic expansion and a shortage of food in many regions. At the same time, we should keep in mind that a decolonisation process was taking place mostly in Africa and Asia. In this context, Theodor W. Schultz proposed, for the first time, the idea of a nutritional transition in his book *Food for the World.*[10] The book summarised the conclusions of a famous meeting held in Chicago before the end of the war in order to discuss the situation of the global food market and the prospects for the production of foodstuffs during the post-war years. This influential

Salute, Malattia e Sopravivenza in Italia fra '800 e '900, Udinde, Forum, 2007, pp. 175-193.

10 Schultz, Th.W., *Food for the World*, Chicago, Chicago University Press, 1945.

meeting was to give impulse to the creation of the Food and Agriculture Organization (FAO).

In this meeting, Frank W. Notestein discussed the importance of the world demographic situation. He focused the challenge on the possibility of a slow reproduction of the Western demographic evolution in other countries and continents by anticipating the capacity to accelerate changes in countries with low economic growth if certain policies were implemented. Based on few demographic records, he identified the demographic situation in different countries, making a projection of the evolution of the population in large regions in the world, as well as the demands for foodstuffs derived from it in future times. The definition of a demographic transition, conceived as a global process, was soon introduced into the academic sphere and served as a tool of analysis for international and national agencies. Initially, mortality was the nuclear factor considered, but fecundity soon occupied the central place, since the need to stop and control the growth of the population in industrialised countries was pressing.

In the early 1970s the idea of an *epidemiologic transition* stressed the importance of concepts such as social dominant diseases, death causes and fertility rates as influential factors for social change.[11] The idea of an epidemiologic and sanitary transition was defined after World War II in industrialised countries, which were characterised by a decrease in overall mortality, child mortality and infant mortality as a consequence of a reduction in infectious diseases accompanied by a rise in life expectancy. Non-infectious diseases and accidents emerged as major social health problems. In societies where traditional plagues had been controlled (mainly through better feeding, sanitation systems, housing and medical preventive technologies), chronic infectious diseases such as tuberculosis, typhoid fever, malaria and venereal diseases were substituted as socially dominant diseases by cancer, heart attacks, strokes and traffic and industrial accidents as main causes of death and invalidity. Obviously, the higher life expectancy had an influence as well on the growing importance of degenerative diseases and vascular accidents.

Epidemiologic and health transitions are considered to be paths followed by all societies, regardless of their pace of evolution. However, they were probably faster on continents other than Europe, as a consequence of the implementation of medical technologies and immunisation campaigns. But predictions failed as a result of the critical

---

11 Omran, A.R., "The Epidemiologic Transition. A Theory of the Epidemiology of Population Change", *The Milbank Quarterly*, No. 83, 1971, pp. 731-757.

ending of the Cold War, and the effects of the globalisation process led to a delay in the evolution of Eastern European countries and to a terrible situation in Africa. A new crisis broke out: new emergent virus diseases, such as AIDS, and life expectancy fell dramatically in wide regions of the planet.[12]

The *nutritional transition* pattern proposed by economic historians and demographers added the crucial importance of nutrition and diets to explain social change. The radical effects of structural and cyclical famines that affected populations during the *Ancien Régime* have been widely acknowledged by traditional historiography. Those famines were the cause of the high mortality rates and the main factor behind the demographic catastrophe, contributing to the stagnant population model. The demographic and epidemiologic transition did coincide with a reduction in hunger and famine, as well as the agricultural expansion and the shaping of a global food market.[13] Records on food consumption, the content and variety of diets, food availability, dietary habits, as well as other aspects such as the height of the population and the labour structure, contributed a great deal of information about the effects of nutrition and diet over the population and the several diseases associated with nutritional deficiencies.

Recent research on the nutritional transition in non-Western countries has shown the quick spread of changes in diet in many countries in Asia, Africa and America. From a purely demographic and economic perspective, any nutritional deficiency, malnutrition, overfeeding, industrial production of foodstuffs and regulation of food quality have become a matter of concern under critical situations in which high rates of demographic growth and nutritional deficiencies threaten millions of lives. Nutrition requires not only a healthy diet based on enough food, but also social, cultural and economic policies.

The evolution of the level of income, and the economic growth experienced by many countries and world regions, are not sufficient arguments to explain the social change identified by historians under the concepts of demographic, epidemiologic, health and nutritional transitions during the second half of the 20th century in Europe. In a complementary way, it is essential to consider, as a main factor, the role of the social agents: international institutions, experts, scientists, practitioners, governments, industry, propaganda, housewives and cooking habits. All of them play a part in the reduction of social

---

12 Barona, J.L., *Salud, tecnología y saber médico*, Madrid, Ed. Ramón Areces, 2004.

13 Popkin, B., *The World Is Fat: The Fads, Trends, Policies, and Products That Are Fattening the Human Race*, New York, Avery-Penguin Press, 2008.

inequalities. The evolution of the levels of income – though an important factor – represents just one of the multiple factors that influence health, nutritional status and diet.

The European pattern of social change that we have named *nutritional transition* adopted different shapes and chronologies in the different countries. In the case of Spain, it achieved a degree of modernisation during the course of the 20th century, consolidating the process of nutrition and diet transition by the 1970s.[14] Other countries went through the process faster. The problems associated with a deficient diet and malnutrition had been overcome, with obesity emerging as a new threat. Like in most European countries, the nutritional transition from scarcity to overfeeding started in the 1920s and 1930s. But in the case of Spain, chronic malnutrition affected large sectors of the population as a consequence of the Civil War (1936-1939) and the post-war years.[15]

In the late 1940s the nutritional landscape of the Spanish population was still a poor one, as we shall discuss in a further chapter. A low calorie and protein intake, marked by low quality proteins of vegetable origin and a shortage of calcium and vitamins, made up the overall picture. In this particular case, the decade of the 1950s was a crucial stage. In the late 1950s and early 1960s the *Escuela de Bromatología* [School of Bromatology] in Madrid carried out research into the Spanish diet and concluded that a small part of the population still had an insufficient calorie intake, whilst 40 per cent of the population consumed too many calories.[16] The total protein intake was adequate, mainly of vegetable origin, although significant deficiencies were still present regarding the intake of vitamins.[17] Agricultural labourers and industrial workers were identified as the social groups that had the worst diet. In fact, the rural surveys carried out during the 1960s showed that the consumption of proteins was no longer deficient but in rural areas

---

14 Bernabeu-Mestre, J. *et al.*, "Nutrition and public health in the contemporary Spain, 1900-1936", *Food and History*, No. 6, 2008, pp. 167-192; Moreno, L.A., Sarría, A., Popkin, B.M., "The nutrition transition in Spain: a European Mediterranean country", *European Journal of Clinical Nutrition*, No. 56, 2002, pp. 992-1003.

15 Bengoa Lacanda, J.M., "Historia de la nutrición en salud pública", in Serra Majem, L., Aranceta, J. (eds.), *Nutrición y salud pública. Métodos, Bases científicas y Aplicaciones*, Barcelona, 2006, pp. 52-61.

16 Bernabeu, 2008, pp. 123-132.

17 *Ibidem*.

the majority of proteins were of vegetable origin, a low intake of calcium affecting most of the population.[18]

According to current research, by the end of the 1960s the population in Western European countries was able to meet their energy, protein and most of their micronutrient requirements, and their caloric profile reflected almost perfectly the recommendations of international organisations.[19] Carbohydrates accounted for 53 per cent of the caloric intake, proteins 12 per cent, and lipids 32 per cent. Between 1940 and 1960 the European nutritional picture shifted from the existence of significant nutritional deficiencies caused by the economic crisis, war and post-war periods, with an insufficient protein intake and severe mineral and vitamin deficiencies, to a tendency characterised by an excessive dietary intake of calories, sugar and fats. The situation worsened with the rise of a more sedentary lifestyle and its subsequently reduced energy needs. Meanwhile, the caloric intake increased at the expense of simple carbohydrates, leading to a significant rise in obesity and diabetes. The consumption of meat per person showed the most spectacular increase, particularly pork and poultry.

These changes in the diet of Europeans during the middle decades of the 20th century have been analysed in recent historical contributions, some of them taking into consideration the plurality of agents involved in the nutritional transition process.[20] These include the role played by

18 Graciani, A., Rodríguez Artalejo, F., Banegas, M.J.R., Hernández Vecino, R., Rey Calero, *Consumo de alimentos en España en el período 1940-1988*, Madrid, 1986; Villalbí, J.R., Maldonado, R., "La alimentación de la población en España desde la posguerra hasta los años ochenta: una revisión crítica de las encuestas de nutrición", *Med Clin Barc*, No. 90, 1988, pp. 127-130, p. 128.

19 Grigg, D., "The nutritional transition in western Europe", *Journal of Historical Geography*, No. 22, 1995, pp. 247-261. For Spain see Cussó Segura, X., Garrobou, R., "La transición nutricional en la España contemporánea: las variaciones en el consumo de pan, patatas y legumbres", *Investigaciones de Historia Economica*, No. 7, 2007, pp. 69-100, p. 97.

20 Cussó Segura, X., "Estado nutritivo de la población española, 1900-1970: análisis de las necesidades y disponibilidades de nutrientes", *Revista de Agricultura e Historia Rural*, No. 36, 2005, pp. 329-358; Cussó Segura, X., Garrobou, R., "La transición nutricional en la España contemporánea: las variaciones en el consumo de pan, patatas y legumbres (1850-2000), *Investigaciones de Historia Económica*, No. 7, 2004, pp. pp. 69-100; Langreo, A., Pujol Andreu, J., "Evolución económica agroalimentaria", *Como vivíamos: alimentos y alimentación en la España del siglo XX*, Madrid, 2007, pp. 41-66; Nicolau Nos, R., Pujol Andreu, J., "Los factores condicionantes de la transición nutricional en la Europa Occidental: Barcelona, 1890-1936", *Scripta Nova: Revista Electrónica de Geografía y Ciencias Sociales*, No. 12, 2008, pp. 256-265.

living conditions,[21] research on anthropometric indicators,[22] cultural factors such as body image or the impact of education, advertising and propaganda,[23] local and state policies, institutional strategies and other studies addressing issues related to food policy.[24]

This recent research gives an insight into the effects of industrialisation, increasing urban growth, women's entry into the labour force and evidence of the changes in dietary habits. The availability of foodstuffs varied widely as a consequence of technological innovations and industrialisation in agriculture. Milk, chocolate, oil, wine, fruit and vegetables and other products all added to the growing impact of the food industry.[25]

The previous arguments show that nutrition has increasingly become an interdisciplinary field of historical research. Traditionally, it was oriented in two main directions. One regarded several aspects of public health, considering the population's nutritional state to be the most important issue. From this perspective, the content of the diet in rural and urban contexts, its change and evolution, and the detection of malnutrition and deficiency diseases, have contributed to the understanding of the *nutritional transition* and its demographic and epidemiologic impact. From this viewpoint, the production, circulation and spread of scientific knowledge, and the role of expertise and the nutritional education of the population, clearly became more and more

---

21 Simón Pérez, H.J., Escudero, A., "El bienestar en España: una perspectiva de largo plazo, 1850-1991", *Revista de historia económica*, No. 2, 2003, pp. 525-566.

22 Martinez Carrión, J.M., "Biología, historia y medio ambiente: la estatura como espejo del nivel de vida de la sociedad española", *Ayer. Revista de Historia Contemporánea* (monographic issue on*: "Naturaleza y conflicto social")*, No. 46, 2002, pp. 93-122; Martínez Carrión, J.M., "El nivel de vida en la España rural. Siglos XVIII-XX. Nuevos enfoques, nuevos resultados", in Martínez Carrión, J.M., Pérez Castejón, J.J. (eds.), *El nivel de vida en la España rural, siglos XVIII-XX*, Alicante, 2002, pp. 15-72; "La Historia Antropométrica y la historiografía iberoamericana", *Historia Agraria*, No. 19 (monograph number 47).

23 Velasco, C., Rodergas, R., "Los productos alimenticios y la publicidad", *Como vivíamos: alimentos y alimentación en la España del siglo* XX, Madrid, 2007, pp. 119-138.

24 Bernabeu 2008; Barciela López, C., *Ni un español sin pan: la Red Nacional de Silos y Graneros*, Zaragoza, 2007.

25 Guillem-Llobat, X., "Food quality controls in the European Periphery. Valencian scientists and laboratories in the late nineteenth century", in Simon, J. *et al.* (eds.), *Beyond Borders: Fresh perspectives in history of science*, Cambridge, Cambridge Scholars Publishing, 2008d, pp. 301-324; Guillem-Llobat, X., "Losing the global view in the establishment of new limits to food quality. The regulation of the food market in Spain (1880-1936)", *Food & History*, No. 6, 2008e, pp. 215-246.

important, especially in terms of the history of public health.[26] This trend included not only health and demographic features, and social and institutional spheres, but also the role of cultural habits and social values from a more dynamic and anthropological perspective.

The other main historiography trend comes from economic history and focuses on agricultural policies, food production and consumption, distribution and availability of foodstuffs and their influence on the economy, trade and the market.[27] This orientation also included research into socio-economic factors,[28] standards of living, the role played by food and nutrition in the diet,[29] studies of anthropometric indicators such as a synthetic index of well-being that tries to express the quality of the nutritional state,[30] or analyses of the influence of socio-cultural factors, such as body image or the impact of advertising, among others.[31]

---

26 Barona, J.L., "Nutrition, knowledge, and action. International trends and social policies in Spain, 1931-1944", in Andresen, A, Groenlie, T. (eds.), *Transferring Medico-Political Knowledge in 19th and 20th Century Europe*, Bergen, Stein Rokkan Centre for Social Studies, 2007, pp. 91-108; Borowy, I., Grüner, W.D. (eds.), *Facing Illness in Troubled Times. Health in Europe in the Interwar Years 1918-1939*, Frankfurt, Peter Lang, 2005; Cura, M.I. del, Huertas, R., *Alimentación y enfermedad en tiempos de hambre. España, 1937-1947*, Madrid, CSIC, 2007; Kamminga, H., Cunningham, A., *The Science and Culture of Nutrition (1840-1940)*, Amsterdam, Rodopi, 1997.

27 Caplan, P. (ed.), *Food, Health and Identity*, London, Routledge, 1997; in Daunton, M., Hilton, M. (eds.), *The Politics of Consumption: Material Culture and Citizenship in Europe and America*, Oxford, 2001; Davis, R., Wheatcroft, S., *The Years of Hunger*, Basingstoke, Palgrave, 2004; Slater, D., *Consumer Culture and Modernity*, Cambridge, 1997; Smith, D.F., "The rise and fall of the Scientific Food Committee during the Second World War", in Smith, D.F., Phillips, J. (eds.), *Food, Science, Policy and Regulation in the Twentieth Century. International and Comparative Perspectives*, London, Routledge, 2000; Steckel, R.H., Rose J.C. (eds.), *The Backbone of History. Health and Nutrition in the Western Hemisphere*, Cambridge, Cambridge University Press, 2002; Trentmann, F., Just, F. (eds.), *Food and Conflict in Europe in the Age of the Two World Wars*, New York, Palgrave, 2006.

28 Cussó Segura, X., "Estado nutritivo de la población española, 1900-1970: análisis de las necesidades y disponibilidades de nutrientes", *Revista de Agricultura e Historia Rural*, No. 36, 2005, pp. 329-358; Cussó Segura, X., Garrobou, R., "La transición nutricional en la España, pp. 69-100; Langreo, A., Pujol Andreu, J., "Evolución económica agroalimentaria", *Como vivíamos: alimentos y alimentación en la España del siglo XX*, Madrid, Lunwerg, 2007, pp. 41-66; Nicolau Nos, R., Pujol Andreu, J., "Los factores condicionantes de la transición nutricional en la Europa Occidental: Barcelona, 1890-1936", *Scripta Nova: Revista Electrónica de Geografía y Ciencias Sociales*, No. 12, 2008, pp. 256-265.

29 Simón Pérez, H.J., Escudero, A., "El bienestar en España: una perspectiva de largo plazo, 1850-1991", *Revista de Historia Económica*, No. 2, 2003, pp. 525-566.

30 Martínez Carrión, J.M., "Biología, historia y medio ambiente: la estatura como espejo del nivel de vida de la sociedad española", *Ayer*, No. 46, 2002, pp. 93-122;

At the same time, the diversity of experience and the importance of the local context have been shown to be among the most significant features of the variability in the nutritional transition process. In addition to anthropometric studies intended to show the relationship between height, weight and the environmental conditions that determine nutrition,32 the differences that had long been observed between urban and rural settings were noted as indicative of wider access to food in urban centres. Difficulties were also reported in the consumption of animal proteins, particularly milk and dairy products, in some European regions.33

Nutrition and Organic Development

Going back to the anthropometric approach, a lot of historical literature has outlined the links between nutrition, health and body height.[34] From the mid 19th century onwards physical anthropologists, general practitioners and paediatricians applied anthropometric measures in order to lay out standards of human development.[35] At the end of the 20th century economic historians developed a new methodological orientation: *anthropometric history*, taking human height as an indicator of wellbeing and social development. The industrial revolution contributed towards changing the social circumstances, the economy, the environment, housing, habits, diet, working conditions; and all of these elements became influential factors

---

Martínez Carrión, J.M, "El nivel de vida en la España rural. Siglos XVIII-XX. Nuevos enfoques, nuevos resultados", in Martínez Carrión, J.M, Pérez Castejón, J.J. (eds.), *El nivel de vida en la España rural, siglos XVIII-XX*, Alicante, Universidad de Alicante, pp. 15-72.

31 Velasco, C., Rodergas, R., "Los productos alimenticios y la publicidad", *Como vivíamos: alimentos y alimentación en la España del siglo XX*, Madrid, Lunwerg, 2007, pp. 119-138.

32 Beneito, A., Puche Gil, J., "Creixement econòmic i desenvolupament fabril en Alcoi, 1840-1915: Misèria fisiològica sota l'esplendor industrial?", *La societat industrial al País Valencià*, Alcoi, 2008.

33 Nicolau Nos, R., Pujol Andreu, J., "Variaciones regionales de los precios de consumo y de las dietas en España, en los inicios de la transición demográfica", *Documents de Treball* (UAB. Unitat d'Història Econòmica), No. 29, 2005.

34 Tanner, J.M., "Growth as a mirror of conditions in society", Lindgren, G. (ed.), *Growth as a mirror of conditions in society*, Stockholm, Stockholm Institute Education Press, 1990, pp. 9-70; Steckel, R.H., "Stature and the standard of living", *Journal of Economic Literature*, No. 33, 1995, pp. 1903-1940; Bodszár, É., Susanne, Ch. (eds.), *Secular growth changes in Europe*, Budapest, Eötvös University Press, 1998.

35 Barona, J.L., "Defining patterns of normality in children's health 1914-1945", Bergen, Bergen Workshop History of Medicine and Health, 2011.

for bodily development.[36] From this bio-somatic perspective, the achievement of a balanced diet, based on the regular consumption of energy and nutrients, influenced body size and height.[37] Alleging that the demographic transition had caused fertility to fall, and that the epidemiologic phase had put an end to avoidable premature deaths, anthropometric historians argued that the nutritional transition had led to an increase in the size of the European population of more than ten centimetres on average in the 20th century.[38] Nevertheless, anthropometric models show that this increase did not follow a linear tendency. On the contrary, some periods of height decrease and impairment have been associated with agricultural crises, demographic pressures and degraded living conditions in unhygienic industrialised areas – among other negative factors influencing the start of the modern economic growth.[39]

Establishing statistical relations between body height, level of income, education and life expectancy, anthropometric history has proposed quantitative parameters to assess biological wellbeing.[40] It argues that a high level of income, a positive environment and a healthy lifestyle correlate positively with height, education and longevity, but negatively with infant and child mortality. In addition to genetic inheritance, anthropometry has shown that changes in height over several generations express a tendency related to nutrition during childhood and adolescence.[41]

---

36 Komlos, J. "Anthropometric history: an overview of a quarter century of research", *Anthropologischer Anzeiger*, No. 67, 2009, pp. 341-356; Steckel, R.H., "Heights and human welfare: Recent developments and new directions", *Explorations in Economic History*, No. 46, 2009, pp. 1-23.

37 Caballero, B., Popkin, B.M. (eds.), *The Nutrition Transition: Diet and Disease in the Developing World*, London, Academic Press, 2002; Popkin, 2008.

38 One of the first researches on the evolution of height among Europeans based on military records and national statistics was Chamla, M.C., "L'accroissement de la stature en France de 1880 a 1960; comparaison avec les pays d'Europe occidentale", *Bulletins et Mémoires de la Société d'Anthropologie de Paris*, No. 6, 1964, pp. 201-278.

39 Komlos, 2009, pp. 341-356; Steckel, 2009, pp. 1-23.

40 Komlos, J. (ed.), *The biological standard of living on three continental. Further explorations in anthropometric history*, Oxford, Westview Press, 1995; Komlos, J., Baten, J. (eds.), "Recent research in Anthropometric History", *Social Science History*, No. 28, 2004, number 2, special issue, pp. 191-350; Steckel, R.H., "Biological Measures of the Standard of Living", *Journal of Economic Perspectives*, No. 22, 2008, pp. 129-152.

41 Tanner, J.M., *A history of the study of human growth*, Cambridge, Cambridge University Press, 1981.

Nutrition has become a central issue in explaining social development. Economic historians have emphasised that the positive correlation of nutrition with public health improving the nutritional state of the population also reduces the health care budget, improves the perception of wellbeing and increases productivity.[42] From a complementary perspective, the economist Angus Deaton associates the nutritional condition acquired in childhood with mental and physical health, especially for the elderly.[43] Moreover, good health in childhood correlates positively with success in school and better employment.[44] This is something not only assumed by public health experts and economists, but also by governments and institutional authorities.[45]

Since the 1990s economic historians have sampled large amounts of records on soldiers' height as a way of assessing the influence of industrialisation, migration and periods of crisis upon the standard of living. Although conscription started in the 18th century, paleontologists and physical anthropologists have studied much older bodies.[46] Due to limitations related with the sources, most of this research refers to adult men, with records on women's and children's height being much scarcer. This failure was more evident until women appeared in schools, universities, hospitals and prisons, the specific places where human measurements were taken. Some of the women's records are socio-economically biased, since the main purpose of taking measurements was to see if the evolution of height in women followed the same tendency as that of men.[47] Several aspects, such as being a housewife or

---

42 Pollit, E., Gorman, K., Engle, P., Rivera J., Martorell, R., "Nutrition in early life and the fulfilment of intellectual potential", *Journal of Nutrition*, No. 125, 1995, pp. 1111-1118.

43 Deaton, A., "Height, health, and development", *Journal of Economic Literature*, No. 41, 2003, pp. 113-158; Deaton, A., Arora, R., "Life at the top: the benefits of height", *Economics and Human Biology*, No. 7, 2009, pp. 133-136; Casse, A., Paxson, Ch., "Stature and Status: Height, Ability, and Labor Market Outcomes", *Journal of Political Economy*, No. 116, 2008, pp. 499-532; Casse, A., Paxson, Ch., "Height, Health and Cognitive Function at Older Ages", *American Economic Review*, No. 98, 2008, pp. 463-467.

44 Martínez Carrión, J.M. "El estado nutricional en la Europa contemporánea. Una visión desde la historia antropomètrica", in Bernabeu-Mestre, J., Barona, J.L. (eds.), *Nutrición, Salud y Sociedad. España y Europa en los siglos XIX y XX*, Valencia, PUV/SEC, 2011, pp. 93-132.

45 Christopher Wanjek, *Food at work: workplace solutions for malnutrition, obesity and chronic diseases.* Geneva, International Labor, Organization, 2005.

46 Steckel, R.H., Rose, J.R. (eds.), *The backbone of History. Health and Nutrition in the Western Hemisfere*, Cambridge, Cambridge University Press, 2002.

47 Harris, B., "Anthropometric History, gender and the measurement of well-being", in Harris, B., Gálvez, L., Machado, H. (eds.), *Gender and Well-Being in Europe.*

a working woman, as well as the unequal distribution of foodstuffs in the diet of the family members, can introduce relevant differences. The father's preferential position as the active worker and breadwinner earned him a number of benefits in the household's distribution of foodstuffs, such as more meat, eggs and animal produce than other members of the family. Similarly, boys were positively discriminated against in relation with girls. Thus, men's height integrated more external influences than in the case of women, and was therefore more likely to be negatively affected under extreme circumstances, as has been described in situations of extreme malnutrition in internment camps.[48]

Anthropometric research has also confirmed the biological influence of social inequalities. Nutritional deficiencies were frequently caused by poverty and exclusion. General practitioners knew very well that poor nutrition led to infection and therefore medicine created the category of the pre-tubercular child, a clinical prototype common among peasantry and poor working classes in industrial areas. Until the end of the 19th century a low height in urban suburbs populated by low class non-qualified workers was attributed to chronic malnutrition. Bodily measurements were substantially better among qualified workers and the middle and upper classes.[49] At the beginning of the 19th century the poor members of the *Marine Society* in London were 130 cm tall, while the aristocratic cadets of the *Military Academy of Sandhurst* were

Historical and contemporary perspectives, Farnham, Asghate, 2009, pp. 59-84; Guntupalli, A., Baten, J., "Measuring gender well-being with biological welfare indicators", in Harris, B., Gálvez, L., Machado, H. (eds.), *Gender and Well-Being in Europe. Historical and contemporary perspectives*, Farnham, Asghate, 2009, pp. 43-58.

48 Barona, J.L. *The Problem of Nutrition*, Brussels, P.I.E. Peter Lang, 2010; Rebato, E., "Crecimiento: una visión desde la Antropología Física", *Revista Española de Antropología Física*, No. 31, 2010, pp. 85-110.

49 The German case is described in Komlos, J., Kriwy, P., "Social Status and Adult Heights in the two Germanies", *Annals of Human Biology*, No. 29, 2002, pp. 641-648 and Komlos, J., "Height and social status in 18th century Germany", *Journal of Interdisciplinary History*, No. 20, 1990, pp. 607-21; Alter, G., Neven, M., Oris, M., "Stature in Transition: A Micro-Level Study from Nineteenth-Century Belgium", *Social Science History*, No. 28, 2004, pp. 231-47.

155 cm,[50] an evident expression of social inequality. Research has shown that other European countries followed a similar pattern.[51]

The Politics of Hunger in the 20th Century

Many conflicts over nutrition, food and diet during the first half of the 20th century – an exceptional time of crisis and conflict – were influenced by social inequalities, local traditions, cultural values, social norms, state policies and failure in the trade market. The First World War was a breaking point within this context. Food and diet became the site of dynamic rearrangements between the state and new demanding groups in society. Workers' unions, revolutionary movements, consumers and an emergent civil society were linked to social and economic conflicts, changing international views and politics.[52]

As a result, the inter-war years saw a close relationship grow between national social reforms and the global restructuring of the impaired global food system. Improvements in food production – including technical innovations for mass production, new delivery systems and the necessary availability of food recognised as a human right –, together with practical aspects such as food preservation, drew a lot of attention. Cooking traditions, nutritional habits and public health were understood to be a part of a global programme in which the eradication of hunger and malnutrition as a means of improving health, especially among poor and marginalised social groups, constituted an essential element in building up a global civil society.[53]

Therefore, since the start of the 20th century, hunger, nutrition and diet became a major concern for most European governments, civil society, workers' organisations and other social and charitable entities involved in social work. Several factors were central to this process: economic ones such as food production, food industrialisation, distribution and trade, as well as those associated with quality control.[54]

---

50 Floud, R.C., Watcher, K.W., Roderick, C., "Poverty and physical stature", *Social Science History*, No. 6, 1982, pp. 422-452; Roderick, C., Floud, R.C., Watcher, K.W., Gregory, A.S., *Height, health and history: Nutritional status in Britain, 1750-1980*, Cambridge, Cambridge University Press, 1990.

51 Komlos, 1990, p. 621; Komlos, J., Baten, J. (eds.), *The Biological Standard of Living in Comparative Perspective*, Stuttgart, Franz Steiner, 1998.

52 Slater, D., *Consumer Culture and Modernity*, Cambridge, 1997; Trentman, Just, 2006, p. 6.

53 Trentman, Just, 2006, p. 7.

54 Guillem-Llobat, X., Perdiguero, E., "Fighting adulteration in early European food industrialisation. The case of Alicante (Spain)", in Vámos, É. (ed.), *History of the Food Chain. From Agriculture to Consumption and Waste*, Hungarian Chemical

Indeed, the cultural factors influencing local dietaries were also operational, e.g. the symbolic meaning and social prestige of certain foodstuffs, mainly in rural districts and among different social classes and professional groups.[55] In this context, scientific investigations propelled by research on the physiological basis of nutrition and its direct relation to health, nutritional expertise and medical advice played a civilising role.[56] All such factors shaped a network of agencies and mutual influences acting in a dynamic and complex process simultaneously.

On the other hand, a new international scenario was configured in the first half of the 20th century as a consequence of several deep crises. Nutrition, like health itself, became an essential factor for social stability, as it influenced the changing relationships between state, society and individuals. Access to food and the entitlement to health became a basic right inherent to any human being, regardless of their race, class or nationality. Therefore, hunger became a problem to challenge, one that possessed a political, social and moral dimension. The political dimension of hunger as a factor of instability, the health and economic consequences of nutritional deficiencies and malnutrition, and the necessity to produce enough foodstuffs and make them available for all, constituted an immense political challenge. The implementation of this goal became a driving force behind social and economic change. Industrialisation and mass food production opened up a transitional path closely monitored by new regulations, which had to be negotiated, and gave way to new scientific methods of quality control. Traditional production schemes – mainly in agriculture – and old dietary habits were to be transformed, as they were potentially dangerous and could have a negative influence on both health and the economy. Under the pressure of the war and the economic crisis, food production and

---

Society, Budapest, 2006, pp. 33-40; Guillem-Llobat, X., "Industrialització i alimentació en la societat valenciana. El control de qualitat dels aliments (1850-1939)", in Herran, N. *et al.* (eds.), *Synergia: Primer Encuentro de Jóvenes Investigadores en Historia de la Ciencia*, Madrid, CSIC, 2006; Guillem-Llobat, X., "El establecimiento de nuevos límites de calidad para los alimentos en el cambio de siglo (1880-1936)", in Ortiz Gomez, T. *et al.* (eds.), *La Experiencia de enfermar en perspectiva histórica. Actas XIV Congreso de la Sociedad Española de Historia de la Medicina, Granada*, Editorial Universidad de Granada, 2008b, pp. 271-274; Guillem-Llobat, X., "El paper dels laboratoris municipals valencians en el control de qualitat dels aliments (1881-1936)", *Actes del Congrès de la Societat Catalana d'Història de la Ciència i de la Tècnica*, 2000, Vol. 1, pp. 293-300; Guillem-Llobat, 2008c, pp. 301-324.

55 Barona, 2010; Kamminga, Cunningham, 1997.

56 Barona, 2008a, 2008b.

consumption increasingly became a concern for the international agencies and European governments, but also an essential political tool.

In the introductory chapter of the influential essay *Hunger and History* (1990), edited by L.F. Newman,[57] S. Milman and R. Kates start the discussion by proposing to understand hunger in history as the breakdown of the food system, as an entitlement failure connected to the lack of access to food, as well as a hazard or "threat to humans and what they value", a permanently threatening risk. But traditionally, hunger has also been a consequence of maladjustment between population growth and the growth in food production, a perspective that is highly relevant for the long-term analysis of hunger ever since the first approaches by Thomas Malthus and Karl Marx.

This book is the result of research undertaken since 2005 on the history of the links between nutrition and health and their relationship with scientific research, economy and politics. It feeds on the archival sources of international organisations such as the League of Nations, the International Institute of Agriculture, the Food and Agriculture Organization and the World Health Organization. A previous monograph analysed the construction of the problem of nutrition during the inter-war period.[58] The present work explores the role of nutrition in international health and the transfer of scientific knowledge in 20th – century Europe, taking as the main perspective the political economy of scientific knowledge.[59]

Recent anthropological, sociological and cultural studies on food and nutrition have shown that more than a century of increasing nutritional knowledge and dietary recommendations to the European population not only eradicated hunger, but there has also been a considerable rise in the number of overweight people and obesity.[60] Based on this evidence, new research aims to investigate the interaction between science and society and the way in which scientific knowledge is spread and popularised,

57 Newman, L.F. (ed.), Crossgrove, W. *et al.* (ass.ed.), *Hunger in History: food shortage, poverty and deprivation,* Cambridge, Mass., B. Blackwell, 1990.

58 Barona, 2010.

59 It is a part of the research project *Sanidad Internacional y transferencia de conocimiento científico. Europa 1900-1975* [MICINN, HAR2011-23233].

60 WHO's recent report shows that between 20 and 70 % of adults in Europe are overweight: http://www.euro.who.int/en/what-we-do/health-topics/diseases-and-conditions/obesity/news2/news/2010/12/2570-of-adults-in-europe-are-overweight (accessed: 30th March 2011).

and how it influences habits.[61] The negative consequences of the nutritional transition have become a source of concern for nutritionists, physicians, sociologists and political authorities.[62] To throw some light on the phenomenon, an interdisciplinary approach is needed, collaboratively involving science historians, and their discussion on the production of nutritional knowledge, economy historians, sociologists and mass media experts, to clarify the selection and diffusion of information as well as the complex topic of consumption patterns.

Food studies has recently emerged as a new and interdisciplinary approach, which considers that "food touches everything important to people".[63] It has a double dimension, private and social, pointing out the role of agriculture, the food trade and retail sector in economic history, in relation to hunger, social conflict and state intervention in social history, with health and disease in the history of medicine and health, and with marketing, cooking and eating in cultural history.[64] Both in classic social history research and in a growing list of recent emerging approaches, food plays a prominent role.[65] Research on food and hunger has direct connections with numerous aspects of society: suffice it to mention the history of food in relation to prices, purchasing power, work capacities, household expenditure, conspicuous spending, power relations, technological and scientific progress, market regulation, health and disease, fashion, quality control, shopping and prices, import taxes, advertisements, or leisure.

In this book, the subject has been addressed from the perspective of the transfer of knowledge and the international history associated to the historiographical background of the political economy of scientific knowledge. My previous research work concentrated on the construction of the problem of nutrition in the inter-war years and the influence of the international health movement on nutrition and public health in times of crisis.[66] In approaching the complex network around health, nutrition, food production, experimental science, the food trade and patterns of consumption, interactions between the local and the international

61 Scholliers, P., *Food culture in Belgium*, Westport & London, Greenwood Press, 2008.

62 Jaime, P.C., Lock, K., "Do School Based Food and Nutrition Policies Improve Diet and Reduce Obesity?", *Preventive Medicine*, No. 48, 2009, 45-53.

63 Counihan, C., Van Esterik, P. (eds.), *Food and Culture. A Reader*, London/New York, Routledge, 2008.

64 Belasco, W. *Food*, Oxford/New York, Berg, 2008.

65 e.g., De Vries, 2008; Jones, 2010.

66 Barona, J.L. 2010.

context emerged as an inescapable referent.[67] In the very complex historical landscape of the period 1918-1960, interactions between theory and practice, as well as the local, the national and the international, made it preferable to use an approach that integrated all these dimensions. Consequently, this research is oriented towards the analysis of nutrition from a European viewpoint as a paradigmatic case study.

Circulating Knowledge

Historical research about international health in the first half of the 20th century became an emerging field over the past decade. The European Union has configured a favourable framework for cooperation projects, scientific meetings and international networks. This process has also taken place in the case of international health and the transfer and circulation of medical knowledge, regarding the scientific production of knowledge, uses and social practices.[68] Indeed, to understand the international character – as well as the role – of knowledge in various fields, it is crucial to understand how, where and why knowledge is produced, communicated and circulated. It is easy to understand that this is not a question of a singular type of process, but of many: from the centre of scientific breakthroughs to more peripheral areas, between countries and within countries, from the experts to the public, from the laboratories to the market, from the market to the kitchen, through institutional decisions or through the actions of individual actors. The transfer of knowledge, artifacts and practices entails a complex network or system that experienced deep transformations throughout the 20th century. The traditional spaces where knowledge is produced in the Modern Age – universities, academies, research institutes, public laboratories – have lost their exclusivity, getting involved in a wide social network linked to other agents such as trade and commerce, industry and public administration. The science-society pattern, shaped in the 20th century, is absolutely different to that initiated with the Scientific Revolution in the 17th century, and which was still alive and kicking at the end of the 19th century.[69] The evolution of the science-society pattern in the second half of the 20th century makes it extremely important to analyse

67 Barona, J.L., Bernabeu-Mestre, J., *La salud y el estado. El movimiento sanitario internacional y la administración española*, Valencia, PUV, 2008.

68 Networks such as *Phoenix, STEP (Science and Tchnology in the European Periphery), Inter-War Network* are some exemples among many others operating.

69 Pestre, D., *Science, argent et politique. Un essai d'interprétation*, Paris, Les Éditions Quae, 2008.

technoscience as a *system in society*, with the interactions between science, politics and the economy representing an essential approach.[70] The interplay between science, technology and the political economy of knowledge will be discussed in more detail in the next chapter.

One of the general aims of this book is to investigate and discuss the production and circulation of knowledge about nutrition, hunger and diseases associated with chronic and acute malnutrition, the institutions and social groups involved, and the networks of power around the science and technology of hunger and health. The main point is not the reception of scientific knowledge in one direction from the experts to the public: how, when and why knowledge reached the general public. The interaction between hunger, food, diet and health essentially touches the relationship between science and society, assuming that science is not *external* to society, a sort of autonomous and *objective* reference, but a substantial element of it, which requires a historical and sociological explanation.

In recent decades, the interactions between society and science have been addressed in many ways by the social history of science. The sociology of knowledge has also contributed an original approach in this direction. Bruno Latour is one of the predecessors in this respect. He found the inner life of the scientific world, and made an intimate connection between science and social values.[71] Of relevance is the shift suggested by Latour from an *external* science to society, to an *internal* science in society.[72]

Some concepts are relevant to the orientation of this book: the role played by the authority of experts and its social and political use, the regulatory role of the state and international organisations, the changes in the food chain, the plural dietary culture and its transformation under the influence of scientific knowledge, market pressure and political action.

Generally speaking, up until the 1850s private institutions seemed to hold more authority than official ones as far as food was concerned, a situation that changed by 1900, when the general public expected official bodies to provide security by controlling the production, manufacturing, trade and preparation of food. By establishing these

70 Barona, J.L., "Science, Democracy and the Global Market", *Chinese Cross Currents*, No. 7, 2008, pp. 24-40.

71 Latour, B., Woolgar, S., *La vie de laboratoire: la production des faits scientifiques*, Paris, La Découverte, 1979.

72 Latour 1998; Nowotny, H., Scott, P., Gibbons, M., *Re-Thinking Science. Knowledge and the Public in an Age of Uncertainty*, Cambridge, Polity Press, 2001.

links, reference is made to the concept of the *food chain*, which assumes a direct and reciprocal relationship between production, distribution and consumption.[73] In this context, the concept of *dietary culture* emphasises the importance of everyday life: the way people give meaning to objects and foodstuffs, connecting scientific ideas and traditions to daily practices.[74] In addition to medical history, economic history, historical demography and anthropometric history, a cultural perspective has to be integrated in order to analyse hunger and health in times of crisis. This is a recent approach with a solid background, following contributions by Zigmunt Bauman,[75] Ulrich Beck,[76] Michael Gibbons,[77] Bruno Latour,[78] Helga Nowotny,[79] Dominique Pestre,[80] and Alain Touraine,[81] among other influential authors who have opened up new avenues in the history and sociology of science. Hunger, food and health could represent an extremely fruitful topic of research.

Indeed, to analyse the transfer of health and nutritional knowledge, one should consider at least a plurality of aspects, such as the professional dimension of knowledge production, e.g. the role of experts and their importance as agents commissioned to legitimate knowledge and practice. New professional communities grew with a focus on expertise: nutritionists, physiologists of nutrition, clinicians, instructive programmes, vulgarisation campaigns, consumer and professional associations, expert commissions and conferences. Specialised journals were also developed.[82] Another dimension of nutrition is the institutional perspective involving relations and influences among local, national, international institutions and organisms, governments and private laboratories, hospitals, dispensaries, institutes of food and hygiene,

---

73 Belasco, W., Horowitz, R. (eds.), *Food Chains: from Farmyard to Shopping Cart*, Philadelphia, Univerity of Pennsylvania Press, 2010.

74 Appadurai, 1986.

75 Bauman, Z., *Globalization. The Human consequences*, Cambridge, Polity Press, 1998.

76 Beck, U., *What is Globalisation?*, Cambridge, Polity Press, 2000.

77 Gibbons, M. *et al.*, *The New Production of Knowledge. The Dynamics of Science and Research in Contemporary Societies*, London, Sage, 1994.

78 Latour, B., *Politiques de la Nature. Comment faire entrer les sciences en démocratie*, Paris, La Découverte, 1999.

79 Nowotny, Scott, Gibbons, 2001

80 Pestre, 2003.

81 Touraine, A., *Comment sortir du liberalisme*, Paris, Fayard, 1999.

82 Barona, J.L., "Public health expert and scientific authority", in Andresen, A., Hubbard, W., Ryymin, T. (eds.), International and Local Approaches to Health and Health Care, Oslo, Novus Press, 2010, pp. 31-48.

sanitary campaigns, health officers, experts' boards, physicians, nutritionists and others. The plurality of stakeholders intervening in the process involves dynamic interaction between the circulation of knowledge through the networks of experts, local, national and international institutions and conferences, publications, media and the market. From this perspective, the political use of hunger, health and nutritional knowledge is most important. Other specific approaches such as gender, social inequalities and the rural-urban divide could contribute relevant aspects and add to the general picture.

The 20th century was a crucial period for the shaping of an international framework in the field of health, with the creation of public health administrations in Europe backed by local, national and international institutions. The Rockefeller Foundation and the League of Nations gave a boost to public health policies during the inter-war period and the middle decades of the century. New legislation and institutional developments in most states and the creation of committees of experts at influential organisations such as the United Nations (UN), the World Health Organization (WHO) and the Food and Agriculture Organization (FAO) after World War II constitute an unavoidable reference when it comes to analysing the circulation of scientific knowledge on nutrition, hunger and dietary practices and values. Some works have contributed towards research on the United Kingdom, Central Europe and certain peripheral regions such as Latin America. These include: Paul Weindling's work on the Rockefeller Foundation and the League of Nations;[83] Marcos Cueto on the Rockefeller Foundation and the health activities of the Pan-American Health Office (PHO);[84] Iris Borowy's book about the League of Nations Health Organization;[85] the series *Bergen Workshops on History of Health and Medicine;*[86] the orientation followed by the journal *Social History of*

---

83 Weindling P. (ed.), *International Health Organisations and Movements, 1918-1939*, Cambridge, Cambridge University Press, 1995.

84 Cueto, M., *Historia de la Oficina Panamericana de Salud*, Washington, Oficina Panamericana de Salud (OPS), 2005.

85 Borowy, I., *Coming to terms with world health*, Frankfurt, Peter Lang, 2009.

86 Andresen, A., Elvbakken, K.T., Hubbard, W. (eds.), *Public Health and Preventive Medicine 1800-2000*, Bergen, Stein Rokkan Centre for Social Studies, 2004; Andresen A., Grønlie, T., Ryymin, T. (eds.), *Science, Culture and Politics. European Perspectives on Medicine, Sickness and Health*, Bergen, Stein Rokkan Centre for Social Studies, 2006; Andresen, A., Grønlie, T., Ryymin, T. (eds.), *Transferring Medico-Political Knowledge in Nineteenth- and Twentieth-Century Europe*, Bergen, Rokkan Centre for Social Studies, 2007; Andresen, A., Groenlie, T., Hubbard, W., Ryymin, T. (eds.), *Healthcare Systems and Medical Institutions.* Oslo, Novus Press,

Medicine; as well as the international conferences promoted by the *European Association for the History of Medicine and Health*. The STEP network (*Science and Technology in the European Periphery*) is also working on several aspects of the circulation of scientific knowledge.

This book considers hunger in relation to science and health, as a starting point for the analysis of a complex network of elements participating in the economy and politics of hunger. The crossroads between food and health makes concrete the claim that food studies reflect societal evolution. Indeed, bringing together food and health allows us to take into consideration a wide range of aspects such as state intervention, the definition of body standards of health, the design of statistics and social enquiries, political criticism, trends in scientific research, economic calculations, scientists' prestige, people's reactions, the role and use of education, the gender divide and, more particularly, dietary requirements, nutritional recommendations, household schools, and illnesses caused by nutritional deficiency.[87] Considering food in relation to health has yet another great advantage: the constitution of an international context. Scientific production has traditionally had a national basis, but since long contacts between scientists from various countries were manifold and international organisations took the initiative, hunger and health entered the international agenda. International meetings, especially those associated with the notion of "public hygiene" – which included healthy food and food safety – have played a crucial role in the exchange of knowledge since the 1850s. International contexts and international networks have to be incorporated in order to understand the local.

This book also aims to fill significant gaps with regard to the representation, interpretation and application of scientific knowledge on hunger and nutrition in Europe in the 20th century. The research carried out involves the combination of three levels: the production, circulation and social use of knowledge, mainly connected through international political action. It tries to identify the connections between science and society throughout the 20th century, connecting politics (revolutions, Fascism, wars, education programmes) and economics (the crisis in the 1930s, protectionism, rationing) to nutritional science and public health policies.

2009; Andresen, A., Hubbard, W., Ryymin, T. (eds.), *International and Local Approaches to Health and Health Care*, Oslo, Novus Press, 2010.

87 Vernon, J., *Hunger. A Modern History*, Cambridge, Harvard University Press, 2007; Barona, 2010.

A series of contributions have been devoted to the emergence of an experimental science of nutrition. The oldest one, which mostly concentrated on food fraud, was predominant until the end of the 19th century; a great deal of scientific research was focused on calories and vitamins during the early decades of the 20th century. Research on the ideal diet followed, up until the 1980s, and preoccupations with obesity and overweight people emerged at the turn of the century.[88] Along with life scientists' comprehensive research, social, political, economic and cultural historians have contributed to particular fields of dietary knowledge. In this respect, the publication of the collection of essays by H. Kamminga and A. Cunningham (1995) may be seen as a turning point. Research has been conducted in a number of fields focused on the search for the ideal diet,[89] the life and work of scientists,[90] food adulteration,[91] the discovery and physiological research on vitamins and nutrients,[92] the political dimension,[93] as well as the constitution of international nutritional networks.[94] All of this work is of crucial importance, as it provides either a clear outline or precise information, while displaying the richness of historical source material. Therefore, our research goes back to texts that were generated by nutritional

---

88 Schneeman, B., "Evolution of dietary guidelines", *Journal of the American Dietetic Association*, No. 2, 2003 (supplement), pp. 5-9.

89 Neill, D., "Finding the Ideal Diet: Nutrition, Culture and Dietary Practices in France and the French Equatorial Africa, 1890s to 1920s", *Food and Foodways*, No. 17, 2009, pp. 1-28.

90 Pemberton, J., White, J., "The Boyd Orr Survey of the Nutrition of Children in Britain, 1937-1939", *History Workshop Journal*, No. 50, 2000, pp. 205-29; Treitel, C., "Max Rübner and the Biopolitics of Rational Nutrition", *Central European History*, No. 41, 2008, pp. 1-25.

91 French, M., Philips, J., *Cheated not poisoned? Food Regulation in the United Kingdom, 1875-1938*, Manchester, Manchester University Press, 2000; Paquy, L., "Santé publique, repression des frauds et action municipal à la fin du XIXe siècle: le laboratoire grenoblois d'analyses alimentaires", *Revue d'Histoire Moderne et Contemporaine*, No. 51, 2004, pp. 44-65; Guillem-Llobat, 2008a; Scholliers, P., Van den Eeckhout, P., "Hearing the Consumer? The Laboratory, the Public, and the Construction of Food Safety in Brussels (1840s - 1910s)", *Journal of Social History*, 2011, pp. 1143-59.

92 Teuteberg, H.J., "The Discovery of Vitamins: Laboratory, Research, Reception and Industrial Production", in Fenton, A. (ed.), *Order and Disorder: the Health Impications of Eating and Drinking in the 19th and 20th Centries*, East Linton, Tuckwell Press, 2000; Frankenburg, F.R., *Vitamin Discoveries and Disasters. History, Science, and Controversies*, Santa Barbara, Greenwood Press, 2009.

93 Atkins, p. (2004), "The Glasgow Case: Meat, Disease and Regulation, 1889-1924", *Agricultural History Review*, No. 52, 2004, 161-82.

94 Barona, "Nutrition and Health. The International Context during the Interwar Crisis", *Social History of Medicine*, Vol. 21, No. 1, 2008a, pp. 87-105.

researchers in the 20th century and to the large amount of information about nutrition and health produced by the international agencies. Most of this information was the point of departure of reports, surveys and political action. This work analyses the discourse of nutritional knowledge and experimental research, paying attention to the way in which science was produced, written and discussed and how research was reported, taking the trouble of defining new terms and new standards.

In the process of knowledge production it is not only laboratories and national food institutes that play a significant role. A fundamental issue also appears to be the knowledge exchange between specialists and the creation of networks of experts' commissions that have scientific and political legitimacy. In addition, when talking about food and diet, it is essential to uncover the circulation of knowledge between experts, as well as between the experts and social actors: how nutritional science served as point of departure for political action, medical intervention and marketing strategies. During most of the 20th century, we witness a permanent tension between food production and the organising of trade, something absolutely determinant to understanding the limits of the experts' recommendations when their proposals were to be transformed into political actions. The relations between nutritional knowledge and food policies, and their importance for the evolution of war and post-war situations, and the spread among the wider public, seem to be essential to understanding scientific trends from an internal social perspective.

Finally, the social application of nutritional knowledge encompasses several spheres: health and disease; nutritional policies in times of crisis (rationing policies); and public canteens for the groups at risk, such as the unemployed, children, industrial workers, pregnant women, refugees and deprived rural populations. It would also be interesting to find out how nutritional information was incorporated into daily practices.[95] This is the most difficult part, since dietary information and guidelines fall within the context of social norms, habits and beliefs, i.e. within existing culinary traditions. Moreover, while nutritional science and the media changed drastically between 1900 and 2000 in Europe, society did too in terms of family structure, power relations, prosperity, state intervention, education, time management, expectations, etc.

---

[95] Perdiguero-Gil, E., Castejón-Bolea, R., "Popularising right food and feeding practices in Spain (1847-1950). The handbooks of domestic economy", *Dynamis*, No. 30, 2010, pp.141-165; Scholliers, p. (Ed.), *Food, drink and identity. Cooking, eating and drinking in Europe since the Middle Ages*, Oxford/New York, Berg, 2001.

The internal dynamics of the European society needs to be taken into consideration, as this would indirectly uncover the concern of households with food recommendations. Yet, the historical literature shows many research possibilities with regard to *public* kitchens. Of course, these differ from private kitchens (in terms of quality control, cost, tradition, cultural links), but the advantages of using source documents from public cooking institutions are too significant to neglect, while similarities between the two sorts of kitchens undoubtedly exist. European countries established different models of public kitchens, so a comparative approach could be instructive in understanding the circulation of nutritional information, as well as some aspects of the relations between nutrition and health. Public kitchens allow us to make a comparative approach to the social application of nutritional knowledge.

On the other hand, local and national regulations caused hospitals throughout Europe to pay attention to healthy food for their patients, especially from the last quarter of the 19th century. In some European countries, nutritionists and dieticians were trained in hospitals according to the principles of the new science of nutrition and appointed to public canteens, hospitals, schools, prisons and military institutions.[96] Prisons and charitable institutions constitute complementary sources of information as well.[97] Diets in public canteens for workers of large factories are similarly interesting. Investigations into school canteens and other initiatives such as school breakfast and milk distribution have become increasingly important in recent years from a historiographical viewpoint, most likely as a result of the recent intense attention paid to children's history and particularly to children's health.[98] This includes the study of various aspects, such as food in relation to illness,[99] the

[96] Thoms, U., "From Cooking to Consultation: the Professionalization of Dietary Assistants in Germany, 1890 -1980", in Oddy, D., Petranova, L. (eds.), *The Diffusion of Food Culture in Europe from the Late 18th Century to the Present Day*, Prague, Academia, 2005, pp. 107-18; Thoms, U., *Anstaltskost im Rationalisierungsprozess. Die Ernährung in Krankenhäusern und Gefängnissen im 18. Und 19. Jahrhundert*, Stuttgart, F. Steiner Verlag, 2005b.

[97] Thoms, 2005b; Carpenter, K.J., "Nutritional Studies in Victorian Prisons", *The Journal of Nutrition*, No. 136, 2006, pp. 1-8;

[98] Gulberg, E., "Food for Future Citizens", *Food, Culture & Society*, No. 9, 2006, pp. 337-43; Rawlings, E., "Choosing Health? Exploring Children's Eating Practices at Home and at School" *Antipode*, No. 4, 2009, pp. 1084-109; Vereecken, C. *et al.*, "Food Consumption among Pre-schoolers. Does the School Make a Difference?" *Appetite*, No. 51, 2008, pp. 723-6.

[99] Bakker, N. "Fresh Air and Good Food: Children and theAnti-Tuberculosis Campaign in the Netherlands, c. 1900-1940", *History of Education*, No. 39, 2010, pp. 343-61;

practical organisation and the moral implications of school meals,[100] the national social policies for the protection of children and mothers,[101] as well as the way that pupils perceived food and school milk schemes.[102]

Dimensions

The articulation of the previously mentioned aspects into a comprehensive explanation of the political economy of knowledge on nutrition, hunger and health in Europe in the middle decades of the 20th century requires the integration of at least the following elements and perspectives, considered in the present book:

1. A general picture, inclusive of a pattern of interactions between the production of scientific knowledge on health, hunger and nutrition, and its social and political use in the period 1918-1960, taking into consideration the influence of critical factors such as the economic crisis, World War I, World War II, the Spanish Civil War, social revolutions and international tensions in the inter-war period, as well as the Cold War.

Relevant aspects of the problem researched have to be considered and discussed in depth. These include: the discussions about international standards; the agreements on statistical methods and technical surveys; the preparation and discussion of the reports presented to the international agencies and groups of experts on the effects of hunger and malnutrition about certain groups of the European population; and the particularities of the problems affecting the rural population and community nutrition services.

2. It is essential to discuss the concepts of circulation of knowledge and transfer of scientific knowledge within the framework of health, nutrition and diet, and to try to understand the historical background from the perspective of the political economy of knowledge. Households, private kitchens and culinary habits are not considered in this book. Conversely, scientists, nutritionists, industries, politicians,

---

Ryymin T., "Tuberculosis-threatened Children. The Rise and Fall of a Medical Concept in Norway, *c.* 1900-60", *Medical History*, No. 52, 2008, pp. 347-64.

100 Nourrisson, D., "Manger à l'école: une histoire morale", *Food & History*, No. 2, 2004, 227-40.

101 Lyngo, J., "The Oslo Breakfast. An Optimal Diet in One Meal. On the Scientification of Everyday Life as Exemplified by Food", *Etnologia Scandinavica*, No. 28, 1998, pp. 62-76.

102 Atkins, P., "Fattening Children or Fattening Farmers? School Milk in Britain, 1921-1941", *Economic History Review*, No. 58, 2005, pp. 57-78; Atkins, P., "School Milk in Britain, 1900-1934", *Journal of Policy History*, No. 19, 2007, pp. 395-427.

traders, peasants and farmers, as well as particular social groups are to be analysed as the main performers of an active platform trying to influence citizens' behaviour in the context of tensions between scientific knowledge, feeding habits and food availability.

3. An analysis of the clinical, anthropometric, psychological and statistical criteria proposed by institutions, physicians, medical inspectors, authorities, etc., to establish standards of nutrition and patterns of health and optimum diet, including experimental, clinical and statistical strategies to clearly differenciate the healthy citizen from the population affected by deficiency diseases and malnutrition. New categories to identify nosological entities that shared experimental and clinical data.

4. A central aspect of the research involves analysing the dimensions of health problems associated with hunger and deficiency diseases in Europe between 1918 and 1960, to assess the political and economic impact of hunger as a health problem and also the task developed by national institutions (National Food Institutes, National Schools of Health, public canteens, rationing programmes) and international organisations (IIA, FAO, WHO, League of Nations, Rockefeller Foundation) in the establishment of patterns of measure, diagnosis, technological developments and political campaigns of intervention.

5. To understand the social dynamics of the political economy of knowledge and practices related to hunger, diet and health, it is also necessary to analyse the agents that intervene in the process of the transfer and circulation of knowledge, agreements on food safety, and their impact in the production and process of industrialisation of food and in public health.

6. The mutual interaction between national interests and programmes, and international proposals based on technical approaches and expertise with a more global perspective, help identify the problems in the fight against hunger and malnutrition, as well as in the education of citizens.

The far-reaching demographic catastrophe and political and economic international crisis caused by the Great War (1914-1918), and the period of conflicts until World War II, together with the financial and economic recession following the economic slump that started in 1927, transformed the global food market. The restoration of the food chain became a considerable political and economic concern, with clear repercussions on the nutrition and health standards of the European population. This book seeks to throw some light on the importance of hunger, malnutrition and health impairment in this historical context. It will also analyse the implication of the states' governments and international organisations in the creation of a new political and economic order.

The historical analysis of the political economy of hunger and health emerged in Europe in the period 1918-1960, and it requires the following aspects to be taken into consideration:

A cartography of hunger, considering as main sources national and international surveys during the economic crisis, and the war and postwar periods.

The importance, if any, of the international action taken by the international conferences and technical reports of experts of the League of Nations, the International Labour Office, the International Institute of Agriculture, the FAO and the WHO.

The evaluation of the impairment of the health condition of the European population directly or indirectly caused by hunger, a deficient diet and malnutrition, especially in rural areas. The influence of war and the economic crisis of the 1930s were especially important.

The politics of scientific research on nutrition and diet, as well as rationing policies derived from the calculation of the physiological values of the minimum diet and the optimum diet, and the parameters to calculate the dietary standards for families and special groups, such as the unemployed, families at risk of exclusion, pregnant women and babies, soldiers, patients, prisoners, refugees, etc.

It is also extremely important to analyse the consequences of famine and malnutrition in internment, concentration and refugee camps. These closed institutions represented an experimental laboratory for the clinical and experimental analysis of the resilience of the human body under extreme exhaustion.

The strategies of governments (Institutes of Nutrition, National Schools of Health, rationing policies) within a framework of international collaboration (the commissions of nutrition experts of the League of Nations, the OIT, the FAO and the WHO), concurrence and tension.

The historical sources listed in the final chapter of this book, archive documents and printed sources include, *inter alia*:

a) Technical reports, conferences and recommendations of the Commission of Experts of the League of Nations, the mixed committee of the League of Nations, as well as the FAO and the WHO on the state of nutrition of the European population.

b) World Food Surveys and regional reports and conferences promoted by the FAO since the late 1940s.

c) Specific studies on malnutrition and the extent of malnutrition in zones of war and in post-war periods. Particularly important are the reports of experts on the Spanish population during the Civil War, and those that analyse the consequences of hunger and famine in Europe during World War II and the post-war years.

A particular consequence of the transformation in food production and food consumption is the food safety issue associated with the fraud and adulteration of foodstuffs. At the end of the 19th century some international initiatives were proposed with a view to agreeing on a definition of fraud and its scope, and some regulations and methods of analysis were developed and standardised in order to homogenise international strategies of quality control. Apparently, these initiatives reached a new dimension, and more technological tools were developed in the early 20th century, when the first initiatives for the international standardisation of food quality emerged. Some of those initiatives created preferential spaces for the transfer of knowledge between national experts and a diversity of professionals. In that context, France took on a new leadership role in the promotion of the regulation of food safety and powerful private enterprises were set up, such as the Foundation of the White Cross in Geneva.[103]

A New Historical Context

As a result of the analysis of the various factors intervening in the political economy of scientific knowledge on hunger and nutrition mentioned in previous pages, this book offers a general discussion on the plural dimensions of hunger and health during the period 1918-1960. The aim is to show how the idea of a balanced diet and food availability became a central issue for the economy, scientific research and politics in the international agenda, a subject widely discussed in national institutions, parliaments, international organisms and scientific conferences. It also includes an overview of previous research that mainly focused on specific aspects and countries,[104] and it represents a step forward from my previous work on the emergence of the problem of nutrition in Europe.[105] The scientific, political and economic dimensions of hunger and nutrition allowed politicians and scientific experts – dieticians, nutritionists, physiologists and clinicians – to dream

103 Guillem-Llobat, 2008e, pp. 215-246.

104 Kamminga, Cunningham, 1997; Steckel, R.H., Rose, J.C., *The Backbone of History. Health and Nutrition in the Western Hemisphere*, New York, Cambridge University Press, 2002; Vernon, 2005.

105 Barona, 2010.

of a rational solution to the problem through the design of minimum and optimum standard diets for different income groups, professions and ages.

The problem I want to address is how the political economy of scientific knowledge on nutrition involved private and public institutions, international and national agencies, experts and citizens, education, health, politics, scientific rationality and cultural habits. Some aspects were particularly influential in understanding the evolution of the complex network shaped around hunger and health: the impairment of the global food system; the political tensions; the effects of the war and the devastating landscape of malnutrition in internment camps; the clinical and physiological research on the pathological effects of chronic nutritional deficiencies and long standing malnutrition; the rural-urban divide; and the emergence of new groups of population at risk, such as internees, refugees, soldiers, children, pregnant women and prisoners.

What was the role of national and international organisations such as the National Schools of Hygiene and the National Institutes of Food, the League of Nations, the International Labour Organisation, the International Institute of Agriculture, the Food and Agriculture Organisation, the World Health Organisation and the Red Cross? Thanks to their intervention, expert commissions built an international framework, which served to promote the circulation of legitimated knowledge, influencing government decisions, scientists, economists, food producers and the population's habits.

Obviously, the first task was to cope with hunger and its negative effects upon public health. International agencies played an essential role in the establishment of a sort of cartography of hunger, which aimed to assess the dimension of the problem and identify the most affected areas: they promoted technical surveys on the nutritional state of the population in countries and regions; commissioned conferences of experts to implement international standards intended to improve the physiological knowledge of nutrition and the clinical consequences of nutritional deficiencies; checked the nutritional state of citizens (children, workers, soldiers, pregnant women…); and screened rural diets and nutritional habits in all corners of Europe.[106] International historians, political economists and economic historians have mainly examined the problem in terms of the power of interest groups and state strategies,[107] but the role of the international organisations in the impulse

[106] Barona, 2008a; Barona, 2010.

[107] Trentmann, Just, 2006, p. 14.

of experimental science and health policies – the major dimension of the problem – have been scarcely considered.[108] A global perspective should analyse all the factors that came together and influenced one another to shape a political economy of scientific knowledge on health, hunger and nutrition.

The critical period between 1918 and 1960, which was characterised by international conflicts, war and post-war, was a decisive time for the appearance of a new international vision of coordination in many aspects of state intervention. Rather than traditional protectionist-state centred politics on the one hand, and liberal market-based traditions on the other, an alternative emerged that connected elements of the civil society with mechanisms of global governance, including a view of mutual dependence. Historiography has shown that since the end of the 19th century, European countries showed different traditions regarding the global food system.[109] Britain had a predominant free-trade tradition, quite different from protectionist Germany, France and Russia, and far from the more simple and self-sufficient agricultural communities in the Mediterranean area. Other countries, such as Sweden, Denmark, Belgium, the Netherlands and Switzerland, were more market and export oriented. Europe was a plural reality.[110]

Therefore, the role of expert scientists when talking about dietary needs and optimum diet would not only influence nutritional knowledge but also inspire agricultural and health policies. It was the starting point of education and propaganda programmes on cooking and diet composition, aiming to civilise and change the population's traditional habits considered to be pernicious for health. It was also the basis for diet in hospitals, charity meals, prisons, schools and other institutions. Proteins, fats, carbohydrates, nutrients, minerals and vitamins became common language.

A wide programme of intervention around nutrition and health was shaped with a view to disciplining, civilising and changing production and consumption patterns and modifying popular habits. The emergence of hunger as a social problem and nutrition as a scientific field of research contributed to the recognition of the social dimension of the self through the emergence of international and state social policies. Hunger, deficiency diseases, rational diet, healthy cooking, calorie intake, undernourishment and famine appeared as a core political and

---

108 Weindling, 1995; Barona, 2010.

109 Boyce, R., *The Great Interwar Crisis and the Collapse of Globalization*, London, Palgrave Macmillan, 2009.

110 Trentmann, Just, 2006, p. 15; Boyce, 2009.

economic issue and therefore became a central locus of action for social and political stability, programmes of intervention, public health and social modernisation. A well-nourished population was healthier, taller and stronger. Local and international institutions and experts appeared in connection with the social and scientific transformation of nutrition, becoming principal agents for the development of public health and social welfare policies.

The emergence of nutrition as an experimental field of research, as a medical speciality, as an economic and political locus, was immediately connected to market and consumption, but also to cultural and socio-historical factors and to the rise and increasing influence of the state as a social regulator.[111] The international crisis that permanently affected the period studied, and the changing meaning of hunger and poverty as unacceptable social realities on the one hand, and the emergence of new governmental responsibilities in the public administration on the other, were some of the most meaningful factors.[112]

As early as in the second half of the 19th century, social initiatives were put in place in order to fight hunger as an intolerable reality punishing most European countries. These initiatives included: school meals; charity meals for the poor, mothers, women and industrial workers; propaganda campaigns on dietary habits; experimental research on the physiology of nutrition and the clinical definition of deficiency diseases associated with a poor diet; as well as economic and agricultural policies. No specific political ideology monopolised this economic, social and scientific process, which indeed was more broadly related to a generally accepted value of progress and modernity widely spread in most Western societies, excluding hunger and deep poverty.[113]

The new social ethics about hunger and deprivation from the perspective of human rights resulted in practical actions in order to determine minimum and optimum standard diets, reshaped dietary habits, planned agricultural production and implemented rationing policies aimed at designing school and family meals, and discipline citizens via education and campaigns. Hunger and feeding were no longer considered purely private matters, as the diet became a locus for economic, political and medical intervention, as well as a scientific field

---

111 Barona, 2010.

112 Andresen, Grønlie, Ryymin (eds.), 2006; Andresen, Grønlie, Ryymin (eds.), 2007; Baldwin, P., *The Politics of Social Solidarity. Class Bases of the European Welfare State 1875-1975*, Cambridge, Cambridge University Press, 1990.

113 Vernon, 2005; Hendrick, H., *Child Welfare. Historical Dimension, Contemporary Debate*, Cambridge, Polity Press, 2003. Barona, 2010.

of knowledge and a practice associated with trade, public health and disease. All these aspects became responsibilities for the state as the main regulator and guarantor of the rights of citizens. For both national and international organisations, hunger, diet and health encompassed public and individual health, working conditions, agricultural production, clinical screening, social stability and scientific research.[114]

During the 1930s the new culture of nutrition and its health dimension (optimum diet, dietary standards, nutritional deficiencies, malnutrition) entered the international scene.[115] An increasing process of industrialisation of food production took place in order to guarantee the calorie intake and satisfy growing demands. This process became even more evident during the 1940s and the beginning of the Cold War. The regulation of food quality, as well as the scientific patterns for a balanced diet and their adaptation to cultural habits, were strengthened. The physiology of nutrition was considered to contribute more than merely nutritional benefits as, according to the new style of thinking, experts and authorities believed that the diet was to be adapted to scientific patterns on individual needs as a way of improving human development. They showed a eugenic perspective to improve *the race* and overcome long-standing shortcomings and superstitions.[116]

Planning the food market was the starting point. In the opinion of scientists, practitioners, public health experts and some politicians, the science of nutrition was to have a civilising effect upon the population, mainly workers and peasants, mothers and children, prisoners and patients. Knowledge on nutrition was to become legitimated by science and expertise, to be spread from the laboratory to the school, hospital, factory and the kitchen, to influence food production, to improve and rationalise the economy, shape scientific knowledge, change dietary habits and become a technical tool for future generations. As a material instrument of statecraft, as well as a new development for trade and market, the political economy shaped around nutrition was an important tool of power, and most European governments were determined to use it. Indeed, nutritional knowledge had to become quantifiable so that political and scientific initiatives could challenge the international crisis.

---

114 *The Problem of Nutrition. Interim Report of the Mixed Committee on the Problem of Nutrition*, 3 vols., Geneva, Series of League of Nations Publications, 1936 [Technical Report A.12.1936.II.B].

115 Burnet, E., Aykroyd, W.R., 'Nutrition and Public Health", *League of Nations Quarterly Bulletin of the Health Organisation*, Vol. 4, No. 2, 1935, pp. 323-474.

116 Carrasco Cadenas, E., *Ni gordos, ni flacos. Lo que se debe comer*, Madrid, Diana, 1935; Burnet, Aykroyd, 1935.

J. George Harrar, President of the Rockefeller Foundation during the inter-war years, synthesised the complex dimension of nutrition and diet, as the discovery of the calorie as a unit of measurement had led directly to an "informal alliance" of "scientists, farmers, government agencies, educators, and processors" working to fight malnutrition worldwide.[117] The *political economy of nutritional knowledge* pooled, in its public health dimension, national and international efforts during the middle decades of the 20th century. A plurality of actors took part in the process. The point of departure were the activities of the League of Nations' Health Committee, often working in coordination with national schools of hygiene in several European countries in the 1930s, with the technical and financial support of the Rockefeller Foundation, and the collaborative expertise of the International Institute of Agriculture. After World War II the World Health Organisation and the FAO assumed food relief strategies in coordinating policies to fight hunger. But a powerful industry emerged in the meantime, and even though the states imposed regulations and quality control, the power of the industry grew more and more at the expense of the regulatory function of the state.

Hunger and poverty had already reinforced national social and public health dimensions in most European countries during the second half of the 19th century.[118] Consequently, the state participated in the regulation of the social relations affecting labour legislation, the protection of mothers and children, other groups at risk, promoting health and sanitary campaigns, trying to control food quality and fighting adulterations, and promoting school reforms and nutritional education. School medical inspection and school canteens became a tool for medical intervention, checking the new generations within the framework of a eugenic policy intended to improve social hygiene.[119]

Nutrition, food availability and diet became an essential component of the new state policies promoted by social reformers for human improvement. Summer camps not only sought a contact with the healing effect of nature, but also feeding undernourished lower-class children.[120] The first municipal institution for school medical inspection was created in Brussels in 1878[121] and the initiative was extended to most European

---

117 Cullather, 2007, p. 5.

118 Baldwin, 1990; Maurer, D., Sobal, J. (eds.), *Eating Agendas: Food and Nutrition as Social Problems*, New York, 1995; Sen, A.K., *Poverty and Famines. An Essay on Entitlement and Deprivation*, Oxford, Oxford University Press, 1981; Vernon, 2005.

119 Barona, 2011.

120 Bakker, 2010.

121 Barona, 2007b.

countries in the following decades.[122] The First International Conference on School Hygiene was held in Nuremberg (1904), a Second Conference in London (1906) and also in Paris (1906). In April 1912 the First Spanish Conference on School Hygiene took place in Barcelona. It defined the inalienable rights of children, set up a *Liga de Higiene Escolar* [School Hygiene League] and requested the extension of medical inspection to schools. The health-at-school policy also comprised school meals and canteens, which emerged in Europe from the 1860s onwards in the context of a broad debate on compulsory education and an environment in which hunger and its links with health were becoming far more visible.[123]

A second dimension of nutrition in the context of public health comes from the idea that good nutrition is essential for optimum health status, a condition necessary to fight infectious diseases, indeed the main health problem during the first half of the 20th century. Feeding was to be considered the basis of good body development and a healthy state, a source of organic energy and good defences against external aggression, something fundamental when faced with the threat of hunger and starvation.

The so-called organic energy was considered to be essential to the understanding of the spread of infectious diseases such as tuberculosis. The concept of the pre-tubercular condition in children as a predisposition to the disease was related to defective feeding, excessive work, a lack of hygiene and poor living conditions.[124] These elements cause us to argue that before the emergence of nutrition as an experimental field of scientific research, especially in the 1930s, hunger and feeding became a subject for social concern and social action mainly associated with public health and an optimum health status in order to minimise the risk of suffering infectious diseases.

This stage was prior to the emergence of a new science of nutrition based on experimental research on vitamins, organic elements and specific deficiency diseases.[125] The concept of *organic resistance* to infection – a useful concept among practitioners – was directly related to

---

122 Barona, 2010.

123 Hendrick, 2003.

124 Ryymin, T., "Tuberculosis-threatened Children. The Rise and Fall of a Medical Concept, *c.* 1900-60", in Andresen, A., Grønlie, T., Ryymin, T. (eds.), *Transferring Medico-Political Knowledge in Nineteenth- and Twentieth-Century Europe*. Bergen, Rokkan Centre for Social Studies, 2007; Ryymin T., "Tuberculosis-threatened Children. The Rise and Fall of a Medical Concept in Norway, *c.* 1900-60", *Medical History*, 2008, Vol. 52, pp. 347-64.

125 Barona, 2010.

the nutritional state and optimum diet. Poor nutrition was claimed to be the main factor for impaired organic resistance as a previous stage leading to losing the battle against infection. From this perspective, vaccines and medicines were important in fighting tuberculosis and other infectious diseases, and also in preventing contagion. But this was not more important than a good nutritional condition, which was considered to be the basis of a good treatment of any infection. In the late 1920s poverty, the problem of children's health and infectious diseases, as well as the economic crisis, paved the road for a new milestone, namely the big international boost to scientific research on nutrition.

The international will to improve nutrition and public health was even stronger after World War II.[126] International agencies were established in order to fight nutritional deficiencies and malnutrition, such as UNICEF (1947), the WHO (1948), in addition to the FAO (1943).[127] A *United Nations Relief and Rehabilitation Administration*-UNRRA was created to face the tragic effects of starvation and malnutrition in the Netherlands in 1944, with the specific target to offer relief to the liberated countries in Europe. Due to the scarcity of funds, the UNRRA received support from the USA and from nutritional experts who helped in the establishment of rationing strategies and food relief for the affected population in the Netherlands, Poland, Greece and other countries.[128]

From the 1960s new agencies were founded to challenge food conflicts: the World Food Programme (WFP, 1963); the United Nations Development Programme (UNDP, 1965); the United Nations Environment Programme (UNEP, 1972); the International Fund for Agricultural Development (IFAD, 1977), which is closely related to the United Nations System the Consultative Group on International Agricultural Research (CGIAR, 1971).

From 1960 the World Bank and regional banks for development increased their contributions to the modernisation of agriculture and rural development. These strategies were promoted in Europe in the

---

[126] Borowy, I., "Crisis as opportunity: International health work during the economic depression", *Dynamis*, No. 28, 2008, pp. 29-51.

[127] Gilliespie, J.A., "International organizations and the problem of child health, 1945-1960", *Dynamis* 23, 2003, pp. 115-142.

[128] Bengoa Lecanda, J.M., "Historia de la nutrición en salud pública", Serra Majem, L., Aranceta Bartrina, J., *Nutrición y salud pública. Métodos, bases científicas y aplicaciones*, Barcelona, Elsevier & Mason, 2006.

1950s and in other world regions after the 1960s. Underdeveloped rural districts were the focus of most of the efforts.[129]

As reiterated in previous pages, historical research that analyses the various factors behind the changes in the diet and nutritional condition of Europeans has highlighted the importance of taking into account a plurality of factors to explain the nutritional transition. These include the progress in scientific knowledge, changes in public health and hygiene and health educational programmes.[130] In the areas of health care and community nutrition, research has been conducted on the pre-transitional and transitional periods and on epidemiological, clinical and food-diet dimensions after the transition. But it also seems appropriate to delve into this analysis from the viewpoint of the history of health sciences.[131] It should not be forgotten that the discovery of the role of active principles in caloric values and metabolic processes, together with the discovery of vitamins and nutrients, enabled the consolidation of nutritional science as a solid ground during the early decades of the 20th century. As interest in quantitative nutritional values waned amongst public health experts, research increasingly focused on the qualitative aspects of nutrition, which could have implications for the development of chronic disease, quality of life, physical and intellectual potential and longevity. This new knowledge, collectively applied in preventive programmes and public health campaigns, gave rise to a new functional concept termed *community nutrition*, the aim of which was to improve the nutritional state and the health condition of individuals and groups within a community.[132]

---

129 Andresen, A., Barona, J.L., Cherry, S. (eds.), *Making a New Countryside. Health Policies and Practices in European History ca.1860-1950*, Frankfurt, Peter Lang, 2010.

130 Nicolau Nos, R., Pujol Andreu, J., "El consumo de proteínas animales en Barcelona entre las décadas de 1830 y 1930: evolución y factores condicionantes", *Investigaciones de Historia Económica*, No. 3, 2005, pp.101-134 and 127-128; Nicolau, R., Pujol-Andreu, J., "Aspectos políticos y científicos del Modelo de la Transición Nutricional: evaluación crítica y nuevas perspectivas", in Bernabeu-Mestre, J., Barona, J.L. (eds.), *Nutrición, salud y Sociedad. España y Europa en los siglos XIX-X*, Valencia, SEC/PUV, 2011.

131 Serra Majem, L., Bautista Castaño, I., "La nutrición en España"; Serra Majem, L., "Dieta y nutrición", *La salud y el sistema sanitaria en España.* Barcelona, Informe SESPAS 1993, pp. 146-152; Serra, L., Risas, L., Lloveras, L., Salleras, L., "Changing patterns of fat consumption in Spain", *European Journal of Clinical Nutrition*, No. 47, suppl. 1, 1993, pp. 13-20; Moreno, Sarría, Popkin, 2002.

132 Aranceta Bartrina, J., *Nutrición comunitaria*, Barcelona, 2001, p. 3; Bernabeu-Mestre, "Nutrition and Public Health", *Food & History*, 2008.

Likewise, the problems associated with nutrition, which lay behind the high infant and child mortality rates that characterise pre-transitional demographic systems, have also been paid some historiographical attention.[133] It is generally accepted that the 1920s and 1930s constituted a crucial period in the development of public health in European countries. The specific situation in each country cannot be considered in isolation from the international context. On the other hand, mass consumption and new impulses towards industrialisation and urban planning after 1950 resulted in an improved food intake. The diet became more diversified and changes took place both in its composition and in household consumption: meat, eggs, milk, and animal proteins generally became more abundant. Calculations by FAO experts attributed to the European population modern standards with a daily intake of over 3,000 calories per person.[134] In the 1970s Mediterranean Europe had similar parameters to those in Northern and Western Europe before WWII.

In addition to an analysis of the principle elements that shaped institutionalisation processes, such as that of community nutrition, it would seem appropriate to consider the social, cultural, economic and political contexts within which these phenomena occurred, and to analyse the discourses and practices regarding diet and health that existed in the international context, as well as in European societies, in the middle decades of the 20th century.

[133] Bernabeu-Mestre, J., Perdiguero-Gil, E., Barona, J.L., "Determinanti Della mortalità infantile e transizione sanitaria. Una riflessione a partire dall'esperienza spagnola", in Pozzi, L., Breschi, M. (eds.), *Salute, Malattia e sopravvivenza in Italia fra '800 e '900*, Udine, Editrice Democratica Sarda, 2007, pp. 175-193.

[134] Cussó, X., "Transición nutricional y globalización de la dieta en España en los siglos XIX y XX. Un análisis comparado con el caso francés", in Chastagnaret, G., Daumas, J.C., Escudero, A., Raveux, O. (eds.), *Los niveles de vida en España y Fr, ancia (Siglos XVIII-XX)*, Alicante, Universidad de Alicante, 2010, pp. 105-128.

CHAPTER 2

Nutrition and Health: the Political Economy of Scientific Knowledge in the 20th Century

The Political and Economic Landscape

International relations broke down during the inter-war years as a consequence of the chaotic conditions created by the world economic depression. The collapse of the international political system was closely linked to the fall of the international economic system.[1] The consequences were extremely hard for Europe. In 1918 the Entente, together with its associated powers, imposed the Versailles Settlement, according to which Germany lost both territory and population and had to face demands for reparations and take the blame for the Great War. In Eastern Europe, the Bolshevik revolution also created a source of regional instability, while the Anglo-American powers tried to assist in the recovery of Germany, Austria and other countries in Central Europe seriously damaged by the conflict. Under those critical circumstances, the Wall Street crash triggered the onset of the world economic catastrophe. The collapse of trade and the enormous unemployment rates created the right conditions for Hitler to take power, and induced Japan and Italy to start new colonialist expansions. Attempting to avoid a breakdown of the existing fragile order, liberal democracies, mainly Britain and France, encouraged by the USA, implemented an appeasement policy.

The British historian Eric Hobsbawn has qualified the first half of the 20th century as the *Age of Extremes*, a period of revolutions, crises and conflicts in all realms of social life, as well as in the values and referents that define the human condition.[2] Suffice it to mention the impact of the Great War, but also the rise of the worker movement and the revolutionary threat (leading to the Bolshevik triumph and the Soviet revolution), the advent of nationalism and the National Socialist expansion, the clash and tension between the Triple Alliance and the Entente, which divided Europe into two conflicting blocks – the prelude

---

1 Boyce, R., *The Great Interwar Crisis and the Collapse of Globalization*, London, Palgrave Macmillan, 2009.

2 Hobsbawn, E., *The Age of Extremes, 1914-1991*, London, Abacus, 1995.

of the Spanish Civil War, which in turn constituted the preamble to World War II and the failure of negotiation and pacification policies. All these events drew a landscape of conflict, tension, radicalism and political instability in the whole world, but with Europe as the main stage.

Some historical narratives have considered that the outbreak of the war in 1914 certainly resulted in the collapse of the international states' system, but only caused global economic relations to be suspended.[3] Expressed in economic terms, economic historians have argued that the 1920s bore a much closer resemblance to the pre-war period than has been commonly assumed. Historical evidence shows that by the second half of the 1920s world trade and international financial flows were greater than before the war and increasing at twice the rate of national growth.[4] By this time Soviet Russia had reached great international power, while the United States of America (USA) had retreated to its pre-war status as a potentially great nation. Germany had regained its sovereignty to some extent and was already the chief threat to the international states' system, just as it had been before the Great War. According to present political and economic historiography, the decisive turning point was not 1914, as could be easily assumed, but 1927, when the great interwar crisis began, bringing out the collapse of both the global economic and political systems. British protectionism was not the only important element in the picture at the time; the most remarkable feature was the progress made in reestablishing a globalised economy and the expansion of international trade and investment after the Ruhr crisis in 1924. On the contrary, between 1929 and 1933 world industrial production declined by about 37 per cent and world trade dropped by at least 27 per cent (68 per cent in current prices), while agricultural prices fell by 75 per cent from the levels reached in the period 1923-1925.[5]

As a consequence of this exceptionally critical situation, many countries did not resist the temptation to retreat into autarchy, foreign investment ceased sharply and by June 1933 the international monetary system was chaotic. Industrial unemployment reached 22 per cent in Britain, 37.6 per cent in the USA and 44.3 per cent in Germany, where wholesale trade fell below 1914 levels. Exports and steel production experienced a strong reduction of nearly 75 per cent. A similar decline took place among Japanese farmers producing silk for exports. At first France seemed to be the exception, apparently little hit by the slump.

---

3 Boyce, 2009, p. 23.

4 *Ibidem*, p. 3-4.

5 *Ibidem*, p. 4.

Unemployment in France was only 276,000 in 1933, but numerous part-time employees, women and some 2.4 million emigrant workers returned to Spain, Portugal and Italy, and unemployment continued to rise until 1936, reaching seven per cent and accounting for 850,000 registered workers. The economic crisis had increasingly negative consequences among the European population. In those years, peasants living in rural Hungary, Romania, and Asian countries such as India and China faced hunger and starvation.[6]

Prior to the depression, the international markets operated according to a set of rules, restraints and institutions capable of ensuring social, political and economic stability. The framework of regulations and institutions was never done away with, as that would have led to the breakdown of the capitalist system. Central banks and international institutions – such as the Bank for International Settlements (BIS), the International Monetary Fund (IMF), the World Bank (WB) and the World Trade Organization (WTO) – ensured the convertibility of currencies and therefore markets remained open. Before the Great War, Britain provided the key institutions to sustain the global economy: the Bank of England, Lloyds of London, the Baltic Exchange and other financial powers settled in the City of London. Nevertheless, between 1927 and 1929 global economic and political relations became increasingly precarious. Notwithstanding important developments elsewhere, Europe was still the centre and the nucleus of the three great democratic powers: Britain, France and the USA. In the 1920s they accounted for 25 per cent of world economic activity, producing nearly 60 per cent of the world's manufactured goods. Altogether, the three of them controlled 33 per cent of world trade and supplied no less than 70 per cent of manufactured exports. In the period 1924 to 1928 they provided over 85 per cent of the world's capital lending and investment and in 1929 possessed nearly 60 per cent of the world's monetary gold reserves.[7] These records suffice to confirm their international power.

On the other hand, the economic slump coincided with an extraordinarily deep political crisis. Political historians have underlined the repeated efforts made by Britain and the USA to modify the Versailles settlement and accommodate Germany again into the international states' system, something that was in opposition to France's commitment to establishing a global security framework. The consequence was the previously described prosperous world of the early 1920s, but the international political system was exceptionally

[6] *Ibidem*, p. 5-8.

[7] *Ibidem*, p. 10.

vulnerable partly due to the fact that the three victor powers did not agree upon the way of managing the situation. Several European countries remained in conflict with the existing states' system and the winning powers failed to come to terms with the rules for operating the international gold standard, the role and functioning of international institutions and the shaping of a framework for international security. Robert Boyce synthesised the critical situation:

> The conventional narrative of interwar history associates the breakdown of the post-war settlement with the rise of extreme political doctrines, including militarism, aggressive imperialism, communism, anarchism, anti-semitism and above all fascism and its German variant Nazism… and it is true that they made most of the running in the 1930s. But this was not the case in the 1920s or at least until the great crisis began. On the contrary, the dominant political doctrine in this period was liberalism and its economic expression, market capitalism. The three main victor powers were all liberal powers.[8]

Therefore, the key to understanding the origin and consequences of the slump is to recognise the causal connections between economic and political factors. According to Boyce, the great interwar crisis started in 1927, resulting in the collapse of international trade and investment. Unemployment punished millions of citizens, currencies were undermined and banking systems endangered, so the survival of countries depended principally upon their economic relations with other countries. The subsequent crisis was one of the greatest catastrophes in modern history. Its crippling effects devastated the lives of a whole generation.[9]

A meaningful feature to keep in mind is that, as a result of the victory in the Great War of the major Western democratic powers, the world's dominant political ideology was not communism or fascism but liberalism, predominantly in its Anglo-Saxon version. In the political scene, it was manifested in the rejection of the 'old diplomacy' of alliances as well as of the ideal of a balance of power in favour of a 'new internationalism' symbolised by the League of Nations. Notwithstanding the rise of radical ideologies, a closer analysis of international relations shows that until 1927 liberalism remained on the rise and dominated the global economic and political spheres. However, after 1927 international networks weakened, support for globalisation decreased and the great interwar crisis started. In a few years, by 1933-1934, the crisis had brought to a violent close the world's second great

---

8 *Ibidem*, p. 17.

9 *Ibidem*, p. 426.

era of globalisation. In fact, the very real failure of liberalism took place at this moment and hostility to liberalism was increasingly dominant along the 1930s with the growing influence of socialist, communist, anarchist and radical nationalist movements.

In the late 1920s crises occurred in many different regions: the Balkans, Morocco, Egypt, Iraq, China and elsewhere. But the key to maintaining world stability remained the containment of Germany within the context of the European states' system, since only a German crisis was likely to affect the balance of the world's powers. Yet an important stabilising factor was missing: no security system existed for maintaining international order. The USA remained isolationist, demanding the European powers to join its policies in disarmament while refusing to openly support the League of Nations as the international venue for challenging threats of aggression.

Unable to draw the Anglo-Saxon powers into a European framework, France saw no alternative but to engage in direct dealings with Germany in 1924. When the Pan-European Union was founded in April 1924, it reached prominence after its first conference in Vienna in 1926 as the most relevant pro-European organisation between the wars. At the 1925 League of Nations General Assembly, the French minister Loucher – a liberal in favour of eliminating trade barriers – nevertheless defended the view that some government intervention was essential to ensure a 'rational economic system', the only one that could handle the uncontrolled tendency of economic competition to aggravate nationalism and the response leading to a recrudescence of protectionism.

On September 24, 1925, the Assembly of the League of Nations, on the motion of the French Delegation, invited the Council to constitute a Preparatory Committee under the presidency of Georges Theunis. From May 4 to 23, 1927, the International Economic Conference met in Geneva. More than 400 delegates and experts from 50 countries attended, including the USA and Soviet Russia. Representatives of the IIA, ICC and ILO were also present. Britain was still the world's greatest trading nation and at the time suffered from heavy unemployment, apparently due to national protectionism. To most historians, economists and politicians, the 1927 World Economic Conference marked a victory for the liberal approach to international economic relations and a defeat for the regulated French approach. Nevertheless, global economic relations remained precarious. The world economy continued to expand and the Wall Street crash was still six months away. However, by 1928 signs that the era of globalisation was nearing its end were already multiplying.

According to recent research, the great post-war challenge in the late 1920s was no longer to contain Germany in its place, but to persuade Britain to remain involved in Europe. The international context was changing fast, as shown by the previous collapse of continental empires: Russia, Austria-Hungary, Germany and the Ottoman Empire. On the other hand, the emergence of the USA forced a new international forum for negotiation. The US government envisaged the League of Nations not as a forum for world governance, but rather as an agency for the negotiation to contain and pacify Europe. The conventional narrative of interwar history has presented the Anglo-Saxon powers as being committed to appeasement throughout the 1920s as a rational constructive policy further pursued in the 1930s. Some recent research has considered this conclusion a mistake, since Britain and the USA were unwise to encourage the creation of an effective framework of security, this becoming the core conflict with France.[10] The USA and Britain were held accountable for their withdrawal from the security framework agreed at Versailles, just at the end of the Great War, to promote disarmament. However, Britain turned to protectionism after 1927, just when the need for international leadership was greater than ever. In addition, the Japanese, Italian and German initiatives that brought down the global political order in the 1930s intensified and prolonged the economic slump. The disaster reached a climax in 1932, but cooperation among the liberal capitalist powers reached a low point in 1934 when the USA still demanded Germany be relieved of reparation payments to safeguard American commercial credit in Europe. At the time, French diplomacy was more realistic about the situation and accepted the necessity of German integration, but they also worried about the security risks posed by Germany.[11]

Britain's temporising enabled Hitler to occupy the Rhineland and absorb Austria without resistance. Britain's obvious reluctance to extend practical help to Poland or associate itself with the Soviet Union, together with its ambiguity over military cooperation with France and continued pursuit of a settlement with Germany, persuaded Hitler that Britain would not oppose his expansionist ambitions in the East. The French were divided over a confrontation with Germany; the Communists threatened to oppose war once the Soviet Union became Germany's ally in August 1939. But after Germany invaded Poland, the French government declared war. The unfortunate role played by liberal democracies, particularly France and Britain, in the Spanish Civil War

---

10 *Ibidem*, pp. 32-40.

11 *Ibidem*, pp. 32-34.

should be placed and understood in this context. The Anglo-Saxon powers responded very slowly in supporting Europe's democracies and, until Pearl Harbour, the USA authorities restricted all efforts to resupply Britain and France to enable them to contain the aggressor.

The dual political and economic crisis that started in 1927 and culminated in 1933-1934 gave way to a more general crisis affecting imperialism, autarchy, industrialised warfare and genocide, tragic events that lasted for more than a decade, until the final world war conflict. Some historians consider the Great War to be only a hiatus in the great era of globalisation that began in 1815 and continued until 1927. According to this idea, Robert Boyce argues that it makes more sense to see the period between 1927 and 1947 as a deeply critical moment, a single generalised crisis, as this period ended only in 1947 and a new era started. From a politico-economic perspective, the long 19th century was even longer than generally assumed by historiography, spanning to the start of the Great War. Boyce proposed the period from 1815 to 1927.[12]

The fact is that in 1918 Continental Europe emerged from the war in a critical condition. Its political system was threatened and shaken by revolutionary movements and the collapse of four great empires. In addition, the European economic regime was strongly dislocated by the consequences of the war, consumption experienced a critical stage due to inflation and the breakup of what had previously been a highly integrated market. In July 1914 Europe was comprised of 20 independent countries and goods moved easily in between. By the Armistice, it comprised 27 countries of a much smaller size, including 20,000 km of additional frontiers. To revive trade, the protectionist barriers erected had to be pulled down and the narrow bilateral arrangements replaced by multilateral ones. At that moment in time the City of London remained the world's greatest clearing house for capital and credit, and the Bank of England sought to turn the League of Nations Financial Committee into the international agency for setting more convenient rules in a post-war monetary and financial system.[13] However, the situation was changing quickly and during the following decade technology was to revolutionise all dimensions of human communication: aviation, transoceanic cables, short-wave radio and telegraph, telephone lines and films. Thanks to the new technologies, international financial activity and corporate enterprise expanded dramatically. Multinational American firms rapidly extended as a prosperous industry. A global tendency dominated the new industries:

12 *Ibidem*, pp. 62-70.

13 *Ibidem*, pp. 43-47.

electrical manufacturing, office equipment, chemicals, fertilizers, motor vehicles, oil extraction, refining and distribution, mining, metal refining for industrial purposes (aluminium, copper, nickel, lead and zinc).

Economic expansion, technological innovation and new international industries coexisted with a fragile political order and deep social conflicts. Under those hard circumstances, the 1929 economic slump led Britain to drop its commitment to economic internationalism in favour of imperial protectionism. This change in strategy initially brought good results within the framework of the British Commonwealth market, and from the end of 1932 Britain enjoyed sustained economic recovery. On the contrary, France was seriously hit by the depression since 1932 and did not recover until 1938. In the meantime, the League of Nations Economic Consultative Committee called for industrial agreements as a means of reorganising Europe. In 1927 the aforementioned World Economic Conference had endorsed the principle of multilateral conventions as a means of liberalising trade, but failed to give a technical solution to how this could be reconciled with the most-favoured nation principle.

The League of Nations' Economic Committee therefore requested Walter Stucki, the Swiss Economy Minister, to investigate and report on the practical options. In April 1929 he presented a report in which he proposed that the states agree to an exception to the most-favoured nation principle, substituting it with multilateral conventions, as long as they met three main conditions: they had to contribute to the reduction of tariff barriers, have the approval of the League of Nations and be open to all countries to join on a similar basis.[14] Exceptions made room for preferential trade between countries with longstanding historical or geographical links. As a result of this policy, a Nordic clause allowed preferential trade between Sweden, Norway and Denmark; an Iberian clause was established as well between Spain and Portugal; and Baltic, Ottoman and imperial British clauses were accepted. But since the spring of 1929 France – like Belgium and Britain – was fearful of a recrudescence of protectionism and, for a few more months, remained loyal to the idea of European economic integration.

In February 1930 the challenge strengthened Europe's position in the League of Nations. In May 1930, at the 10th General Assembly of the League of Nations, a memorandum was circulated on the construction of a European Federation through the integration of markets. The document called for a common economic policy, industrial agreements, improvements in general infrastructures and coordination of civil works,

---

[14] *Ibidem*, p. 252

as well as cooperation in transport, communications, credit provision, labour policies and migrations. But Europe was simply too divided to take this plan any further, and, from a British viewpoint, France was too powerful and aggressive integration-wise so as to support such a unification programme. British authorities were wary of France as a global power and were confident of Germany coming back to its position in Europe. They did not consider Germany to be a problem but a way of containing the French. Britain promoted the appeasement of Europe through the League of Nations and supported disarmament, having to choose between entering a European federation and remaining the head of the Empire. Indeed, Europe's growth was a threat to the Empire, the maintenance of which required liberal internationalism in both political and economic spheres, and firm opposition to the project of European integration.

As is known, in the Reichstag election of May 1928, when the German economy was still relatively strong, the Left and Right parties did poorly: the Communists obtained 54 seats and the Nazi party only 12, altogether accounting for 14 per cent of parliament. But the situation changed very quickly. Two years later, in 1930, with unemployment soaring above three million, the budget deficit threatening currency stability and the nightmare of inflation growing out of control, the two parties rose to 33 per cent: the Communists obtained 77 seats and the Nazis 107 seats, becoming the second largest party in the *Reichstag*.

On the other hand, since the end of the Ruhr crisis in 1924 until the spring of 1928, Germany enjoyed a period of relative stability and economic growth, although unemployment had grown to 1,188,000, which accounted for 12.9 per cent of the work force in December 1927, rising to 16.7 per cent by December 1928 and 20.1 per cent in December 1929. The political twist represented by Hitler's victory undermined the remaining international confidence in Germany and this in turn intensified the political crisis, the economic slump and the decline. By December 1930 unemployment in Germany had gone up to 4.4 million and to nearly 4.9 million in January 1931, accounting for 34 per cent of the working population.

In the 1930s the economic and political situation became extremely complex in Europe. The 12th annual Assembly of the League of Nations, held in September 1931, saw 50 delegations, a record-breaking figure. Mexico was admitted as a member and Soviet Russia and the USA sent unofficial representatives as observers. But, for the first time since the League's foundation, Britain was not represented in the Assembly by a delegation headed by a minister.

The suspension of the gold standard on September 21, 1931, opened a window of opportunity for Britain to get back its leadership of the international monetary system. The economist John M. Keynes was prepared to accept almost any sacrifice to keep the sterling on the gold standard. He and other prominent British economists and bankers promoted an international currency conference to try to address the economic issues through a combination of unilateral external action, protectionism and imperialism. But at the time Britain was no longer prepared to take the international lead in this field. The British financial system had become extremely vulnerable to the crisis and French newspapers described the situation as *la décadence anglaise*. The global picture was terribly dull. World industrial production declined over 10 per cent between 1929 and 1930, 20 per cent by 1931 and over 30 per cent by 1932. Unemployment rose accordingly to 2.75 million or 15.6 per cent of the industrial workforce in Britain, 2.8 million or 17 per cent in France, 12 million or 36 per cent in the USA and 6 million or 44.6 per cent in Germany. Furthermore, world trade touched a new low, falling to merely 52.5 per cent of the 1929 level.[15]

In 1930 and 1931 the economic crisis in Eastern Europe had drawn the attention of the League of Nations' Economic and Financial Committees, as well as that of the Committee of Enquiry for European Union, created to follow up on the plans for a European Federation. The situation was extremely serious, as the collapse in commodity prices had devastated agrarian countries like Poland, Hungary, Romania, Yugoslavia and Bulgaria, also weakening the precarious economy of Austria and increasing unemployment in Czechoslovakia. The Danube region got divided between French plans and German influence. Moreover, in 1932 a regional initiative was implemented – the Ouchy Convention in Lausanne – by Belgium, the Netherlands and Luxemburg, with a view to reaching commercial agreements and economic cooperation.

The end of World War II marked a new point of departure characterised by the challenge of a redefinition of the international sphere. After 1947 new international institutions were created: the International Monetary Fund (IMF), the International Bank for Reconstruction and Development (central component of today's World Bank), and the General Agreement on Tariffs and Trade (GATT). The British leaders encouraged a unified Europe after the war, but not including Britain itself. The heads of the Labour government did not favour this stance and ordered party members to stay away from the Hague Congress in May 1948, which marked the rebirth of the

[15] *Ibidem*, p. 346.

European movement.[16] Until 1947, American and British assistance to Continental Europe was limited almost exclusively to economic aid.

Only with the onset of the Cold War did the Anglo-Saxon powers join in a framework of security for Western Europe. The first step came with the announcement of the Truman doctrine in March 1947, affirming America's support to countries threatened by 'Soviet-encouraged subversion', followed by the announcement of the European recovery programme or Marshall Plan. Washington now took direct responsibility for Europe's economic stability with a four-year programme of $13 billion, which tried to contribute towards stability. In 1948 came the American decision to confront the challenge of the Soviet Union's blockade of Berlin, and formal negotiations with Canada, Britain and Western European countries for the creation of a North Atlantic Alliance started. The American security guarantee, which required a British commitment, removed the threat overhanging Western Europe's recovery. Therefore, the third great era of economic and trade globalisation began in 1947, bringing economic growth and sustained prosperity to most parts of the world. Although numerous regional conflicts occurred during the Cold War years in East Asia, the Middle East, Africa, the Balkans, southern Caucasus, the superpowers avoided major war and most of the world enjoyed peace.

The present crisis that began in 2007 cannot be understood without regard to its exogenous causes, which some historians identify as weaknesses in the political framework surrounding the markets.[17] An essential element of the political framework is the international institutions created at the end of the Second World War. The importance of these institutions grew in line with the increase in globalisation shaped by Anglo-Saxon ideology. After the end of the Cold War they have declined in representativeness, international respect and influence. The most relevant international agencies such as the World Bank, the International Monetary Fund, the World Trade Organization, as well as other influential groups (G7, G16, G20), and the global structure of the United Nations, have been fought against and discredited by the main powers, accelerating the trend away from multilateralism towards imperialism and bilateral agreements.

Obviously, the current crisis is not the same as that of 1927-1947. Among the more evident differences underlined by experts is the fact that the great interwar crisis began at a time of deflation, whereas the

16 *Ibidem*, pp. 347-349.

17 *Ibidem*, pp. 445-450.

present crisis started at a time of accelerating inflation.[18] A second difference is the greatly enlarged role of the state-public administration in every country since the Second World War, commonly triple of that of pre-war times as a fraction of the national economy. It is the largest employer, one that exerts a stabilising influence on the private sector of the economy. But the most important difference is the contrasting behaviour of the world's powers in the two crises. The Franco-German axis, now a constructive partnership, has contributed to European unity, and the existence of a single currency and the European Central Bank has reduced the risk of individual countries succumbing to speculative attacks. And with the leading developing countries – Brazil, Russia, India and China (the BRIC countries) – widely expected to equal the combined gross domestic product of the original G7 industrial countries by 2040, and exceed it by 409 per cent by 2050, even assuming a slowing of Russian and Chinese growth rates, international tensions seem inescapable.

Nutrition, Health and European Citizenship

Going beyond the purely economic and political perspective, whatever the viewpoint, the first half of the 20th century represented, from a social stand, a critical, contradictory and essential period in the development of the *civilising process* defined by Norbert Elias as one in which external social constraints proscribing behaviours gradually became internalised.[19] He suggested that, in modern Western culture, behaviour associated with the body, as is the case with nutrition and dietary habits, came to be strictly regulated. The *civilising process* can also be interpreted as the genesis of what Alfons Labisch described as the construction of the *homo hygienicus*,[20] basically an expression of the triumph of the ideals and values of urban bourgeoisies. This was therefore the breeding ground for a new concept of citizenship and the

---

18 *Ibidem*, pp. 448.

19 Elias, N., *Über den Prozeß der Zivilisation. Soziogenetische und psychogenetische Untersuchungen. Erster Band. Wandlungen des Verhaltens in den weltlichen Oberschichten des Abendlandes* and *Zweiter Band. Wandlungen der Gesellschaft. Entwurf einer Theorie der Zivilisation*, Basel, Verlag Haus zum Falken, 1939 (Published in English as *The Civilizing Process, Vol.I. The History of Manners*, Oxford, Blackwell, 1969, and *The Civilizing Process, Vol.II. State Formation and Civilization*, Oxford, Blackwell, 1982); Andresen, A. *et al.* (eds.), *Citizens, Courtrooms, Crossings*, Bergen, Stein Rokkan Centre for Social Studies, 2008; Barnes, D.S., *The Great Stink of Paris and the Nineteenth-Century Struggle against Filth and Germs*, Baltimore, The Johns Hopkins University Press, 2006.

20 Labisch, A., *Homo Hygienicus. Gesundheit und Medizin in der Neuzeit*, Frankfurt, Campus, 1992.

spread of civil rights, among which hunger, extreme poverty, avoidable disease, child, infant and birth-related mortality and the abandonment of children drew a universe of intolerable situations. Access to food became an implicit right.[21]

That same period also set a milestone in the cultural scene as a key factor for innovation, *modernity* and *progress*. The new bourgeois society boosted urban culture and cosmopolitanism versus the values of country living; world exhibitions were fostered in major European cities, art avant-gardes and any art movement that broke away from former conceptions and rules were worshipped, and a new model of universal citizenship was implemented. This was in contrast with the impoverished image of the rural world, one that was increasingly considered *backward, non-hygienic and rude*, that is to say, not very civilised, according to urban bourgeoisie standards, and unrefined.[22]

It was amidst this complex historical climate that the Interventionist State strongly emerged as a fundamental regulatory element in conflict management and stabilisation policies. Bourgeois liberalism and democratic ideals had shifted from 19th century *laissez-faire* attitudes that detested the State to active commitment, usually in the form of a *protecting* or *providential State*. The State, as the main guarantor and defender of the *common good*, appeared as an unavoidable means to implement human rights associated with new values of citizenship. The State broke through as a regulating player, controlling people's social life to prevent abuse. It was legitimated as the warrantor of social wellbeing, regulating the economy, encouraging scientific activity and social care programmes, the construction of hygienic housing, cities and clean schools, and the design of new suburbs. The State emerged as the regulator of inequalities and the main advocate of people's rights. As a result, Western countries developed an increasingly strong public administration that dealt with social order, including health and diet, both locally and nationally.

On the other hand, the global dimension of social, political and economic problems demanded the configuration of an international context, one usually employed as a reference for State initiatives that regulated competition between countries and staking the boundaries of the most-favoured nation principle. During the inter-war period, this international framework was focused on the League of Nations, not only

---

21 Andresen, A., Barona, J.L., Cherry, S. (eds.), *Making a new countryside? Health Policies and Practices in European History ca. 1860-1950*, Frankfurt, Peter Lang, 2010.

22 *Ibidem*, pp. 15-20.

to foster stabilisation policies on trade, the economy and political conflicts, but also to play a determining role in international public health and in the emergence of *social medicine*.[23] From a sanitary perspective, a new period started following international health conferences and international meetings on hygiene and demography, tuberculosis, cancer, infant health, vaccines, vitamins and rural health. Via international organisations such as the International Health Board of the Rockefeller Foundation and the Red Cross, philanthropy became very relevant on the international health scene in terms of stimulating cooperation between countries.

New values made hunger, famine and malnutrition a visible problem to address, with multiple dimensions: political, economic, medical, scientific and environmental, affecting millions of people all over the world. Individual human rights and social stability were involved. From a social and historical perspective, nutrition and diet made up excellent ground with multiple dimensions, to explore the genesis of experimental knowledge, the social values and interests involved, as well as the transfer of knowledge and practices to public health, the economy, trade and politics. The exceptional confluence of all such factors influenced the emergence of a political economy of knowledge and actions around hunger and nutrition, the main object of analysis of this book.

The Political Economy of Scientific Knowledge

Numerous elements constitute an essential part of the economy of knowledge in any situation: scientific knowledge and products; the system in which knowledge and products are provided, as well as their public; the definition and role of scientists and technologists as experts; financial support; the legitimating paths; and patents and royalty regulations. Today, all of these elements make up a complex network or operating system. In addition to the traditional sites where knowledge was generated (universities, research institutes, hospitals, public offices and laboratories), during the last decades of the 20th century the *system for the production of scientific knowledge* underwent a profound transformation that involved not only traditional institutions, but also other parties, among them the private industry, trading companies and public administrations. This phenomenon appears to be extremely important for any approach to scientific studies that consider *science in*

---

23 Weindling, P. (ed.), *International Health Organisations and Movements, 1918-1939*, Cambridge, Cambridge University Press, 1995.

society and that analyse the relationship between science, politics and social institutions.[24]

The latest contributions by an influential group of social thinkers, economists, philosophers and historians,[25] have helped conceptualise and make understandable the profound changes that our society experienced from the second half of the 20th century, particularly since the fall of the Berlin Wall. As science and technology form a substantial part of this transformation,[26] some sociologists have taken a step further by analysing the changes in what is called the technoscientific production system.[27]

What is the origin and what have been the main coordinates of the transformation experienced by the relations between science and society? Contemporary historians of science generally assumed that a new *regime of knowledge* emerged over the past three decades, one which is essentially different from that initiated by the Scientific Revolution in early modern Europe. Science changed radically in the context of profound social and political transformation experienced by Western societies during the 20th century, changes that affected the social regulation of knowledge production, circulation and use. From this standpoint, the simultaneous evolution of society on the one hand, and science on the other, have reconfigured scientific practices and institutions into a very different system of relations widely dispersed among a number of agents: universities, innovative companies, private laboratories, financial institutions linked to the market, as well as other social structures that result from collaboration between research bodies and private and public spaces (laboratories, research groups) General agreement has been reached on the fact that actors (researchers, financiers, technicians, administrators) constitute separated groups, have different training, operate according to different interests and show different cultures. Nowadays, innovation and technoscience shape a new political economy of scientific knowledge, being the main source of wealth in developed countries.[28]

---

24 Latour, B., "Essays on Science and Society: From the World of Science to the World of Research?", *Science*, 5361, 1998, pp. 208-9.

25 Among them, Zigmunt Baumann, Ulrich Bech, Jürgen Habermas, Jean Le Goff, Alain Touraine, Joseph Stieglitz and others.

26 Hereinafter I will use the term *technoscience* as a neologism expressing the new reality.

27 The contributions to this field by Bruno Latour, Michael Gibbons, Helga Novotny, John Kriege and Dominique Pestre, as cited in the bibliography, have been widely recognised among academics.

28 Pestre, 2003, pp. 151-155.

While the traditional pattern of organising science was based on a stable academic structure – a hierarchical organisation of work, well established expertise, strong and permanent facilities, public funds and a system arranged into areas of knowledge and stable disciplines – the current model of technoscience production could be described by using the famous expression proposed by Zigmunt Baumann to represent today's society: *liquid modernity* (flexibility), change, adaptability of organisational models to meet the demands of a reality in a continuous process of transformation.[29] Science no longer represents essentially logical or epistemological values. On the contrary, it develops according to social demands and the interests of the stock market or the capital gain business. Obviously, the financing of science in more technologically developed countries depends not only on public authorities; it is now increasingly supported by private initiatives. The new model requires collaboration and the coinciding interests of researchers, professional groups, entrepreneurs, lawyers, public demands, the market and politicians. The complex dimension of scientific production and its size can be easily perceived if we consider controversial issues such as genetically modified food production, the industrialisation of foodstuffs, research, the production and marketing of large-scale vaccines, the search for solutions to climate change, energy production, engine design, the effects of electromagnetic waves upon human health, reproductive technologies, stem-cell regenerative medicine, as well as a long list of topics that represent the most relevant challenges of today's world.[30]

As a counterpoint to the complex current network of relations, many social scientists believe that science was characterised in the past by the autonomy of research as a system of knowledge production, depending exclusively on the logic of scientific research, the interests, judgements and methods of experts, and the intrinsic value of scientific knowledge in itself, regardless of the interests and social demands of dominant groups. This vision of science in the past shows little criticism of the rhetoric that has traditionally represented science as an independent entity, giving knowledge an intrinsic value that does not require social legitimacy. However, the history of science shows that at least from the starting point of the so-called *scientific revolution*, all contributions are formally or informally subjected to a plurality of social evaluations, whether or not they are technically suitable, positive for the future, cost

29 Bauman, Z., *Globalization. The Human consequences*, Cambridge, Polity Press, 1998.

30 Barona, J.L., *Salud, tecnología y saber médico*, Madrid, Ed. Ramón Areces, 2004.

effective or timely to solve a problem. All of these conditions obviously depended on cultural, social and economic factors, always having to justify rational consistence and efficiency in the context of a social and economic system, which gave scientific products significance and suitability.

The transcendence of the techno-scientific activity is unprecedented, as many current environmental, human, political and economic challenges depend on it: stopping the deterioration of the environment, using genetically modified organisms, assisted reproduction, stem cell culture in regenerative medicine and reproductive technologies, waste treatment, and many others. Technoscience has generated interdisciplinary areas of action which are based on collaboration between scientists with different expertise to resolve technical problems, as happened in the mid 20th century with issues such as new materials science or computer science applied to medical diagnosis, but sometimes trying to tackle issues of a greater magnitude and dimension with regards to industrial policy, health and economic impact. The sociological analysis of the relationships and influence between technical and scientific networks, the industry, economy growth and social policies are of great interest in understanding today's society and explaining social change. After all, we must admit that ever since the 1980s there has been a change in the production of scientific knowledge and its relations with the productive system and the structure of society itself. The production of knowledge and the production of wealth are now closely related, constituting an inseparable binomial. Western citizens have developed a particular culture of science and have a different perception of the capacity of technoscience to affect human life and transform the world in a positive sense, even if new risks are involved.[31]

However, the idea that science before the past few decades was pure and independent from the economy, politics and social interests would not stand up to a history test. History of science has shown that since the beginning of the Modern Age in the 16th and 17th centuries, science has always supported the army and contributed to the wealth of nations and empires, closely linked to politics. From the outset, modern science has developed techniques, instruments, objects, weapons and devices that have contributed to the practical domain, to political or military control and to the construction of the prevailing order in the world. Moreover,

---

[31] Beck U., *Risk Society: Towards a New Modernity*, Newbury Park, CA, Sage, 1992; Beck, U., "From industrial Society to the Risk Society: Questions of Survival, Social Structure and Ecological Enlightenment", *Theory, Culture and Society*, No. 9, 1992, 97-123

since the late 19th century, scientific communities have been grouped into a wider range of academies, associations and societies, creating legitimacy through the role of expertise, establishing networks and conferences, sharing laboratories and technologies. At the beginning of the 20th century, science was more than just academic science enclosed by university structures. The technological change experienced by the new economy based on chain production in the globalised 1920s – including the production of cars, aeroplanes, electrical devices, atomic energy and so on – was essentially based on scientific research. A wide and diverse range of public and private laboratories, hospitals, museums and workshops served the economic expansion and the massive production of artefacts.

Although it seems difficult to speak about public funding during the first decades of the 20th century, the emergence of a providential state, together with universities, scientific associations, public and private laboratories, shared their space with scientific military academies, societies for the advancement of science or technical schools and industries. Royal protection was essential as well for the development of natural science at the beginning of the modern age, and the new technologies (navigation, the military, mining and agriculture) represented an essential contribution in the process of colonial expansion of European monarchies around the world between the 15th and 20th centuries.

However, since it is clear that the technoscientific systems in place in the 16th century and in the second half of the 20th century are neither the same nor comparable, it is convenient to establish a new periodisation based on the idea of *science in society*, different from that which has so far been traditionally based mainly on the history of the evolution of scientific ideas.

As a starting point, the concept of *regime of knowledge* has been proposed in research about certain trends in the sociology of knowledge. Other sociologists and historians have talked about a *system of production of scientific knowledge* and technological artefacts. Pure sciences and humanities initially shared the same intellectual context. But in the 16th and 17th centuries astronomy, navigation, cartography, artillery, military architecture, construction tools and machines, natural philosophy, anatomy, chemistry, natural history – alongside colonial expansion and other matters and social changes – led to a reversal of classic science into new ways of relating to nature and the manner in which scientists traditionally explored the world. The so-called *Scientific Revolution* – a controversial concept from different points of view, and something that cannot be discussed in depth here – in fact represented a methodological change that prioritised experimental empiricism, but also a big transformation in the social dimension of science and in the social use of machines and artefacts derived from scientific knowledge. Examples that show the important role of science and technology at the start of colonisation include the vacuum pump, the art of machine building, the construction of botanic and acclimatisation gardens, alchemical laboratories for liquors and scents and perfumes.[32] Later, in the 18th century, natural history, agriculture, chemical laboratories and physics cabinets proved that knowledge and actions resulting from good scientific practice were associated with an adequate organisation of the social body.

During the 19th and 20th centuries the academic superiority of scientific knowledge over the technoscientific practices of other social groups (workshops, laboratories, chemistry, meteorology centres) was demonstrated. Steam engines, railways, the telegraph, the chemistry of dyes and textiles, electricity or the radio, are examples of emerging forms of interaction between the industry and academic science, which would later reach a much more meaningful dimension with the use of nuclear power and the aeronautical industry. The period from the late 16th century to the early 18th century was marked by the goal to intervene in nature and dominate it. There was no pure science on the margins of social dynamics in a different context dominated by trade and economic, military or political interests.

Scientific change in this period was a result of many factors that converged to transform the global system of knowledge production and its methodologies. Speakers from a variety of institutions – not only from universities, but also religious groups such as the Jesuits, military academies, scientific travellers, naturalist institutions (botanical gardens, gardens of acclimatisation, departments of natural history), physics cabinets, chemical industries and small public and private laboratories – weaved a particular network of science production and knowledge circulation. A number of social actors took part and stimulated scientific activities: courts, monarchies and aristocracies, commercial companies, entrepreneurs and financiers, scientists, theologians, naturalists, doctors, politicians and philosophers. Knowledge and *ingenium* constituted an inseparable binomial, and the same applied to empirical observation and the experimental method (*experimentum*) and the increasing role of expertise.

---

[32] Moran, B.T., *Patronage and Institutions: Science, Technology and Medicine at the European Court, 1500-1750*, Woodbridge, Suffolk, Boydell Press, 1991; Rossi, P., *I filosofi e le machine 1400-1700*, Milano, Feltrinelli, 2002.

From the *science in society* perspective, the production of knowledge is structured in a particular way in each historical period, but it is always consistent and integrated into the socio-cultural system, never mind the *regimes of scientific knowledge* or *systems of scientific knowledge*. Both concepts are based on the observation that modern science was never an independent reality, a purely coherent system of statements of a cognitive dimension that possess autonomous dynamics from the social context and stable over time. Science and scientific practice have been concentrated across a set of relationships and production techniques, instrumental calculations, metaphors, methodological standards, moral behaviour and, in pluralistic settings, laboratories, universities, conferences, professional associations, as well as economic, political and legal institutions. Every historical period and socio-political context articulates all of these elements in a specific way, making science a form of institutionalised social practices of production and technical management and policy. The functional dynamics of institutions, the methods of validating knowledge and the practical behaviour of researchers are the result of social, economic, political and ideological factors. The notion of system of knowledge, regime of knowledge or system of knowledge production refers to a network of institutions, ideas, beliefs, practices and regulations, showing the social, political and economic boundaries of scientific practice. It represents *a set of institutional commitments* that depend on a plurality of logics typical of various historical forms of society and values.

Since the late 19th century science adopted a new reality as a social institution, covering new areas of production and new modes of action. Universities were open to more technical approaches and industry started to exert more influence. The scientific work was closely tied to mass production, influenced by market dynamics and, as expressed by Max Weber, to what could be called *bureaucratic rationalisation*. The laboratory, as a major site of production of scientific knowledge, became an organised and hierarchical institution, establishing new forms of labour division and specialisation, and giving social importance to the figure of the expert, as is obvious in medical specialisation or in industrial laboratories. Science was accepted and promoted by the state in a context of international rivalry and war risk, to the point of becoming a key element in the politics of the nation-state. Think of the health system, the national institutes of hygiene, such as the Pasteur Institute in Paris or the Robert Koch Institute in Berlin, or the *Junta para Ampliación de Estudios e Investigaciones Científicas* in Madrid. Consider the expansion of provincial health laboratories, national food institutes, the Radium Institute, as well as many other scientific institutions that contributed to the wealth of nations in the early decades of the 20th century and to people's health and reinforced national identities.

The new historical context stimulated the social use of scientific knowledge and the development of new tools and international standards for the industrial production of scientific products (vaccines, vitamins, hormones, medicines...). It also increased the size of scientific and technological businesses, marking the origin of a new technoscience industry that emerged as a multinational economic driver already in the inter-war years, with specific applications such as electrification, the telephone, drinking water, sanitation supplies, electricity, vaccines and vitamins. Science and technology became the spinal cord of modernity in the process of urban transformation and had a growing presence in the economy, international trade and industrial development. Electricity applications, bacteriology and serology, the physics of radiation, among many other scientific fields, made up the basis for many practical domains, such as industry, the army, communications, transport and innovation in domestic affairs.

A transformation in governance practices also occurred and the management of scientific activity multiplied the areas and spaces of knowledge production. The ways in which knowledge was legitimated and appropriated diversified and new interaction and negotiation dynamics between scientists appeared, via conferences, professional associations and specialised publications, modifying and amplifying the social structure of science. Involving the transformation of scientific practices and the emergence of a new technoscientific system closely rooted in the economy, this intense process of science reconstruction was closely linked to new organisational structures with a social, economic and political dimension.[33] The state played a new role, expanding its functions in the promotion of science as a tool to stimulate progress and modernity, a structural reform involving public administrations, which gave the state unprecedented prominence in the social dynamics.

The national reconstruction that took place in Europe between 1870 and 1960 gave new legitimacy to the state as a social agent intervening in scientific, technological and sanitary developments. Science, technology and health were considered again a greater good for citizens and an emergent field for business and economy growth. Becoming the primary, most important stakeholder, the state had to regulate and promote the interests of national defence, as well as the economic, political and military applications of science. A strong and providential

---

33 Pestre, 2008, p. 47.

state therefore emerged as the manager and regulator of social relations, applying expertise and scientific knowledge to integrate workers and peasants to reduce inequalities, and to dismantle worker revolutions; it was a state that managed economic growth, living conditions and people's health by means of scientific indicators, epidemiological records, economic calculations and vital and social statistics. Western countries participated in this tendency most actively. The state apparatus was used in science and industry to improve the economy, the health standards of the population, living conditions in urban and rural areas, as well as design hygienic houses for workers and prepare for war. In the first half of the 20th century, technoscience was basically at the service of the State.

The former world, under a Westphalian balance of power between nations, and regulated by elected or representative parties that collectively defined the priorities (for science, industry, or the redistribution of services and wealth) gave way, at least in part, to global or planetary systems mainly regulated by markets and other partially new forms of 'governance'. One should, however, keep in mind that the major states still played a pivotal role in geopolitical relationships – this being particularly clear when one investigates the great national innovation systems in the principal powers.[34]

In such a controversial period, technoscience achieved great importance as a tool for the State as policymaker, to serve the public good, ensure order and national power and create the conditions for national stability. It was a wide and complex programme based on the commitment of the social classes under the hegemony of the State. The crisis of the 1930s further strengthened the role of the government in social and economic activities. Liberalism and the market were adapted and took advantage of the growing importance of the providential state. A sort of social agreement for the population's welfare and social assistance transformed the State into the only power to counterweight the threat of war, social crisis and conflicts.

From the perspective of the contribution of science to economic growth, the productive system also renewed practices, structures and objectives during the first half of the 20th century. Numerous things were developed: mass production; new production lines based on Fordism and Taylorism as productive ideologies (driven by the massive sales of advertising policies); product standardisation; and new patterns of industrial production and labour organisation. Technoscience was called on to play a growing role in the materialisation of modernity and

---

34 *Ibidem*, pp. 181-190.

innovation. Throughout the 20th century economies based on the knowledge of laboratory technicians became widespread and fundamental for economic planning. The transformation of economic structures also implied a crisis for family businesses without any planning. The middle decades of the 20th century saw a movement of social transformation that leaned on experimental science, technology, social science research and management, which led to a redefinition of the social function of science and technology, opening up new links with the economy and the market. In certain fields, this was the origin of an economy of knowledge, driven by the latest communication technologies.

It can be generally accepted that until the last quarter of the 20th century some balance existed between open and public science driven by universities, large foundations, national laboratories and other public institutions, and science produced by private companies. The equilibrium was based on coordination through circulation and exchange between the two areas, state universities operating as intermediary agencies and strong entrepreneurs of science. There was also a balance between science as an independent project in the hands of university scientists, basic socialisation rules as state institutions and industrial research focused on producing benefits in relation with market competition. This balance was reflected in regulations and patents.[35] In this context science contributed to the rationalisation of Western societies and to the construction of national states through national science, as an element of industrial management and government in macroeconomic administration, public health or military organisation.

Between 1870 and 1940 industry grew spectacularly based on scientific knowledge: the pharmaceutical laboratories; the National Institutes of Bacteriology; telegraphy and electricity companies; radio channels; the industrial production of food; and the film industry. The new industries were based on new laboratories, technical institutes such as the Radium Institute, the Pasteur Institute, the National Bureau of Standards (USA), the Curie Laboratory, National Institutes of Health, the Institute for Health and Tropical Medicine and National Institutes of Physics. National agencies and research laboratories sponsored by the state or local authorities were the main driver and the source of funding. It is easy to understand that the beginning of the technoscientific industry in the late 19th century was not an isolated event, since it was being set up at a time in which the nation-state experienced a transformation, as discussed above. This helps us gain an insight into the

35 *Ibidem*, pp. 142-150.

fact that the new economies based on scientific research contributed to constructing national ideologies, reinforced by the historical discourse and the material power of science and technology. This is evident with the Spanish crisis following the 1898 military defeat and also with Nazi Germany. Science meant wealth and power.

The laboratory became the key space for the production of knowledge. Professional scientists, now enjoying an expert status, also became key legitimating actors. Scientists were no longer sheer scholars or intellectuals; they also acquired recognised expertise and monopolised professional fields. Science and experts' activity became a part of the industrial context and an ideological agent in the nation-building process. National science and technology reached similar importance to that of the national army or the national economy. A long list of scientific, economic and political dimensions make nutrition, hunger and health a paradigmatic case study, along with numerous other aspects: agricultural innovation, food production, nutritional science, education in nutrition, nutritional habits, calorie and nutrient analysis, the patterns for an optimum diet. There is also the rationing of diets, the definition and limits of malnutrition, the clinical effects of nutritional deficiencies, experimental nutrition science, the food industry and the food chain.

World War I prompted greater economic planning, new forms of rationalisation of production and new scientific applications (vaccines, detection of attacks, etc). At the same time, the pressure of the labour movement and the fear of communist expansion posed a threat to liberal industrialised societies. Liberal reformism invented social security systems that went beyond traditional paternalism in addressing disability, death, sickness, unemployment, hunger and old age. Social protection systems were based on varying forms of insurance, representing a new corpus of values around the concept of citizenship and civil rights, a form of collective solidarity increasingly coordinated by the *welfare state*. The new ideology promoted common good as the highest value and a sense of belonging to a community. This mentality reflected the great pillars of the new nation state after the decline of the old empires: the right to education, health, housing, food, etc. The implementation of the welfare programme was only possible thanks to a political economy based on scientific and technological progress. More than a bilateral relationship between the individual and society, the new political culture promoted identification with the community; a culture of analysis and planning linked to the State as a governing agent and a regulator.

Access to foodstuffs and a sufficient calorie intake, a healthy life, social wellbeing, and health care constituted essential values in the programme. Among those called on to implement it were reformist national elites, political national authorities and international networks – mostly promoted by the League of Nations, the Rockefeller Foundation and later on by the international bodies created within the orbit of the UN. The two world wars and the Spanish Civil War had brought about unprecedented opportunities and exceptional crises. The idea of progress and modernity was built around scientific and technological development that had specific goals, prospective reports, a solid analysis of the situations, meetings of experts and action plans. This wide programme required a strong state administration and technically well-trained experts. The period that spanned between the Cold War and the first oil crisis in the early 1970s was characterised in most Western countries by the construction of the *welfare state* and grounded on a strong and efficient public administration. Trade, education, culture and health converged in a socially constructed idea of progress and community commitment. The state, through public policies, implemented the dynamics that brought the working classes to configure new middle classes, far from the situation of the *proletariat* and its traditional claims for a social revolution. In Western Europe the Nation-State operated as social regulator, intervening in the economy and redistributing goods and services in a system of social protection. This was based on taxation to redistribute the proceeds among all social sectors for public benefit.

Under these circumstances, the technical capacity for the material handling of physical and biological entities was to be strengthened. Atomic nuclei, molecules and genes became fields of technological development, and collaboration between university laboratories, national research entities and industrial and private research institutes gave birth to new technologies such as the laser, those derived from atom physics, electromagnetic wave applications, high precision instruments and many others, which contributed to medicine and communication technology, and improved daily living conditions. Technoscientific development became the cornerstone of the economy, progress, modernity and national power, encompassing numerous products: the telephone, the telegraph, the radio, refrigerators, washing machines, cars, planes, high-speed trains, television, followed by electronics, aerospace devices, computers, satellites, etc..

Hunger at the Crossroads

The expansion of liberal democracies in Western countries since the second half of the 19th century contributed to transforming the social role of the state, particularly in areas such as education, transport, communication, infrastructures, health care and social assistance.

Gradually, since the early 20th century, the state emerged as the social guarantor of civil rights and citizens' wellbeing and as a regulator of social inequalities. State and collective interests were identified as being the same thing. The state therefore assumed the responsibility of organising and directing the future of the nation. It created a rational bureaucracy and intervention policies, taking on the political and intellectual project of the Enlightenment ideology of achieving social justice.

Among the strong elements in this construction process was the new cultural, social, political and economic significance of hunger, food and diet. With the right to being healthy considered an attribute of citizenship, the right to decent and sufficient food came next. A poor diet was deemed to be the threshold of infection, and so microbes and foodstuffs drew the attention of physicians and hygienists. The confluence of such a wide range of elements helps us understand the interest in identifying deficiency diseases and in defining the concept of deficiency disease, *undernourishment and malnutrition*, according to scientific parameters.

Due to its multiple dimensions affecting agriculture, the economy, health and war, *diet* and *nutrition* became a central issue in Europe between 1918 and 1960. A first aspect to consider is the *political and military dimension* of hunger. In times of crisis and war, it was urgent to ensure a minimum diet for the whole population and, in particular, to avoid famine in specific risk groups: children, mothers, pregnant women, elderly people, patients, soldiers, refugees, prisoners and unemployed workers. Secondly, the *economic dimension* of the food supply became especially relevant as a result of the deterioration of the global food system, which had been built up in the second half of the 19th century. War conflicts and the 1929 economic and financial splash caused food production and food trade to collapse worldwide, with terrible consequences in the 1930s, leading to World War II. In a purely commercial sense, the crisis of the global food system did not only result in scarcity and a high cost of living but also gave way to protectionism and the return of protection in domestic markets. All such factors encouraged the growing industrialisation of more and more foodstuffs (milk, chocolate, oil, sugar, bread, etc) as opposed to traditional manufacturing. The food industry demanded the regulation and control of production processes, strict surveillance of fraud and adulteration, and the control of additives, colourings and preservatives, as well as hygienic conditions in the final foodstuffs for the consumer at the end of the chain. Basically, new rules were needed to stake the boundaries of what was permissible and what was unacceptable in human diets, a debate whose backdrop was the natural/artificial divide.

The cultural dimension of hunger and nutrition soon emerged from the economic, sanitary and political importance. Hygienists and politicians became aware of the deep differences in dietary and cooking habits and traditions that were not only due to the level of income. Cultural habits also influenced dietary differences between cities and the countryside in the same country and between European regions. It was necessary to analyse nutritional needs in age groups and according to gender, for manual and factory workers, farmers and more sedentary professionals. This need prompted surveys and reports that intended to map nutrition and hunger, to be used as a basis for political action, rationing policies, health care and social protection.

Scientific knowledge – the new experimental science of nutrition – was to become the cornerstone of a healthy diet and the reference for food production and consumption. That required solid physiological grounds at the laboratory in relation to calorie coefficients, the need for nutritional principles, tables of foodstuff values in calories, nutrients, vitamins and minerals. The parameters of the *optimum diet* and the requirements of the *minimum diet* had to be accurately defined to be able to apply this knowledge to rationing strategies in times of war and scarcity. That was also essential for the organisation of food relief. In turn, the establishment of physiological standards of nourishment had to determine the boundaries of normality and pathology, defining the concepts of food deficiency, undernourishment and malnutrition.

The figure of the *nutrition expert* (dietician, nutritionist) stood out in the challenge of establishing physiological, clinical or anthropometric exploration methods to conceptualise and delimit all types of deficiency diseases and malnutrition in children and adults. In this way, during the inter-war period, hunger and nutrition opened up an avenue for the medicalisation of diets, the spread of medical knowledge, the development of a powerful food industry and international food trade networks.

In sum, *hunger, nutrition* and *diet* were closely linked to the new social construction of health as a human right, and reached economic and political importance in order to harmonise food production, trade and demands, since dietary habits brought to light traditions that were contrary to the new logic of nutritional science and the evolution of the food market.

Once the parameters of the problem of nutrition had been set, an economic and political strategy had to be put forward in order to resolve it. Obviously, the answer was to build a new system of scientific knowledge production and to transform social practices; a new culture was needed in food and consumption, in the regulation of what could be eaten, and in the redefinition of the social and cultural meaning of food.

This strategy was mainly promoted by international organisations and by the states both from local and national levels and with a multidimensional focus on the transformation of the food production system, the regulation of industrial production and the control of quality, fraud and adulteration.

Collaboration between national and international institutions was essential. National governments coordinated public policies according to international standards. The League of Nations Health Committee, the International Institute of Agriculture, the Food and Agriculture Organization, the World Health Organization, the International Labour Organisation and the International Health Board of the Rockefeller Foundation worked together to play a major role. Joint Expert Committees on Nutrition worked for decades to establish physiological standards for food and patterns for a healthy diet, surveying the nutritional state of the population, changing dietary habits and fighting malnutrition and nutritional deficiencies in many parts of the world. International trade had to be rebuilt and substantially transformed and the exceptional situation caused by the war confronted. Diet habits also had to be changed on the basis of scientifically defined patterns, and health levels had to be improved by means of a balanced diet.

The foundations of this new social, political and economic architecture were found in the onset of a new experimental science of nutrition based on exact physiological concepts (calorie, nutrient, protein, etc) that enabled scientists to draw the border between health and pathology. That was the main argument that legitimated experts and the creation of international commissions of nutrition experts and conferences to discuss different aspects of the subject. The tragic aftermath of the world wars, the Spanish Civil War, the famine crisis in the Netherlands, Poland, Russia and Greece, urged an international response and provided an excellent testing ground for the new science of nutrition.

The international construction of a political economy of hunger and nutrition gathered momentum between 1918 and 1960. International intervention took on the form of a network of expert commissions drawn from national and international levels. Their work was mainly focused on the following practical programme:

1. Implementation of surveys and reports on diet and food consumption habits in different European countries and on the specific consumption of meat, rice, milk, fresh vegetables, fruit or sugar. They also included studies on specific social groups such as pregnant women, children, industrial workers, peasants or the unemployed. This work was encouraged and supported by international organisations and philanthropic groups.

2. Implementation of public health strategies by national schools of hygiene, aimed at training health professionals as nutrition specialists, and programming information campaigns for the population to change their dietary habits. Basically, the goal was to educate according to the scientific principles of nutrition.

3. Development of empirical methodology based on the research undertaken by specialists in food surveys, with a dual orientation: social surveys and studies on dietary habits, and clinical exploration methods to assess the health condition of the population.

The starting point of the latter was experimental physiology, complemented by anthropometric, clinical and physio-pathological studies. They intended to identify, with scientific-experimental parameters, the nutritional state of individuals and populations, identifying the presence of deficiency diseases such as beriberi, pellagra, scurvy, neuropathies due to nutritional deficiencies, as well as different malnutrition levels.

Such an ambitious programme made necessary the validation of empirical methodology and required an agreement concerning the standards of proteins, fats, carbohydrates, vitamins and minerals in a balanced daily diet. Experimental research was called on to lay down the *standards for adequate nutrition*, and a new language also emerged from the new experimental science: *optimum* and *minimum* diets were typified; the protection of food was defined and supplementary foods classified; calorie methods and energy coefficients were established; dietary standards for specific populations were recommended; and nutritional values and principles, basal metabolism, calorie requirements, family coefficient scales in rationing were standardised and applied in rationing policies.

A large body of experimental knowledge started to be developed as a basis for the clinical categorisation of undernourishment, malnutrition and obesity, as well as a range of new clinical entities associated with specific deficiencies of one or more nutritional principles. This was the starting point for political action, economy planning and industrial production. As a regulating, stabilising, disciplining and civilising agent, the State – assisted by large international corporations, international agencies and philanthropic organisations – promoted community nutrition policies and trained nutritionists to become experts. It also organised campaigns from the sections of food hygiene and community nutrition of the National Schools of Hygiene and the National Institutes for Mother and Children Care with a view to influencing mothers and modifying cooking traditions, given that women are the main channel of diet information and practices within the family. From the second half of the 1930s Institutes of Food Hygiene sprang up across Europe with a view to implementing rationing policies in times of crisis, war and post-war years.

During the middle decades of the 20th century, nutrition concentrated on a series of aspects that made it an expression of the emergence of experimental knowledge, its circulation and transfer into social practices. The nutritional status of the population was not traditionally a matter linked to the political economy or state policy. Conversely, hunger was connected to poverty, and nutritional habits were considered part of a culture, a reflection of income and social status, lacking any moral or sanitary implications.[36] It was the advent of the state as a social regulator in the complex situation of the first half of the 20th century that placed hunger and feeding at a complex crossroads at which citizenship, culture, economy and health played a meaningful role.[37] Food availability became a challenge in many regions for most citizens. Shortages and famines, fears of deprivation and food regulations were a common European experience during the period 1918-1960. Market and food production, nutrition and conflict stressed the emergence of a global food system starting in the late 19th century, which suddenly experienced a deep crisis in the following years in an era of wars, increasing intervention by the state and rising economic nationalism.

---

36 Vernon, J., "The Ethics of Hunger and the Assembly of Society: The Techno-Politics of the School Meal in Modern Britain", *American Historical Review*, No. 110, 2005, pp. 693-725.

37 Barona, J.L., "Rural Life and the Problem of Nutrition. Technical Approaches by the Nutrition Committee of the League of Nations", in Andresen, A., Gronlie, T., Ryymin, T. (eds.), *Science, Culture and Politics. European Perspectives on Medicine, Sickness and Health*, Bergen, Stein Rokkan Centre for Social Studies, 2006, pp. 201-214; Smith, D.F., Phillips, J. (eds.), *Food, Science, Policy and Regulation in the Twentieth Century. International and Comparative Perspectives*, London, Routledge, 2000; Vernon J., 2005; Barona, J.L., "Nutrition and Health. The International Context during the Inter-war Crisis,' *Social History of Medicine*, No. 21, 2008, pp. 87-105.

CHAPTER 3

The Production of Scientific Knowledge and Social Practices: the International Response

The political, demographic and economic consequences of the Great War during the following decades were an immense threat to international stability. Food had already been included on the agenda of international meetings of experts and social movements before the First World War, stretching from malnutrition and relief, the feeding of children and pregnant women, to adulteration and the search for a healthy, balanced diet. In the 1920s there was a shift away from charitable relief to a more professionalised and scientific approach to nutritional relief.[1] The International Labour Organisation [ILO] and the League of Nations' Health Organisation placed the emphasis on the production and use of scientific knowledge. They became international transmitters of new nutritional knowledge, as well as places from where reformers put pressure on their national governments to raise minimum standards and social benefits.[2]

New Experts and New Institutions in the Fight against Hunger

Since its foundation, the League of Nations got involved in health problems. Its Council drew up a scheme for a Health Organisation as early as in February 1920. Several steps forward led to the constitution of a Health Committee (Geneva, August 1921) and a cooperative strategy with the *Office International d'Hygiène Publique*, in Paris, the International Labour Organisation [ILO] and the International Institute of Agriculture [IIA], in Rome.[3] A *Health Committee*, an *Advisory Council*, and a *Health Section of the Secretariat* constituted a complex administrative framework devoted to the coordination of an ambitious programme in international health. The series of *Annual Reports*, the

1 I have analysed these activities in more detail in my book Barona, 2010.

2 Trentmann, Just, 2006, pp. 29-30.

3 Dubin, M., "The League of Nations Health Organization", in Weindling, P. (ed.), *International health organisations and movements, 1918-1939*, Cambridge, Cambridge University Press, 1995, pp. 56-80.

Bulletin of the Health Organisation, the *Annual and Monthly Epidemiological Reports*, the *Weekly Epidemiological Records* (Geneva), and the *Weekly Fasciculus* (Singapore) summarised the main trends of intense activity in international health.[4]

The first technical reports by the Health Organisation of the League of Nations date back to 1926, with a wide range of documents on nutrition-related aspects.[5] All of them emphasised the importance of developing a science of nutrition as a point of departure, to challenge the nutritional requirements of the global population. These scientific studies had to have both a social and experimental orientation, and include standardising methods to study dietary needs, the links between nutrition, agriculture, the economy and public health, especially in rural areas, statistics in countries and regions, as well as reports on the real feeding restrictions in Europe and the diseases caused by them. Meaningful players such as John Maynard Keynes, Jean Monnet and Albert Thomas, all advocated intervention in food production and consumption as one of the best alternatives to tackle economic instability.[6]

Most of the technical and social studies of nutrition in the 1920s and 1930s focused on European countries (Czechoslovakia, Denmark, France, Great Britain, Hungary, The Netherlands, Romania, Spain, Portugal and Sweden).[7] Europe was the centre of the crisis. The

---

4 A summary of the activities developed by the League of Nations can be found in "Bibliography of the Technical Work of the Health Organisation of the League of Nations, 1920-1945", *League of Nations Bulletin of the Health Organisation*, Vol. 11, 1945, p. 6.

5 Boxes in the Archive of the League of Nations (Geneva) containing specific information on nutrition include R.6133 to R.6140. Some internal reports related to the period 1928-1937 (R.5865-5866) are devoted to nutrition. See also Saiki, T., *Necessity of the Study of Nutrition*, Geneva, League of Nations, 1927. Document R.5910 analyses food supplies, reparation and distribution (1929). It also included some other internal documents on food supplies: preparations alleged to contain vitamins (1929-1932) and food supplies, standardisation of vitamins (1930-1932) (Documents R.5921 y R.6078-79). Documents R.5935 and R.6009 (1932) were entirely devoted to food supplies, production and distribution of vitamin standards. Document R.5936 contains an *Étude de l'état alimentaire* (1932-3) and also several *Études sur la meilleure utilisation, pour l'alimentation des budgets réduits* (1932-3).

6 Barona, 2010.

7 Milk and Milk Products in Sweden (Studies on nutrition), 1926, (Document C.H./Com.Exp.Alim./5: Divers/I); Moerkeberg, H.C., *Meat inspection in Denmark and Inspection of Milk in Danemark*, 1924, C.H./E.P.S./49; Mackenzie, M.D., "The Administrative Machinery by which the Adequate Nourishment of the Poor is Ensured in Great Britain", *League of Nations Quarterly Bulletin of the Health Organisation*, 1933, Vol. 2, pp. 333-352; [McDougall, E.J.] "Rural dietaries in

consequences of war, international conflicts and financial chaos could explain a concern basically focused on European regions.

The emergence of a science of nutrition, based on experimental principles, involved, on the one hand, expertise based on new methods and, on the other, technologies to survey and evaluate the nutritional condition of the population and its impact on public health. Moreover, it required political measures to rearrange agriculture and commercial networks, as well as education to change the population's negative habits. The huge impact of malnutrition and deficiency diseases associated with dietary problems during the post-war years gave scientific authority to nutritionists. They increasingly had a scientific approach based on experimental research on bodily energy needs and on the physiological contribution of vitamins, minerals, proteins, carbohydrates and fats. Politicians and economists turned their eyes to the new science of nutrition as a starting point of a steady solution.

In 1925 a proposal from the Yugoslav delegation to the Assembly of the League of Nations requested the Health Committee to study "the methods to be recommended in the interests of public health for the regulation of the manufacture and of the sale of food products". Shortly after, in 1926, the Health Organisation published a collection of memoranda on the physiology of nutrition and its clinical meaning.[8] In 1927 the specialist on the physiology of nutrition T. Saiki gave several lectures on nutrition in the USA, Argentina, Brazil and Chile under the auspices of the League of Nations. In 1926 and 1927 the League of Nations' Health Organisation promoted a visit by Egerton Grey, a professor at the University of Cairo, to Tokyo. He published an internal report about *The Food of Japan* following the visit.[9]

During the 13th session of the Health Committee held in 1928, Léon Bernard, a delegate of the French Government, asked for nutrition to be included into the Committee's work programme. As we know, the situation became more urgent and dramatic the following year. Based on its interest in nutrition, a collective tour of the Health Committee to the

Europe", *Bulletin of the Health Organisation*, 1939, Vol. 8, No. 3, pp. 470-497, [C.H./Com.Exp.Alim./59, 25 p.]; Muehel, W., "Ill effects of food restrictions in Europe, 1940-1944", *League of Nations Bulletin of the Health Organisation*, 1945-1946, Vol. 12; *Nutrition in various countries*, Series of League of Nations Publications, Geneva, 1936. [Technical Report A.12(b).1936.II.B]; "Report on Bread in several European Countries", *League of Nations Bulletin of the Health organisation*, 1939, Vol. 8, pp. 498-55.

8 Saiki, T., *Progress of the Science of Nutrition in Japan*, Geneva, League of Nations, 1926. It was followed by Saiki 1927.

9 *The Food of Japan*. Internal report. Archive of the League of Nations Doc CH 861.

USA took place in 1931 in order to study the supply of milk; a year later the Government of Chile requested collaboration from the League of Nations to carry out a study of popular nutrition in Chile.

In 1932 general concerns arose about the consequences of the crisis and, as a result, the 19th session of the Health Committee undertook a study on the effects of the economic crisis on public health, with particular reference to the undernourishment conditions caused by the recession. Two conferences of experts were convened in connection with the studies on nutrition. The first one was the Experts Conference held in Rome in September 1932 and the second one was held in Berlin in December 1932. Against the backdrop of these two conferences, there was an implicit call for experimental science and technical expertise to consider the principles of an adequate diet as a means to overcome the economic crisis.[10]

By 1932 the problem of nutrition was fully integrated in the international agenda due to exceptional circumstances. In accordance with the recommendation of the Berlin Conference and the invitation of the Council of the League of Nations, the Health Organisation and the International Labour Organisation pooled their efforts to study the most suitable methods for safeguarding public health in times of depression. A Joint Conference of Experts in Sanitary Administration and Social Insurance promoted by the League of Nations and the International Labour Organisation, including members from Belgium, the United Kingdom, Czechoslovakia, France, Germany, the United States of America and Yugoslavia, met on two occasions under the chairmanship of M.G. Cahen-Salvador, a State Councillor in Paris.[11]

A couple of years later, in September 1935, the General Assembly of the League of Nations, having considered the subject of nutrition in relation to public health and the effects of improved nutrition on the consumption of agricultural products, urged Governments to examine the practical means of securing better nutrition and invited the Health Organisation to continue and extend its work on nutrition in relation to international public health.[12] Furthermore, it requested the Council to instruct the technical organisation of the League of Nations, in

---

10 Information about these conferences in *Quarterly Bulletin of the League of Nations*, Vol. I., 1932-1933, No. 3 and Vol. II, 1933, No. 1.

11 "Report of the Health Organisation for the Period October 1932 to September 1933. IV. Economic Depression and Public Health", *League of Nations Quarterly Bulletin of the Health Organisation*, 1933, Vol. 2, pp. 529-535.

12 *The Problem of Nutrition. Interim Report of the Mixed Committee on the Problem of Nutrition*, 3 vols., Geneva, Series of League of Nations Publications, 1936 [Technical Report A.12.1936.II.B].

consultation with the International Labour Office and the International Institute of Agriculture, to collect, summarise and publish information on the measures taken in all countries for securing improved nutrition. The Assembly also proposed to appoint a Committee, including agricultural, economic and health experts, instructed to submit a general report on the whole question.[13]

Some months before, in June 1935, the 19th session of the ILO had voted in favour of a resolution that unanimously recognised that adequate nutrition was essential for the wellbeing of workers and their families. Similarly, the resolution admitted that large numbers of people in many countries were not sufficiently nourished. The ILO resolution stated that an increase in consumption of agricultural foodstuffs would help to raise the standards of living and relieve the depression in agriculture. The ILO Conference requested the Governing body to continue investigations in collaboration with Health and Economic Organisations of the League of Nations, the IIA and others.

As a consequence of the international organisations' agreement on the wide dimension of the hunger problem and the necessity of collaboration, a mixed technical commission was founded and held in London between November 25 and 29, 1935. The mixed commission had to prepare a "Report on the Physiological Basis of Nutrition".[14] This report was of a preliminary nature and therefore included a general assessment of the nutrition issue, embodying suggestions by the Mixed Committee to the Assembly and giving an overview of the problems involved. Three more volumes reported on the physiological basis of nutrition, according to the Technical Commission of the Health Committee and the state of nutrition in various countries. The volumes summarised the available data delivered by governments that replied to the Secretary-General's Circular letter of November 30, 1935. It contained a survey of popular dietaries since the war and a summary of statistical materials. The last part included statistics of food production, consumption and prices in several countries.

The Mixed Committee consisted of experts representing not only the League of Nations but also the International Labour Office and the International Institute of Agriculture, which means that access to foodstuffs and the fight against hunger was given worldwide priority in

13 *Ibidem*, 1936, p. 7-8.

14 "Report on the Physiological Bases of Nutrition by the Technical Commission of the Health Committee in the meeting held in London, November 25-29, 1935", *League of Nations Quarterly Bulletin of the Health Organisation*, 1936, Vol. 5, No. 3, pp. 391-415.

the international policies of the 1930s. The Mixed Committee was especially concerned with the nutritional needs of the lower-income sections of the community – children and the unemployed – and sought to ensure an adequate food supply, particularly of protective foods, at prices affordable by all social groups. A main challenge was the safeguard of the interests of producers as cornerstones of the system. Therefore, improving the marketing and distribution of foodstuffs and reducing their costs both in the cities and in industrial and rural areas was necessary, encouraging collaboration between cooperatives and other forms of producers' and consumers' organisations.

Nutrition and Public Health

In 1934 the Health Committee of the LoN was preparing a three-year programme. E. Burnet and W.R. Aykroyd were entrusted with a series of enquiries in different countries – the United Kingdom, France, the United States, Denmark, Sweden, Norway and the Union of Soviet Socialist Republics – on institutions linked to nutrition policies.[15] Burnet and Aykroyd's report emphasised the importance of international economic conditions and income differences across social groups in relation to adequate nutrition. "The general problem of nutrition as it presents itself today is that of harmonising economic and public health development".[16]

The report by Burnet and Aykroyd was published at a time when the social problems of housing and nutrition were definitely occupying the foremost position in public health. Continuing the work carried out by the Rome and Berlin Conferences, the report addressed the preoccupations arising out of the protracted economic depression. The report contained the essential elements for a general discussion of the practical problems of nutrition in relation both to public health and to economic recovery. It was used as a basis of discussion when the delegations of 12 governments at the 16th Assembly of the League, held in September 1935, requested that nutrition be placed on the agenda. Indeed, the discussion in the 2nd Committee of the Assembly was introduced by Mr. Bruce, the Australian delegate, who stressed the necessity of harmonising agriculture and public health in the interest of the latter. An increasing consumption of protective foods was presented as a remedy for malnutrition, and also as some help towards facing the agricultural crisis. Bruce called for a change in State protective

15 E. Burnet and W.R. Aykroyd report was summarised in the *Quarterly Bulletin of the League of Nations*, 1935, Vol. 4, No. 2, pp. 323-474.

16 *Ibidem*, p. 394.

subsidies, so they could be used to increase consumption rather than restrict production.

Lord de la Warr, a representative of the United Kingdom delegation, presented a report to the Assembly, considering the subjects of nutrition in relation to public health and the positive effects of improved nutrition on the consumption of agricultural products in such a difficult context. Consequently, the Assembly of the League of Nations adopted a resolution inviting the Health Organisation to continue and extend its work on nutrition in relation to public health. It instructed the technical organisations of the League of Nations, in consultation with the International Labour Office and the International Institute of Agriculture, to collect, summarise and publish information on the measures taken in all countries for securing improved nutrition. It also appointed a committee that included agricultural, economic and health experts and instructed it to submit a general report on the whole question to the next Assembly.[17]

At the same time, the International Labour Office, which had been informed of the general plan of action contained in the Burnet and Aykroyd report, gave proof of its interest with collaborative participation. The Mixed Advisory Agricultural Committee (a board that ensured liaison and cooperation between the ILO and the IIA) and the International Committee for Inter-Cooperative Relations (a private organisation that liased between farmers' and consumers' cooperatives) had expressed their desire to cooperate on research into the question of the nutrition of workers. Therefore, during the critical decade of the 1930s, a network of international organisations agreed on the search for expertise to tackle the crisis, taking the population's nutrition as a main tool.

In 1930 the Polish expert of the League of Nations Health Committee, Witold Chodzko, the Head of the National School of Hygiene in Warsaw, summed up existing fears regarding poor nutritional conditions in the rural areas of most European countries.[18] A month later, the League of Nations Health Committee appointed a Sub-Committee on Rural Health, consisting of the Spanish expert Gustavo Pittaluga as president, Witold Chodzko, Gerard Fitzgerald, Carl Hamel, Alberto Lutrario, Ludwik Rajchman and Frank Boudreau. They represented most of the national schools of health in European countries,

[17] *Ibidem*, 1935, p. 395.

[18] Chodzko W., *The Rural Centre for Public Health and Social Welfare and the Improvement of Rural Health Conditions, Sixteenth Session of the Health Committee*, Geneva, League of Nations, 1930.

where public health experts established links with national public health policies.

At the end of the 19th International Labour Organisation Conference (June 1935), the following resolution was unanimously adopted:

> Seeing that adequate nutrition, both in quantity and in quality, is essential to the health and well-being of the workers and their families;
>
> And seeing that, in various countries, evidence has been brought forward to show that large numbers of persons both in town and country are not sufficiently or suitably nourished;
>
> Seeing, moreover, that an increase in the consumption of agricultural foodstuffs would help to raise standards of life and relieve the existing depression in agriculture:
>
> The Conference welcomes the attention drawn by the Director in his report to the problem of nutrition and requests the Governing Body to instruct the Office to continue its investigation of the problem, particularly in its social aspects, in collaboration with the Health and Economic Organisations of the League of Nations, the International Institute of Agriculture and other bodies capable of contributing to its solution, with a view to presenting a report on the subject to the 1936 session of the Conference.[19]

Nutrition was present in every international event during that period. The 22nd Assembly of the League of Nations held in October 1935 recommended the circulation of Burnet and Aykroyd's report to national administrations. Political and sanitary measures pointed out the necessity of instructing medical practitioners, public health workers and the public in the field of nutrition. A resolution was adopted, asking the Technical Commission on Nutrition to select a list of questions, to be classified by order of priority, as a basis for the work to be carried out in cooperation with the other international institutions. The members appointed to the Technical Commission on Nutrition were: A. Durig (Austria); E.P. Cathcart, E. Mellanby and J.B. Orr (United Kingdom); M.J. Alquier, A. Mayer and L. Lapicque (France); F. Bottazzi (Italy); A. Höjer, C. Schiötz and L.S. Fridericia (Scandinavian States); B. Sbarsky (USSR); and E.V. McCollum, M. Swatz Rose and W. Sebrel (USA). H. Chick (London) was also invited to participate, since he was the technical secretary of the International Conference on Standardisation of Vitamins.

---

19 Burnet, Aykroyd, 1935, pp. 395-396.

Nutritional Status: Health, Physiology and Clinics

The League of Nations' Health Committee set up an Advisory Commission on Nutrition in 1932. It was committed to tackling the most important challenges involved in the scientific definition of malnutrition: promoting the standardisation of methods used in dietary studies and establishing optimum and minimum diet standards according to the physiological contribution of vitamins, minerals, fats, carbohydrates and protein requirements. Such big commitments were to be accompanied by other challenges such as: the discussion of guiding principles for a healthy human diet; the spread of clinical methods to determine the state of nutrition in school children; the establishment of patterns of nutritional requirements at all ages; the identification of specific diets for those sectors of the population on small incomes; and the implementation of surveys on the state of nutrition in every country, particularly in rural areas. This was an ambitious and long-term programme that required technical and methodological agreement among all the active countries in the League of Nations' Health Committee.[20] The international response promoted by the League of Nations required, as a first condition, the creation of a fully legitimated international group of experts. Then, a series of meetings, conferences, technical documents, scientific articles and regional surveys would produce an assessment of the situation as a point of departure for further strategies based on the coordination of national and international action.[21]

It was hoped that following the dissemination of new scientific knowledge about nutrition and its influence on social practices, substantial changes would take place in all the aspects involved. The *Final Report of the Mixed Committee of the League of Nations on Relation of Nutrition to Health, Agriculture and Economic Policy* (1937) marked the culmination of the nutritional programme against international under-consumption. Increasing the consumption of "protective" foods was a dual strategy intended to tackle malnutrition and agricultural depression. This reference report stressed the need for governments to take the lead in raising public awareness on nutrition,

20 Barona, 2010, pp. 28-32.

21 *Introductory note on the work accomplished (History and method)* by the League of Nations up to October 1935 (Nutrition), 12 p.

and established the centrality of consumption for global trade and agriculture improvement.[22]

National and international organisations recognised the nutrition problem as affecting both industrial and agricultural countries even before the 1929 crash. During the early 1930s defective nutrition was not only limited to areas hit by the economic crisis, such as impoverished urban communities and depressed agricultural regions. The awareness of such a situation prompted regional surveys and made the new scientific concepts more trustworthy as key political tools to overcoming the crisis.

Scientific research led to the search for a formula regarding the *optimum standard of human diet*. Experimental physiologists identified a total of 12 inorganic mineral elements that play an important role in human nutrition. This meant that their absence definitely produced deficiency diseases. Then there were the vitamins, which were considered to exert a great deal of influence on health. At least the lack of any of nine of those inorganic elements was experimentally and clinically associated with definite deficiency diseases, defective nutrition or malnutrition. The primordial objective was not to prescribe a single type of diet for all the peoples of Europe, but to promote agricultural production to provide the most efficient food supply, taking into consideration the population's traditional dietary habits. Children's health was considered to be the kernel of the problem of nutrition and therefore education and instruction had to become the main instrument of intervention. Science and medicine asserted their authority, since "ignorance of the principles and main features of the modern science of nutrition is one of the commonest causes of deficiencies in nutrition".[23]

Social, sanitary and cultural implications became the focus of the work to be done regarding specific information to health professionals, doctors, hygienists, and public health nurses, as well as on the instruction of the general public in schools and associations through pamphlets, propaganda, films, posters, pictures and lectures. At the same time, economic and agricultural aspects of the problem revealed the need for a policy of nutrition and social welfare at a national level, within the framework of international coordination. Indeed, nutrition had become an essential part of public health work. Gradually, under the pressure of circumstances, governments were to adopt measures of

22 *Final Report of the Mixed Committee of the League of Nations on Relation of Nutrition to Health, Agriculture and Economic Policy*, League of Nations, Geneva, 1937.

23 *The Problem of Nutrition*, 1936, pp. 20-21.

protection and assistance with regard to the food supply, and legislation on food quality, consumption and food codes.[24] These aspects firstly called for action on a national level, but also required international cooperation, something indispensable for the efforts made to improve workers' nutrition to be in harmony with the needs of the world economy.

The diversity of surveys, reports and features aimed at assessing the nutritional state of the European population contributed a large amount of information for experts and authorities. Unfortunately, most of the work carried out in different countries and presented in international expert conferences and meetings was not suitable for comparison because of a lack of methodological agreement. Standards were to be defined in order to solve this particular problem.

Physical standards was the technical name given to anthropometric, clinical and physiological methods used to assess the population's nutritional condition. These methods were employed to identify people suffering from nutritional deficiencies or malnutrition and considered by the experts to be in need of dietary treatment. Experimental research on nutrition during the Inter-war period required the assistance of some systematic clinical screening in order to assess the effect of dietary regimes on the human condition. The problems of establishing satisfactory dietary and physical standards were intimately interconnected, since the ultimate proof of a satisfactory diet was its positive effect on the organism and the health status.[25]

The complexity of factors intervening in human dietary systems and organic nutrition soon gave way to the methodological problem of establishing global standards for an adequate diet. General agreement had not been reached either on the boundaries of *malnutrition* nor on the methods to identify it in individuals under scrutiny. Physical standards were applied to determine children's normal development, since school medical officers requested simple working methods that could be applied to large groups of children to enable them to spot those suffering from weakness, retarded development and malnutrition.[26]

Nutrition is connected to the right functioning of every tissue, organ or system of the body and every aspect of human physiology had to be taken into account to determine the *global state of nutrition* of an

---

24 *Ibidem*, 1936, p. 66.

25 Burnet, Aykroyd, 1935, p. 336.

26 Barona, 2007a, pp. 93-96; Perdiguero, E. (ed.), *Salvad al niño. La protección a la infancia en los países de la Europa mediterránea*, Valencia, Seminari d'Estudis sobre la Ciencia, Universitat de València, 2005.

individual. However, the expression *nutritional status* also included different and more restricted meanings, and at the time referred to the amount of flesh covering the skeleton. The equivalent of the German term *Ernährungszustand* was the perspective adopted by some Anglo-American experts. Generally speaking, three different methods of assessing the state of nutrition were mentioned. One was the comparison of certain measures to a standard; another one was the assessment of the state of health and development based on clinical screening; and the last one was a more refined clinical test to detect physiological problems and early deficiency diseases.

Starting with a general check-up, *somatometric* screening aimed to classify the subject according to a type. Height and weight were recorded next to determine an index based on the height-weight-age ratio. Although it was recognised that the height of a child depended on heredity aspects, faulty feeding could influence it if prolonged. Since a child's stature is so variable that single comparisons with standards made no sense, height gain rates and regularity provided useful information, even though growth was not a uniform evolving factor.[27] The weight gain rate and the height-weight ratio were often used in assessing the nutritional status. The so-called *indices of nutrition* were formulated by establishing more complicated relationships between height, weight and other bodily measurements, although, concerning children, some experts preferred a simple comparison between the individual's weight and the average height for an age. Four diagnostic elements were graded in clinical exploration: complexion, fat, water content in tissues and muscle condition. Other methods involved measurements of arm, chest and hip girths.

A great deal of work was devoted to finding out how clinical methods helped to detect children's nutritional status. Obviously, the state of a schoolchild was directly related to his/her health condition; therefore, not only physical characteristics were to be studied but also the general functions of the body.[28] To do so, a complete study would require laboratory techniques, not easily available and expensive to run on large groups. Some experts proposed *clinical methods* only, including careful examination of external features, a series of body measurements and the general examination of organs and systems.

---

27 Burnet, Aykroyd, 1935, p. 360.

28 Nobécourt, P, Vitry, G.P., "Clinical methods for determining the state of nutrition in school children", *League of Nations Quarterly Bulletin of the Health Organisation*, Vol. 5, No. 3, 1936, pp. 544-548.

Since malnutrition impaired many organic functions, the Conference of Experts in Nutrition convened in Berlin in 1932 proposed a number of tests on *physical efficiency and fatigability.* Some were especially devoted to the early detection of vitamin deficiency, although the clearest evidence of a defective diet, a poor nutritional state or malnutrition was deficiency disease.

In order to solve the crucial problem of establishing guidelines to make the diversity of surveys, reports and features aiming to assess the nutritional state of the European population comparable, the experts' committee on nutrition of the League of Nations requested E.J. Bigwood, a professor at the University of Brussels, to propose some guiding principles and methods for research. In 1938 his proposal was presented to the commission of experts, who agreed on the final wording of Bigwood's *Guide*, which was published shortly after and submitted to the Conference of Representatives of the National Nutrition Committees in October 1938 for its approval.[29] In the meantime, the Secretariat collected data on the state of nutrition of populations living in rural regions of Europe to form preparatory documentation for the 1939 *Rural Life Conference*. Such data was considered to be of great value, particularly when dietary surveys and nutrition assessment were combined with information on the general conditions of public health.[30]

The Physiology of Nutrition and Optimum Diet

From physiological rationality, the diet had to supply the necessary substances for the growth and repair of the organism, as well as energy for the production of animal heat and organic work. Experimental science was to be the necessary basis of any practical action.[31] Experiments with animals seemed to be useful to clarify fundamental aspects of human nutrition, but only the screening of humans and the analysis of clinical data could contribute to establishing specific standards for humans. During World War II human experiments were made, not only in the camps but also in some reputed laboratories.[32]

There were, however, a number of facts that were firmly established. The organism needed to be supplied daily with a certain quantity of food energy that could be evaluated in terms of calories and, from the

29 Bigwood, E.J., Guiding Principles for Studies On the Nutrition of Populations. Technical Commission on Nutrition, Health Organisation of the League of Nations Geneva, 1939 [C.H.1401; C.H./Com.Exp.Alim./50(2)].

30 Barona, 2010.

31 Burnet, Aykroyd, 1935, p. 334.

32 We shall comment upon those experiments in a further chapter.

beginning of the experimental science of nutrition, a considerable amount of information on calorie requirements was increasingly available. It was accepted that food factors such as vitamins and mineral salts were essential to health but, at the same time, it was also clear that they did not affect the fundamental problem of energy needs. The daily diet had to yield protein, fat and carbohydrates, with their proportion varying according to circumstances. On the other hand, small amounts of minerals were also considered necessary, the most important being phosphorus, calcium, iron and iodine, as well as vitamins and other essential factors.[33] Energy needs are met by fats, carbohydrates and proteins, the latter having the additional function of building new tissue for the growing animal and of repairing tissue wastage in the adult.[34] In addition, experimental research on the physiology of nutrition had stressed the great importance of other essential elements, such as vitamins and minerals, which were also deemed indispensable. The lack of those elements or their defective presence in dietaries was related to deficiency diseases and children's organic development.

Physiologists in previous decades had generally devoted their attention to the establishment of minimum dietary requirements.[35] Such was also the usual standpoint of governments and administrations when called upon to fix the rations for workers, feed large numbers of soldiers and civilians in wartime, assist the unemployed and their families and establish school meals and public canteens. Minimum dietary requirements were the keystone. Nevertheless, the idea of an *optimum diet* was developed during the Interwar period and brought into preeminence as a more meaningful concept. An optimum diet was one that provided for the full development of the individual for efficiency without exhaustion and resistance to disease.[36]

Diseases such as scurvy, rickets, beriberi or pellagra were identified as being associated with deficient nutrition. Therefore, nutrition was to become an essential factor to enjoy optimum health, a condition necessary to fight infectious diseases. Since the late 1920s malnutrition, poverty, children's diseases and economic crisis paved the way for a

---

33 Burnet, Aykroyd, 1935, pp. 323-474.

34 *The Problem of Nutrition*, 1936, p. 32.

35 Livi-Bacci, M., *Population and Nutrition: An Essay on European Demographic History* Cambridge, Cambridge University Press, 1991.

36 *The Problem of Nutrition*, 1936, p. 53.

new field of action, and the idea of a *standard for adequate nutrition* was widely accepted as a starting point for future policies.[37]

According to the *London Report*, a dietary standard had to take into account energy demands, the proportion of protective foods and mineral and vitamin requirements.[38] Once those general aspects were clearly determined, further research was to focus on specific problems such as nutritive needs during the first year of life and infancy. Since a common methodology was needed in order to allow comparisons, the Technical Commission on Nutrition of the League of Nations shaped some guiding principles for experimental research and social surveys.[39]

The notion of *optimum diet* had been introduced at the beginning of the 20th century, based on physiological research into calorie intake and expenditure, and protein, fat, mineral and vitamin requirements. Foodstuffs were classified into two main groups: *protective foods*, such as milk, eggs, meat, cheese, vegetables, potatoes and cod liver oil; and *supplementary energy-yielding foods*, such as cereals, fats and sugar. A new *calorie method* was then introduced to calculate individual needs according to tables based on *energetic quotients* so that calorie requirements could be assessed to ensure the healthy development of the human organism. The calorie represented a universal value to measure nutrition.[40]

The Mixed Technical Commission on Nutrition of the League of Nations, the International Labour Organisation and the International Institute of Agriculture convened in London in November 1935. A preliminary "Report on the Physiological Basis of Nutrition" (1936) was published, including an interim report with their suggestions.[41] Edward Mellanby presided over the Technical Commission and R. Cathcart, an expert on quantitative methods in nutrition, chaired the sessions. Participants included physiologists, clinicians and statisticians. Evidence on vitamin deficiency diseases (scurvy, rickets, beriberi, pellagra) reinforced the scientific project of reaching a universal standard for an optimum and minimum diet. The London Report made room for the concept of *dietary standards* that took into account protective foods, energy, mineral and vitamin requirements, and their proportion in the main foodstuffs, although it seemed impossible to establish exact

37 Burnet, Aykroyd, 1935; Caplan, P. (ed.), *Food, Health and Identity*, London, Routledge, 1997.

38 *The Problem of Nutrition*, 1936.

39 Bigwood, 1939.

40 *Ibidem*.

41 Archive of the League of Nations, Document C.H.1197.

normal standards of health and physical development in order to stake the boundaries of the pathological. Empirical research and clinical observation showed that borderline conditions between health and pathology existed and they were hard to detect and define. The same applied to discussions about the validity of the so-called *indices of nutrition*, which mainly applied to children and were used to determine underdevelopment, insufficient nutrition and those pre-clinical states traditionally conceptualised as *weakness* and *consumption.*

The League of Nations' Technical Commission on Nutrition submitted a report to the Health Committee in April-May 1936 and to the General Council in May 1936. The Health Committee suggested further work to attain practical effects in different countries, with specific research on food requirements during the first year of life and the implementation of social policies to scientifically assess the nutritional state of children, pregnant women, workers and, ideally, the whole population.[42] Technical aspects of research had to be covered and conceptual agreements reached, such as coefficients for calculating calories and proteins according to age and sex, particularly regarding maternity, infancy and periods of organic growth and convalescence.

The information sent by national boards was studied by the Technical Commission in its 2nd session held in Geneva between June 4 and 8, 1936.[43] The main point on the agenda was a critical review of the *London Report* on the physiological bases of nutrition, to oversee the progress of studies on the problems recommended in it, followed by some specific topics, such as milk consumption, physiological properties of milk, assessment of children's nutritional condition, as well as the means to prevent, identify and cure malnutrition. The main difficulties emerged from the need to establish fixed standards for the optimum diet. Since health and nutrition were closely related, a distinction could be made between primary malnutrition due to a defective diet and secondary malnutrition resulting from illness.

When meeting in March 1937, the Technical Commission on Nutrition of the League of Nations was composed of 16 members, with E. Mellanby as President. Some specific commissions devoted to technical studies were integrated with national representatives.[44] The

---

42 "Report on the Physiological Bases", 1936, pp. 391-415.

43 "Report by the Technical Commission on Nutrition on the work of its second session held in Geneva, June 4th to 8th, 1936", *League of Nations Quarterly Bulletin of the Health Organisation*, 1936, Vol. 5, No. 3, pp. 416-426.

44 League of Nations, Health General, R. 6133, Registry No. 8A, 21287, 20883. 1933-1939. Nutrition. Technical Commission on Nutrition. Reports, printing. Archives of the League of Nations.

Spanish representation was entrusted to the *Real Academia de Medicina* in Madrid.[45] Two main topics drew attention; the first one was related to energy, protein and fat requirements associated with calorie production and consumption in the light of the influence of climate on dietary requirements, and the second one focused on mineral and vitamin requirements. Physiological conditions such as pregnancy and lactation, and age groups – childhood and adulthood – were specifically discussed.

What constitutes a balanced diet? Answering this general question meant specifying the human requirements of calories, fat, proteins, vitamins and minerals, and establishing the right proportions in which the various nutritional factors had to be combined. The nutritive value of food was to be the basis for dietary standards as the starting point for further practical action; they allowed experts to gauge the value of the diet of individuals or social groups, making it possible to draw up dietary schedules for those communities or social groups that had no choice, such as armies, people in institutions, schoolchildren and prisoners. They were also used as the basis of large-scale wartime rationing schemes and as a starting point for future agricultural policies.

Human calorie requirements were investigated by direct and indirect calorimetric methods to determine the energy output of subjects at rest or performing various kinds of work. Experimental conditions provided data for the establishment of quantitative standards of food intake. Another method consisted of assessing dietary requirements by means of the observation of what healthy individuals consumed under various conditions and performing different kinds of work.

The basal metabolic rate of an average European citizen was considered to range from 65 to 75 calories per hour, the energy exchange being lower during sleep and considerably higher during physical activities. The increase in energy exchange in relation to the basal metabolism, which takes place during the execution of different tasks, was carefully investigated in the laboratory. As a result, it was possible to put together an energy budget for an average individual for an average day, which was found to be about 3,000 calories per day. This figure was widely used in practical dietetics, put forward as a standard by the Advisory Committee on Nutrition of the British Ministry of Health, and accepted by V. Tyzska, one of the most influential German specialists.

A crucial point was the acknowledgement that energy requirements varied enormously according to the type of work done, from about 6,000

45 It consisted of three members: Teófilo Hernando, E. Suñer and J. Murillo, director of the Institute for the Control of Food and Medicines.

or 7,000 calories in the case of a lumberman to 2,200 for a sedentary worker.[46] The energy requirements of children and women were considered to be lower than those of an adult man. Both statistical and calorimetric data regarding caloric intake and requirements were registered for both sexes and age groups as the basis of *scales of family coefficients*, which calculated the needs of children and women in terms of an average man, the latter being taken as the standard. More than 20 different scales of family coefficients were proposed. Such scales allowed the establishment of a *consumption unit* in terms of which the requirements of the entire group could be calculated. The scales of family coefficients were essential to finding out family dietary habits, comparing the total food intake with other families.[47]

The Expert Committee on Nutrition convened by the League of Nations in 1932 produced the following scale:[48]

Calorie Coefficient by Age and Sex

Age	Male	Both sexes	Female
0-2		0.2	
2-3		0.3	
4-5		0.4	
6-7		0.5	
8-9		0.6	
10-11		0.7	
12-13		0.8	
14-59	1.0		0.8
Over		0.8	

1.0 = 3,000 calories

This international proposal was widely employed to make results easily comparable. The first serious attempt to set up a dietary standard was made by Carl von Voit in his book *Food and the Principles of Dietetics* (London, 1927). Using a calorimeter, he calculated that a man

46 Burnet, Aykroyd, 1935, p. 339.

47 Bigwood, E.J., Roost, G., *L'alimentation rationnelle et les besoins énergétiques d'une population ouvrière*, Bruxelles, Université Libre de Bruxelles, Institute Solvay, 1934, 256 p.

48 *Quarterly Bulletin of the Health Organisation of the League of Nations*, Vol. 1, 1932, p. 480.

weighing about 70 kg and doing moderate work needs 3,055 calories, 118 g of protein, 58 g of fat and 500 g of carbohydrates every day. Other standards proposed by experts on physiology of nutrition, such as Atwater, Rubner and Hutchinson, did not differ significantly.[49]

Heated discussions on the optimum protein intake took place during the 1930s. Even among experimental scientists, some advocated a high intake while others emphasised restricted consumption. To some extent, contradictory clinical evidence about the effects of high-protein diets on the kidneys heated the debate. Some experiments had shown that diets containing 30% of protein produced signs of kidney damage in rabbits and human beings. But those results had been criticised, with allegations that experimental diets were incomplete regarding dietary components other than protein. In most of such experiments, the proportion of protein in the diet greatly exceeded that in the ordinary, freely chosen diets of Western societies.[50] Physiologists, on the whole, agreed on the fact that societies with a high protein intake have a better organic development than those with a lower one, but no inference could be drawn as to the optimum protein consumption.[51]

In their report, Burnet and Aykroyd (1935) proposed the following standards:[52]

Standard dietaries put forward by various authorities as being suitable for the average individual:

	Protein	Fat (g)	Carbohydrates	Calories
Voit	118	56	500	3,055
Rubner	127	52	509	3,092
Atwater	125	125	450	3,520
Advisory Committee (British Ministry)	100	100	400	3,000
Playfair	119	51	531	3,140
Tyszka	80-100	60-80	500	3,000

As a general principle, no diet was deemed adequate by physiologists unless it contained enough mineral elements present in human tissues,

49 Aykroyd, W.R., "Diet in relation to small incomes", *League of Nations Quarterly Bulletin of the Health Organisation*, 1933, Vol. 1, pp.130-153.

50 Burnet, Aykroyd, 1935, pp. 342-343.

51 A wider discussion about the optimum protein intake in Barona, 2010, pp. 67-70.

52 Burnet, Aykroyd, 1935, p. 348.

those minerals taking part in metabolic actions and needing to be replaced by nutrition. Mineral deficiencies could also produce diseases. Calcium and iron were soon identified as a causal factor for diseases such as anaemia, osteoporosis and other deficiencies, and iodine deficiency was associated with goitre and cretinism. The consequences of phosphorus, calcium, iron and iodine deficits were immediately investigated and the dietary amounts of those minerals estimated. A diet rich in cereals was considered poor in phosphorus, while the absence of vitamin D was a complementary factor for rickets. The estimated amount of phosphorus in the diet was around 1.30 g per day for the average adult, the needs of growing children being relatively higher. Most Western dietaries contained sufficient amounts of phosphorus. Calcium was considered to be the inorganic element, which contributed the most to body weight, since over 99% of organic calcium is in the bones.

Experts on the physiology of nutrition linked vitamin D with the metabolic use of calcium and they therefore argued that calcium intake was especially important when the intake of vitamin D was very small, as was the case in wintertime or in countries where the sun seldom shone. The physiological effects of iron had been less investigated than the previously cited minerals although its deficiency was associated with some types of anaemia. Public health campaigns to prevent goitre were carried out in Las Hurdes, a depressed rural area in Spain, Switzerland and some areas of the United States: iodine compounds were administered to schoolchildren and sodium iodine was added to table salt.

An International Vitamin Conference, attended by a wide group of experts in the physiology of nutrition, was held in London in June 1931 under the auspices of the Standing Commission on Biological Standardisation of the League of Nations' Health Organisation.[53] A further report was published in 1934 on the international adoption of standards and units for vitamins A, B1, C and D. The conference was chaired by E. Mellanby (League of Nations) and the participants were: J.C. Drummond (League of Nations); H.von Euler (Stockholm); L.S. Fridericia (Copenhagen); B.C.P. Jansen (Amsterdam); P. de Mattei (Pavia); E.M. Nelson (Washington); E. Poulsson (Oslo); Randoin (Paris); Steenbock (Madison); Szent-Györgyi (Szeged); Chick (League of Nations); and Aykroyd (LoN, Geneva). Other delegates were: H. Brorw (Toronto); K.H. Coward (League of Nations); H.H. Dale (League

[53] "Second Conference on Vitamin Standardisation", *League of Nations Quarterly Bulletin of the Health Organisation*, Vol. 3, 1934, pp. 428-440.

of Nations); P. Hartley (League of Nations); E.M. Hume (League of Nations); A. Jung (Basel); Ch. Lormand (Paris); Rafael Méndez (Madrid); A. Morton (Liverpool); R.A. Peters (Oxford); O. Rosenheim (League of Nations); M. Tsurumi (LoN, Japan); T.A. Webster (League of Nations); and S.S. Zilva (League of Nations).

A report published in 1937 by the Technical Commission on Nutrition of the League of Nations summarised the available knowledge regarding mineral and vitamin requirements, proteins, fats and nutritional requirements in the first year of life. The report also touched upon the nutritive value of milk and referred to some nutrition surveys on food consumption and some methods to assess the nutritional condition of infants and adolescents.[54] A table on the nutritive value of foods included milk, cheese, eggs, liver, fatty fish, green vegetables, raw fruits, butter, cod-liver oil, yeast, meat, root vegetables, legumes, cereals (bread, rice, nuts), sugar, jam, honey, margarine, olive and vegetable oil.

In August 1938 the Technical Commission on Nutrition of the League of Nations met in Geneva.[55] The experts convened under the chairmanship of Sir E. Mellanby, Secretary-General of the Medical Research Council, London.[56] In an extremely critical period, due to the economic slump and international tensions, the experts discussed the nutritive value of different cereals according to the degree of milling, the influence of climate on food requirements and the extent to which diets in common use fell below the standards recommended in the *Report on the Physiological Bases of Nutrition.* As bread played a prominent part in nutrition, particularly in rural areas, and since its composition widely varied across European regions, a special study on the composition and preparation of bread was considered indispensable. This research was formerly conducted by E.J. McDougall, a member of the Imperial

54 "Report by the Technical Commission on Nutrition on the Work of its third session, held in London from November 15th to 20th, 1937", *Bulletin of the Health Organisation*, Vol. 7, 1938, pp. 460-502.

55 "Technical Commission on Nutrition. Report by a Special Committee which met in Geneva from August 22nd to 24th, 1938", *Bulletin of the Health Organisation*, Vol. 7, 1938, pp. 667-678

56 The participants were: W.R. Aykroyd, Director of the Nutrition Research Laboratories, Conoor, India; E.J. Bigwood, Professor of Physiology, University of Brussels; L.E. Booher, Chief Food and Nutrition Division Bureau of Home Economics, US Department of Agriculture, Washington; H. Chick, Head of the Division of Nutrition, Lister Institute, League of Nations; L.S. Fridericia, Professor of Hygiene at the University of Copenhagen; A. Mayer, Professor at the *Collège de France*, Paris; J.B. Orr, Director of the Rowett Institute of Animal Nutrition, Aberdeen; participating also as observer: W.Ph. Kennedy, Professor of Physiology at the Royal College of Medicine, Baghdad.

Bureau of Animal Nutrition at the Rowett Institute (Aberdeen) and the Basle Institute of Physiology.

The Committee also requested an advisory opinion concerning the feeding of refugees in countries where whole population groups were threatened with acute malnutrition, or with actual famine. Considering all these important topics, a summary of the meeting's agenda was drafted. Food requirements for infants and those on small incomes represented a particular source of concern. When considering special dietary needs for different social classes and age groups, expectant and nursing mothers occupied a central place for "although it is true that our knowledge of feeding in pregnancy and lactation is elementary, it can be said with some assurance that, in regard to the health of both mother and offspring, an increase in the protective foodstuffs would have a large effect in eliminating many of the ills of pregnancy".[57]

Most paediatricians agreed that breastfeeding was the best option for nourishing an infant, but its health, diet and development had to be supervised because "the causes of infant mortality… made it clear that the pernicious combination of poverty and ignorance was largely responsible for the malnutrition of infancy, as, indeed, for that seen in other stages of human life".[58] Gastrointestinal disturbances and other diseases in mothers during lactation could induce vitamin deficiency, affecting the child's health. Concerning early childhood and preschool and nursery age: "There is a great need to maintain the resistance of children at the highest possible level against the ravages of the infectious diseases to which they will be exposed…"[59] For the poorer social groups, who could not easily afford fresh cow's milk or dried milk preparations, breastfeeding had many advantages and minimised the risk of infection, but attention had to be paid to the fact that the quality of the mother's milk depended on the quality of her diet to a certain extent.

In the 1930s *artificial* feeding and the so-called *humanised* dried milks had improved, a growing industry was expanded and those substitutive products were well accepted both by physicians and mothers as a way to complement or replace breastfeeding without risks to the infant's health.[60] Some research on mortality and morbidity was conducted on a large sample of infants under care at the Infant Welfare Society of Chicago. A total of 48.5% received breast milk only until

---

57 *The Problem of Nutrition*, 1936, p. 39.

58 *Ibidem*, p. 43.

59 *Ibidem*, 1936, p. 44.

60 Burnet, Aykroyd, 1935, pp. 401-402.

month nine, 43% were partially breastfed and 8.5% were fed on cow's milk mixtures. All the groups received accessory food including orange juice, cod-liver oil and cereals at certain ages. These are the mortality and morbidity results for the three groups:[61]

	Breastfed	Partially breastfed	Artificially fed
Percent total	48.5	43.0	8.5
Morbidity	37.4	53.8	63.6
Total mortality	6.7	27.2	66.7

Breastfeeding was associated with higher standards of health in this group of 20,000 children, although other factors could have influenced the figures.

As a result of the 1929 economic crash, a great deal of the population in most European countries saw their income fall. The situation affected the availability of foodstuffs.[62] The relationship between income, expenditure and adequate nutrition in poor families, whether employed or unemployed, became of interest for public health experts, social workers and politicians.[63] Subsequently, with the new international situation and the rise in social problems related to diet, community feeding became a reality. The Spanish Civil War was an exceptionally critical domain, soon followed by World War II.[64] Community feeding developed an essential social task, since a meaningful part of the population received their meals in residential institutions, armies, hospitals, sanatoria, prisons, asylums, schools and similar institutions. Health authorities became engaged in ensuring satisfactory diets and public health officers assumed the supervision of institutional diets. An increasing section of the population asked for food relief. Several systems for the provision of cheap meals appeared or extended previous experiences in most countries. In France, the *soups populaires* and the *fourneaux économiques* were extended. In Germany, *Caritas*

61 *Ibidem*, p. 402.

62 Rotberg, R.I., Raab, T.K., *Hunger and History. The Impact of Changing Food Production and Consumption Patterns of Society*, Cambridge University Press, Cambridge, 1985.

63 Aykroyd, 1933.

64 Cura, M.I. del, Huertas, R., *Alimentación y enfermedad en tiempos de hambre. España, 1937-1947*, Madrid, CSIC, 2007; Barona, J.L., Perdiguero E., "Health and the War. Changing schemes and health conditions during the Spanish Civil War", *Dynamis*, 2008, Vol. 28, pp. 103-126.

Association lent its kitchens to volunteers in 1932 in cities such as Cologne, to provide meals for thousands of people. In Britain, the provision of meals through central city kitchens, traditionally used for school meals and nursing mothers, was extended. In some cities like Birmingham the *Citizens' Society* founded a number of canteens in occupational centres run by the unemployed.

Community feeding was conceived as one of the great public services when based on scientific grounds by national institutes of nutrition. Nevertheless, industrial and mass food production was considered by the experts to be a real risk for the quality of foodstuffs and the preservation of their physiological properties. Food industries were held responsible for the partial, total elimination or destruction of *vitamins*.

Rural Dietaries and the Problem of Feeding Habits

A specific report on food habits in rural populations in Europe was prepared by the experts' commission on nutrition of the League of Nations' Health Organisation. Rural health, dietaries and living conditions became a source of interest in times of crisis. According to all surveys, rural communities and dietaries were extremely different in the varied rural areas of Europe, although they showed certain common characteristics when compared to urban dietaries.[65] The chief characteristic of rural diets was monotony, since the average peasant household only used a limited number of foodstuffs. From a nutritional point of view, this was clearly a disadvantage: in a more varied diet, there was less risk of being deprived of one or more essential foods, particularly minerals and vitamins. In rural communities, seasonal variations were considerable, but day-to-day dietaries often lacked variety for most of the year.

The improvement in communications and means of transport was indeed an advantage for food trade and commercial distribution, but at the same time it might imply a nutritional disadvantage for primitive isolated rural areas in as much as they allowed the selling of their products in towns. This meant that certain foodstuffs traditionally consumed were being kept for sale and not eaten at home. McDougall's report attributed to this reason the fact that the level of consumption of animal foodstuffs was reported to be higher in certain poor parts of Europe than in more developed neighbouring areas. It was not ignorance but economic necessity that prevented peasants from eating the meat, eggs and dairy products they produced. In most districts these foodstuffs

65 [McDougall, E.J.], 1939.

were considered a luxury and only prosperity introduced them into peasantry dietaries.[66] Nevertheless, local tradition played a meaningful role and this important factor was frequently overlooked in most of the expert reports. Goat or sheep-milk cheese was eaten in poor rural areas whereas in more developed ones the cheese products were usually sold in towns.

Again, education was pointed out as the key element to improving rural nutrition. Quite often, when talking about dietaries and food consumption, popular culture and scientific knowledge confronted one another. McDougall's report on rural dietaries stated that: "The majority of rural housewives in Europe know little or nothing of the principles of nutrition, and they might frequently be able to feed their families more adequately if they knew the relative value of different foodstuffs".[67] Yet, cultural habits relating to the consumption of certain foods varied considerably across countries and regions depending on availability, religious beliefs and local traditions. During the interwar period many Western countries started campaigns to instruct the rural housewife, who was considered to be the keystone to changes in traditional habits that were incompatible with new scientific ideas.[68]

Apart from education as a tool to change habits, state relief in the form of food supplies was often given to destitute rural families in many European countries after the 1929 crisis. School meals and public canteens for unemployed and poor people spread in many rural areas in Europe. However, two levels of action orientated political strategies. The first level was linked to the urgent need to overcome shortages, inadequate dietary habits and nutrition deficiencies. But this was not enough, because the economic dimension of severe deficiencies in rural nutrition could only be tackled by agricultural and economic readjustments, both nationally and internationally.

Some exceptions were reported for mountain regions of the Balkans, Sub-Carpathian Russia and Scandinavia, where cereals could not be easily grown and the diet was made up of whatever variety of vegetables could be produced (potatoes, beans, etc) and animal foodstuffs available. Since these foods were usually more expensive than cereals, these populations were frequently underfed, unless some complementary income was found or state relief was provided through special means such as large amounts of cereals.

66 *Ibidem*, p. 475.

67 *Ibidem*.

68 *Ibidem*, pp. 474-475.

According to McDougall's report, the preponderance of cereals in the rural dietary was most marked in Central, Eastern and South-Eastern Europe, where the cereal provision of energy was estimated to be 80% to 90% of the total diet.[69] His report concluded that the high proportion of cereals intake decreased as the peasant population became more prosperous, and had been substantially reduced in Western and Northern Europe for a number of agricultural and climatic causes. On the other hand, in those European regions identified by nutritionists as "the more primitive areas", cereals were not only eaten as bread but also simply ground to a rough meal and cooked with water as groats, porridge, polenta or cakes.[70]

The second most important foodstuffs in the rural areas of Europe were some vegetables of a high energy-providing value. In rural Ireland, Poland or Germany, potatoes were even more important in the diet than cereals, while in the Balkan Region and Central Europe, beans constituted a regular source of calories in the rural dietary, according to data in McDougall's report.

Less homogeneous seemed to be the amount and varieties of meat eaten from one region to another. The consumption of meat was said to depend on the prosperity of the peasantry and on cultural habits, but the importance of certain animals for human survival in many rural districts is well known. Some of them delivered milk, wool and other goods fundamental for rural families. In other cases, animal products were important in the rural economy, as well as in rural dietaries. The case of Spanish peasantry and farmers in relation to pork consumption is paradigmatic. The so-called *matanza* [slaughter of the pig] constituted a big feast, an essential event in many rural districts, associated with old traditions and probably religious beliefs. One should conclude that the insistence of nutritionists on the lack of meat consumption among poor social groups in rural districts is not always acceptable; sausages, most animal viscera and organs, blood and intestines were present in popular rural dietaries in different ways and proportions. Animal products were not always a luxury for many peasants in Southern Europe; medical topographies and official reports confirm this fact.

However, McDougall insisted on the idea that poorer farmers in the poorest parts of Europe would only have meat on feast days, just a few times a year, while the more prosperous peasants in those poor regions used to eat it once or twice a week. This was probably true for meat, but not for all animal produce that provides animal proteins. On the

69 *Ibidem*, p. 470.

70 *Ibidem*, p. 471.

contrary, he reports that in the most prosperous areas of Western Europe the poorest peasants ate meat once a week, while prosperous farmers had two or three meat meals daily. Was it mainly a matter of prosperity? He stated: "The consumption of milk also varies enormously from one part of Europe to another. In Finland and Latvia, the rural population is reported to drink a litre of milk per head per day, while in Hungary, Romania and Yugoslavia there are districts where peasant families drink practically no milk at all".[71]

Indeed, not only McDougall's report but also other nutritionists insisted on the idea that production and consumption were sometimes dissociated. The case of milk was frequently mentioned because it was reported that peasants who produced milk, butter and cheese regarded these products primarily as market goods and not as essential foodstuffs for their own families. McDougall cited the striking example of Danish farmers producing butter for export and buying margarine for their own consumption. In many rural areas, milk was considered an essential foodstuff for newborns and infants, but was absolutely absent from an adult's diet. Due to the insistence of rural doctors and hygienists on the benefits of milk consumption, a widely extended popular belief was reported in Spanish rural districts that associated milk with a medical product, a sort of medicine for sick people, rather than a foodstuff.

Surveys and reports by hygienists and nutritional experts showing evident deficiencies in rural dietaries put some questions to historical evaluation. Cultural habits were seldom positively considered as a fundamental element of rural dietaries. Science and culture clashed and scientists labelled any idea or practice that was contradictory to the new scientific discourse as *ignorance.* To what an extent were experts legitimated to talk about ignorance as a main cause of nutritional deficiency, especially when cultural habits were the principal tool for survival in traditional societies? Was it really a lack of scientific knowledge or was it cultural habits and economic necessity that prevented peasants from having meat, eggs and the dairy products they produced? In most cases, certain products were not included in traditional rural dietaries and it seems reasonable to wonder if such foodstuffs were considered to be a luxury or simply they were not part of traditional family cooking. Was prosperity really the path for the introduction of new foodstuffs into the peasantry dietary? Undoubtedly, cultural habits played a major role. But popular customs were often put down to *ignorance* if they did not fit with experimental approaches. McDougall remarks that such valuable foodstuffs as whey and blood

[71] *Ibidem*, p. 472.

were wasted in certain areas while consumed in others. It is remarkable how new scientists identified science as knowledge and considered culture and popular habits on the side of ignorance, illustrating the authoritarian mentality of the positivistic approach of trying to civilise the ignorant.

Other factors were also considered in nutritional surveys in relation to the urban-rural divide. Rural dietaries tended to be affected by much greater seasonal dependence than in urban areas, because most peasant families relied on what was grown locally and urban areas received goods from different places. In those cases, the diet used to be at its best in late summer and autumn, a period in which a wide variety of fruit was available and cereals, vegetables, eggs and dairy products were more abundant. During this period, the diet of peasants was almost ideal, particularly in areas where milk was abundantly drunk. Fruit and vegetables were eaten in adequate amounts; milk and meat products were easily available. Just the opposite was true in spring in Central and Eastern rural Europe; it was during this season that most health problems associated with the diet appeared, such as pellagra, scurvy, night blindness, rickets and others. During the hard periods of the year, rural diets tended to be deficient in fruit, fresh green vegetables and animal foodstuffs. In addition, religious fasting further impoverished the winter diet, as no animal products were eaten and the global intake of proteins decreased.[72] According to the expert's approach, to increase the consumption of fresh fruit and vegetables, it was necessary to learn how to preserve them for winter use, avoiding much of the crop being wasted. The conservation of fresh foodstuffs became an important challenge for many rural areas.

McDougall's report coincided with other experts in the idea that the only special advantage of rural dietaries over urban ones was that food in the countryside was usually consumed in fresher, more natural condition, something important for cereals "which are usually eaten as highly refined white flour in the towns, while in most parts of Europe the rural populations still eat whole-grain cereals".[73] The difference between refined and wholemeal flour was undoubtedly considered of great nutritional significance, especially in rural regions, where bread and other forms of cereal food formed the basis of the diet. Nutritionists knew that the proportion of minerals and vitamins decreased largely in refined white flour, something that might not be important in urban varied diets but, on the contrary, it was probably meaningful in the more

72 *Ibidem*, p. 470 passim.

73 *Ibidem*, p. 474.

restricted rural dietaries. In many cases, nutritionists shared a critical and suspicious attitude towards the quality control of industrialised food at a time when a debate was open on the use of colourings and other additives that required further regulation.[74] Among other losses, minerals and vitamins were considered by some physiologists to be lost as a result of industrial processing. This would not be important in urban and more varied diets but, once more, it could be a serious threat in the more restricted rural diets.

One of the main sources of confrontation between popular habits and the new expertise was the feeding of specific groups of the population, such as infants, young children, and pregnant and nursing mothers. Although infants were usually breastfed longer in rural areas than in towns and cities, experience showed that rickets was widespread in most rural regions. This paradox was explained by hygienists, who considered it a consequence of deficiencies in the mother's diet, which was too poor to provide the child with the necessary minerals and vitamins. Once more, this was seen as a sign of the mothers' ignorance of nutritional needs in pregnancy and lactation. "It has been found in Greece and Yugoslavia that prolonged breast-feeding, which is the usual practice of peasant mothers, rather increases than prevents the amount of rickets in the children, showing that the diet of the nursing mother is seriously deficient".[75]

Despite the availability of milk, eggs, meat and vegetables, experts blamed mothers: they were unaware of how important it was to increase their intake of these foods. McDougall stated: "Amongst the slightly older children also, wrong feeding is probably more common in the country districts than in the towns, due to greater ignorance, as well as to lower purchasing power".[76]

The concern about deficiency diseases in the rural areas mainly appeared in the 1930s as a consequence of the international crisis. Not many dietary surveys could give exact figures to estimate whether the intake of vitamins and minerals was enough to meet physiological requirements, but certain signs of shortage of one or more vitamins could explain the symptoms of deficiency diseases frequently reported

---

74 Guillem-Llobat, X., Perdiguero, E., "Fighting adulteration in early European food industrialisation. The case of Alicante (Spain)", in Vámos, É. (ed.), *History of the Food Chain. From Agriculture to Consumption and Waste*, Hungarian Chemical Society, Budapest, 2006, pp. 33-40

75 *Ibidem*, p. 474.

76 *Ibidem.*

amongst rural populations in many parts of Europe.[77] Nutritional deficiencies and malnutrition were indeed a threat for the new generations, and the new science of nutrition supported by state policies posed a sort of eugenic issue, a strategy to improve health and organic development.

In the Muslim rural communities of Yugoslavia, where women used to live a secluded life, some cases of osteomalacia and osteoporosis had been reported, reflecting a shortage of vitamin D and calcium in the diet and a lack of exposure to sunlight. These cases were probably even more frequent in towns than in rural districts. Pellagra cases appeared every spring in rural areas of Romania, where maize was the staple foodstuff. Once more, pellagra cases were easily avoidable; they indicated a dietary deficiency that could be prevented simply by improving dietary habits.

The availability of foodstuffs in rural areas, as well as farm and agriculture production, was important. But, for the experts, education became the keyword, the eligible and most prominent method to change habits and subsequently improve rural standards of nutrition. Spreading scientific knowledge among the rural populations would help to eliminate bad habits. Now and again popular culture and the experts' scientific knowledge clashed. McDougall's report stated: "The majority of rural housewives in Europe know little or nothing of the principles of nutrition, and they might frequently be able to feed their families more adequately if they knew the relative value of different foodstuffs".[78]

In fact, cultural habits attached to the consumption of certain foods varied considerably in different countries and regions. Milk could be considered a valuable foodstuff, being drunk by old and young, or, on the contrary, discarded for adults and only given to very young children and invalids. Some peasants did not grow vegetables for their own use while others grew and ate a variety of vegetables – even in the same or very close areas – and thereby the latter escaped pellagra and other deficiency diseases. Experts concluded that ignorance in the rural population was a serious waste of potential foodstuffs in rural communities and this should be resolved through education. Once again, cultural habits were confronted: whey was used as pig feed or thrown away in some rural areas, while in others the peasants would take it home for cooking, adding valuable minerals to their diet. The animals' blood was thrown away after slaughtering and the blood was made into sausages or drunk as soup.

---

77 *Ibidem*, pp. 474-475.

78 *Ibidem*, p. 477.

Education was called upon to rationalise feeding habits and therefore help to prevent such a loss of valuable foodstuffs. "Education in the feeding of infants and growing children would also be of immense value in most villages of Europe, for it is here that ignorance is the greatest danger to health".[79] Many European countries realised the urgent need for education to change rural dietaries and started campaigns to instruct the rural housewife. This was one of the most frequently recommended strategies.

Apart from education, in areas where peasants did not have sufficient land to produce all the food a family needed, or enough money to buy an adequate diet, planned assistance from the state was required to procure a healthy diet. State relief in the form of food was often given to destitute rural families during the big crisis and in war and post-war years. Rationing standards for families and individuals and the scheme for a minimum diet was also based on expert work on the physiology of nutrition. Country children were sometimes given free or very cheap meals at school or in public dining rooms. Famine and malnutrition required immediate, urgent action, yet the experts agreed that "these relief measures only touch the fringe of the problem and offer no real solution".[80] The background – the economic dimension of the serious deficiencies in rural nutrition – could only be improved through agricultural and economic readjustments, both nationally and internationally. The complexity of the problem was discussed in the *Final Report of the Mixed Committee on Nutrition* (1937), which considered nutrition in relation to a wider perspective, including agriculture and economic policy.[81]

Agriculture at the Service of Nutrition

The inter-war crisis forced the state to play an important, active role in improving the availability of foodstuffs for the lower-income sections of the community. In some countries this was done through unemployment insurance policies, minimum wage laws, old age pensions and other social services that made the income of the working classes more secure against cyclical fluctuations.[82] A decline in the average size of the family added to the general rise of national revenues, a further argument to support the redistribution role of the State.

79 *Ibidem*, p. 476.

80 *Ibidem*, p. 477.

81 *Final Report*, 1937.

82 Trentmann, Just, 2006, *Introduction*, pp. 1-12.

Controlling agricultural prices to guarantee the availability of farming produce to all the population was essential to political economics.

In addition to economic and technical factors, consumer education also played an important part in overcoming the crisis; the *new science of nutrition* had disseminated among an ever-increasing portion of the population knowledge on the nutritive values of foods. For those that could afford a liberal diet, an abundance of green vegetables, fruit and milk was considered to be more important and richer as a source of mineral matter than wheat bran and wheat germ. Another example used by nutritionists to show the harmful effects of prejudice and ignorance was the decreased consumption of skimmed milk, not substituted by whole milk as desirable, but by a reduction of total milk consumption to the extent that in certain countries and social groups milk was not considered a foodstuff but a medicine.

The core question was to determine to what extent agriculture production had adapted to changes in demand. Changes were expected to occur gradually as the newer knowledge of nutrition was disseminated among wider groups of the population: the general income rose, private diet habits changed and special actions were taken by the states to improve the nutritional conditions of particular groups of the population. There was a direct relationship between changes in consumption habits and changes in the demand, which in turn required changes in production and the food supply. Two main words were uttered by both experts and economists: adjustment and adaptation.

In attempting to define the effort of adaptation required in the important field of agriculture, emphasis was placed on two points. First, nutrition policy did not involve a rapid transformation in the existing structure of national agricultural systems. Second, as nutritional policy moved towards its objective of an adequate diet for all, an increase in the demand for all classes of agricultural products was predicted. The demand for protective foods was expected to rise more than the demand for those chiefly consumed for their high-energy value.

But in times of crisis the main concerns were not only the changing habits and energy requirements of the population. The first aim of nutrition policy was to ensure that all sections of the population could afford a sufficient amount of calories. The main tendencies observed suggested that for a long time to come, taking the world as a whole, the increase in the demand for energy-bearing foods among populations suffering from malnutrition would counterbalance the fall in the demand for cereals. It was clear, therefore, that nutrition policy by no means required a drastic shift from the production of energy-bearing foods to the production of protective foods, nor did it require that agriculture should produce protective foods in advance of the market.[83]

Agricultural adaptation was essential for tackling the complex situation of nutrition, health and the economy, but important obstacles had to be removed for agriculture to be adapted to the new consumption trends and demands. Special attention had to be paid to the importance of natural conditions and agricultural productive systems in each country. A great deal of capital was needed and the international financial situation was not optimistic at all. On the other hand, culture and tradition played a central role in dietary habits, which appeared to be a factor of deep concern in terms of reaching the hard target of adapting production and habits to scientific patterns. More pragmatic obstacles were to be mentioned too: a low level of agricultural technique and the lack of an efficient transport system for commercial networks, since the perishability of certain protective foods made it difficult to ensure availability to all potential consumers.

During the post-1929 crisis period, some national and international agencies certainly made attempts to overcome some large hurdles and assist agriculture in its task of adaptation. Now and again governmental policy and state social programmes became very important, since changes in production, the evolution of agricultural prices and the links between income and nutrition habits were crucial aspects of the problem.[84] In some countries legislation was enacted,[85] as economic depression and the agricultural crisis hindered the availability of food and a price reduction policy was recommended. The prosperity of farmers, peasants and agricultural workers was considered to be an essential element in any policy intended to improve nutrition. Even agricultural practices had to be adapted to meet the new requirements.

As far as the demand tended to be transferred from energy-producing foods to protective foods, the prices of these two categories did not fail to adjust themselves in the same proportion. This adaptation had to act, in itself, as an effective regulator of production. In conclusion, the experts found good reasons to believe that the trend of dietary habits towards a larger consumption of protective foods, particularly in Western countries, would coincide with a parallel evolution in agricultural production, which would in all probability benefit the rural

83 *Final report*, 1937, pp. 160-163.

84 *Ibidem*, p. 173.

85 "Report on the Physiological Bases", 1936, p. 66.

populations of the various countries, and might also greatly contribute to a resumption of normal economic relations between the nations.[86]

Concern was expressed about the steps to be taken to meet the nutritional needs of the lower-income sections of the community, to ensure an adequate food supply at prices within the reach of all classes. This safeguarded the interests of producers and improved and reduced the cost of marketing and distribution of foodstuffs both in industrial and rural areas, encouraging collaboration between cooperatives and other forms of producers' and consumers' organisations. An international food policy also involved the international unification of the technical control of foodstuffs, setting up standards of reference and specifications for grading foods of all kinds according to quality. A coordination of the work of different authorities affecting nutrition and food control was necessary and national statistics on food supply and consumption had to be improved. The International Institute of Agriculture was requested to collect information regarding supply, national consumption and prices.[87]

The IIA in Rome contributed fundamental materials and provided information on the consumption of foodstuffs, as well as on trends in production, prices and consumption, particularly milk and fresh vegetables in large cities. The international programme also collected data on the financial aspects of assistance to national agriculture in various countries, and studied wholesale and retail prices, particularly of protective foods, relating prices to trends in production and consumption in different countries.[88]

The enormous differences in the diet of western countries were not considered to be accidental but a consequence of local traditions and the changing structure of the labour system. A main tendency was the reduced use of muscular energy as a result of increased mechanisation in industry and agriculture, and a reduction in the hours worked.[89] Improvements in housing were considered a way to reduce the amount of food required to keep the body at a constant temperature. The use of automobiles and rapid transport that reduced the amount of walking meant that less energy would be spent. Changes in the nature of work and life in modern societies had resulted in changes in food requirements.

---

86 *Ibidem*, p. 95.

87 *Ibidem*, 1936, pp. 97-98.

88 *Nutrition in various countries*, 1936, p. 269.

89 *Ibidem*, pp. 267-270.

Obviously, during the Depression years, European agriculture had to adapt to new realities. As general income rose, special action would have to be taken to improve the nutrition of particular groups. Changes in consumption habits implied changes in the demand and required transformations in the production and food supply. In attempting to define the effort of adaptation required for agriculture, particular attention was paid to two points: nutrition policy should not involve a rapid transformation in the existing structure of national agricultural systems and, as nutritional policy moved towards its objective of an adequate diet for all, an increase in the demand for all classes of agricultural products was expected.[90]

The prosperity of farmers, peasants and agricultural workers was therefore considered an essential element in policies directed towards improved nutrition, but agricultural practice had to be adapted to meet the new requirements.[91] Considering the negative effects of the Depression and the agricultural crisis on the nutritional state of the population, one important method of making food available at reduced prices was that of reducing the services provided by the distributor and considering the positive influence, in this field of action, exercised by producers' and consumers' cooperatives. In many countries, these organisations achieved considerable success in their endeavours to reduce the cost of goods to the consumer.[92]

From the political perspective, improved nutrition had to yield immediate general benefits to agriculture and fishing. Better nutrition implied an increase in demand for foodstuffs, which meant greater agricultural activity. Certain adjustments in agricultural production would be required: "While national agricultural systems will thus benefit by the growth in the demand particularly for the more perishable protective foods, countries producing for export will benefit, as the primary needs of the poorer classes for energy-producing and less perishable protective foods are more adequately satisfied".[93] Adaptation in industry, commerce or agriculture also required financial support by national and international agencies and the stimulus of agricultural cooperation. The state had an important role to play facilitating the adaptation of agriculture to changes and so the problem of nutrition suddenly became a matter of state.

---

90 *Final report*, 1937.

91 *The Problem of Nutrition*, 1936, p. 84.

92 *Ibidem*, p. 83.

93 *Final report*, 1937, p. 45.

In this critical context, tensions between economic agents, states and experts were expected to come into play. No specific references were made during the big depression to the influence of black markets, a problem that became increasingly present in the war and post-war years. While individual countries were absolutely free and autonomous to make decisions about their own commercial interests and policies, experts and international agencies called for one basic principle to be universally accepted: that adequate nutrition was the main factor determining all policies.[94] Due to its worldwide dimension, the problem of hunger, nutrition and food production required international collaboration and consultation through national boards and international agencies. From an international perspective, "the malnutrition which exists in all countries is at once a challenge and an opportunity: a challenge to men's consciences and an opportunity to eradicate a social evil by methods which will increase economic prosperity".[95]

Mixed committees that included representatives of the League of Nations, the International Labour Office and the International Institute of Agriculture gave nutrition policies priority in the 1930s. They presented recommendations to the governments encouraging further scientific research with a view to ascertaining the optimum standards for each individual country. They emphasised the importance of updating information in the teaching of medical students, practitioners, officers and district nurses, and of following a vigorous policy of education for the general public. The experts required support not only for scientific research but also in promoting the application of modern nutritional science in social practices. This was to be for the benefit of the different age and occupational groups of the population, as well as for facilitating international cooperation in that field. Fighting malnutrition had to become an international commitment led by the United Nations.[96]

---

94 *Ibidem*, p. 50.

95 *Ibidem*, p. 53.

96 *Ibidem*, pp. 54-56.

CHAPTER 4

Defining Risks

Peasants, the Unemployed and other Risk Groups: the Effects of War and Depression

The critical situation of the food supply and the poor nutritional condition of Europe's population dated back to the Great War years. It became a chronic problem in the 1920s, getting worse during the 1930s economic crisis and reaching dramatic levels at certain moments and in certain regions during World War II and the post-war period. Specific regions suffered from acute critical problems of starvation and malnutrition and the general picture was further aggravated during the war and post-war years in the 1940s and early 1950s. The high cost of food in Europe cast a very dark shadow and, according to the specialists, chronic hunger threatened Europe's health after the Great War.[1]

In a paper published in 1922, the Catalan physiologist August Pi i Sunyer compared the prices of basic foodstuffs in Berlin, Barcelona and other European cities with the level of income and concluded that European people were much poorer in 1922 than in 1914. Making a comparison between the average income and market food prices, Pi i Sunyer determined the threshold of poverty, identifying it in those sectors of the European population that had to spend 70% of their income on food. He estimated that in Barcelona in 1922 "reducing the food expenditure under 1.75 pesetas per person per day is certainly the way towards insufficient nutrition..."[2] In the early 1920s the victims of poor nutrition were counted by the millions in Russia, China, Germany, Austria, the Balkan countries and Poland, and in Spain certain rural districts like *Las Hurdes* showed the ravages of poverty on health and physical development in many population groups, especially those living in the countryside in a situation of semi-exclusion.[3] The social

---

1 Pi i Sunyer, A., *El hambre de los pueblos*, Conferencia dada en la Academia de Medicina en 29 de enero de 1922, Barcelona, Asociación instructiva de obreros y empleados municipales, 1922.

2 *Ibidem*, p. 23.

3 *Viaje a las Hurdes. El manuscrito inédito de Gregorio Marañón y las fotografías de la visita de Alfonso XIII*, Madrid, El País-Aguilar, 1993.

and medical perception that a deep crisis resulted from a poor diet alarmed politicians and put European states into action to assess the situation and define risks.

Laboratory and clinical research in the 1930s made it clear that the health of a nation was closely bound up with the state of nutrition of its population. It seemed therefore important to discover what kind of food the unemployed millions, with an income reduced to a very low level, were able to buy as a consequence of the international crisis. While very few studies of the dietaries actually used by unemployed men and their families had been made in previous years, sufficient data existed to enable certain inferences about nutrition in lower income groups.[4] Specialists in the new experimental physiology of nutrition adapted calorie requirements to the new critical situation.

A sedentary worker was supposed to need from 2,200 to 2,400 calories a day. This was estimated by subtracting from the 3,100 calories needed by an average worker the 800 calories demanded by an average day's work. Therefore, during the period of unemployment, calorie needs could be reduced by 27% for workers and around 8% for the entire family. Based on the food expenditure and income figures of a number of unemployed families collected by the German *Statistisches Reichsamt*, evidence of undernourishment was found for 1927, a year of relative prosperity, but the financial position of the unemployed steadily worsened ever since. A 19% fall in the cost of living and a 25% drop in food prices had taken place between 1927 and 1932, the situation being described as a hidden famine.[5] An estimate of the state of nutrition among the unemployed in Germany, which was based entirely on official figures relating to allowances and market prices, slightly over-accentuated the seriousness of the situation, since only 45% of the available income went to food. If unemployed families spent this proportion of their income on food, the number of calories purchasable would be about 532 to 1,140 per day for children and 840 to 1,800 for adults. Some detailed dietaries regarding unemployed families in Germany provided evidence of the difficult situation: in three meals out of four, very little other than coffee and bread with margarine or jam

4 "The Economic Depression and Public Health, Memorandum prepared by the Health Section. III. The Nutrition of the Unemployed", *League of Nations Quarterly Bulletin of the Health Organisation*, Vol. 1, 1932, pp. 443-457.

5 *Ibidem*, 1932, p. 448.

was eaten. The midday meal usually included a greater variety of foodstuffs: soup, potatoes, green vegetables and sometimes meat.[6]

In Britain, technical reports for 1932 showed that the total income of the unemployed just about covered the necessary food expenditure, but the safety margin was very small. At the time, the situation in Germany was comparatively worse. Food availability was a central factor from the perspective of both domestic and foreign affairs. According to the British Ministry of Health, "the diet in the households of the unemployed men comprised little beyond white bread, butter or margarine, potatoes, sugar, jam, tea and bacon in limited quantity: although meat was seldom eaten, fresh milk was not seen and the usual milk was skimmed condensed. Fresh vegetables other than potatoes were seldom eaten".[7]

Such disproportion between the income of the unemployed and their necessary food expenditure existed in many other European countries. The general awareness of a loss of quality in the nutrition of European citizens was inevitably raised, the resulting tendency being a growing consumption of cheaper vegetable foods at the expense of milk, meat, eggs and butter. This tendency had to be counteracted by mass production in order to meet an urgent demand for very cheap animal foods.

According to international expert surveys, in the Far East, Tropical Countries and Colonial territories dietary standards were not essentially different from those of Western countries. Since a scientific approach was based on the idea that physiological standards were universally applicable, dietary habits were basic for assessing the nutritional state of the populations. Research work on nutrition in the Far East prompted the study of the nutritive value of local foodstuffs, the diet of the different population groups, their state of nutrition and the incidence of diseases caused by dietary deficiencies. In order to carry out diet surveys for different population groups, data had to be calculated not only in terms of nutrients and food factors (calories, nutritional principles, vitamins, minerals, etc) but also in terms of real foodstuffs consumed: in terms of diet. In any case, such investigations were expected to come up with a definition of the problem and therefore encourage the consumption of certain products: under-milled rice, red palm oil and others. As a complementary option, feeding experiments on human groups were suggested by nutritionists.

6 Report by Lehmann in 1931, included in "The Economic Depression and Public Health", 1932, p. 452.

7 *Ibidem.*

The League of Nations' Technical Commission on nutrition underlined the importance of relying on natural local products, but they also agreed that certain population groups could benefit from the distribution of pure and concentrated vitamins, provided these could be obtained cheaply in large quantities. Yeast, a product rich in nitrogenous elements and B group vitamins, was considered to be of particular value in correcting deficiencies in the diets of tropical and Eastern populations. Something similar was said about mineral elements, which could be supplied cheaply to schoolchildren and groups suffering from a deficiency of these elements. One of the most important defects of the so-called *poor rice-eater's diet* – a problem identified in some Asian regions – was precisely calcium shortage.

Raising education standards and giving specific instruction on the principles of nutrition was considered necessary for all social classes as an essential instrument to improve dietary habits in each country. In 1938 circumstances were very critical in Europe. For two years Spain suffered the shortages caused by the civil war, and a severe restriction of foodstuffs aggravated the nutrition problem in many other European countries to the extent that emergency measures by governments against famine as a real threat were needed. National institutes of food had been created in most countries to coordinate food policy, to address trade and improve availability. Under those circumstances, the League of Nations' Technical Commission on Nutrition took on the task of implementing a dietary standard aimed at ensuring an optimum degree of nutrition. On the other hand, the approach to famine relief was largely dependent on local circumstances. In this regard, important factors had to be taken into account, such as the relation between available funding and the numbers to be fed, food transport and storage, fuel supply, etc. As a consequence, several programmes to prevent famine were proposed by the Technical Commission, according to the special peculiarities of the countries. The evolution of the work done by the Technical Commission and its field of implementation took a shift at the end of the 1930s, from a scenario in which *optimum diet* was the aim – in a wide project involving agriculture, health, experimental research and politics – to quite a different one threatened by malnutrition and famine.

Coping with Nutritional Deficiencies and Malnutrition

A diet mainly composed of bread, potatoes and margarine, and comparatively lacking in eggs, butter, milk and green vegetables was considered incompatible with optimum health at any age, the latter two foodstuffs being identified as *protective*. Such a diet was deficient in protein of high biological value, in vitamin A and other vitamins and calcium.[8] On the other hand, the falling consumption of milk was considered to be serious deprivation for children. It was seemingly important to realise that the dietary value of animal food bore little relation to their commercial quality and cost, both elements being affected by shortages and inflation. Consequently, various food-deficiency diseases, such as scurvy, beriberi, and hunger oedema, were apt to occur in those people who, while consuming a deficient diet, were forced to make severe physical efforts. The problem deserved to be carefully studied, both from a national and international point of view, involving factors not only of an economic, social, political and agricultural nature, but also of a dietetic and hygienic type.[9]

A general feeling spread among the population about the economic depression that affected the whole world. It not only undermined the social foundations on which the life of nations were based, but also involved serious dangers for people's physical and mental health and for the survival of millions. The progress made in medicine and hygiene in previous decades was also being threatened. According to the report of the League of Nations' Health Organisation for the yearly period October 1932 to September 1933, deficient nutrition affected more than 50 million people. Enquiries into the state of nutrition among the unemployed were underway in various countries and, as we know, a conference was convened in Berlin in December 1932.[10] Indeed, in an investigation of the effects of the depression on public health, consideration had to be given to a wide range of aspects, particularly the intensity of the economic crisis, its duration and extent. Working conditions and the cost of living had to be considered, to assess the influence of a plurality of factors on death and morbidity rates. To evaluate the real dimension of the threat, collecting evidence through official statistics was the best way of mapping the situation and planning a solid programme of action.

An important aspect was the efficient organisation of health care in every nation. Several political testimonies in different countries reported that it was not rational, complete or economical, with the cost of medicines representing a very large item in the expenditure incurred by medical care providers. The seriousness of the crisis and its influence on

8 *Ibidem*, p. 456.

9 *Ibidem*, p. 473.

10 "Report of the Health Organisation for the Period October 1932 to September 1933. IV. Economic Depression and Public Health", *League of Nations Quarterly Bulletin of the Health Organisation*, Vol. 2, 1933, pp. 529-535.

the impairment of economic and social conditions brought to the forefront the idea of compulsory sickness insurance, a possibility that was generally regarded as the most rational method of organising the protection of the working classes against sickness and the risk of malnutrition. In fact, the cost of hospital treatment was one of the most important items of expenditure in some states and therefore governments started to introduce a financial approach to the health care system, considering the idea of exact budgetary calculations, uniform methods and daily costs based on rationalisation. It is worth noting the impairment of the social and health situation of the European population and the growing regulatory intervention of the state as main factors leading to the establishment of national health services in many European countries and not only the pressure of socialist, working class unions and political parties.

A strong link between the experimental science of nutrition, public health, economy and politics was established in the period. Experts in the physiology of nutrition and public health authorities reinforced liaison, as during the inter-war crisis public health work on nutrition was an extremely important part of public health activity. The threat of malnutrition became a serious social and economic issue and, as such, concerned politicians, economists, agriculturists, and social workers as much as it concerned health professionals. Nutrition deficiencies emerged as a new factor for what was perceived as *racial degeneration*, therefore nutrition, food and diet opened up an avenue to medicalisation and to the spread of medical knowledge as a way to rationalise social relations. Social hygiene was based, in a sense, on a right diet for everyone.

Scientific and medical research showed that the food consumed by the organism was not only important for providing energy. The physical state of the organism largely depended on its nutrition and had a bearing on immunological reactions. From the last decades of the 19th century physiologists such as Claude Bernard had insisted on the importance of nutrition as a fact of *organic synthesis*, which meant the perpetual creation of what he conceived to be a living organism's *internal environment.* Other researchers, such as the American physiologist Walter Cannon, conceptualised this internal balance as *homeostasis*. At the beginning of the 20th century it was generally believed that the dietary requirements of human beings were satisfied so long as they had enough to eat, and therefore any illness suffered by those who were not hungry would be ascribed to causes other than the diet. Infectious diseases represented the main problem and microbes were held responsible. However, a few decades later, it was accepted that the adequacy of a dietary depended on a number of factors and mere quantitative sufficiency was considered compatible with a whole series of qualitative defects, any one of which might produce the most serious physical consequences. In the late 1920s poverty, children's infectious diseases and the economic crisis paved the way for a new field of action. Nutrition and infection were the main references.

On the other hand, experimental and clinical research had proved that an insufficient diet leads to serious diseases like rickets, scurvy, beriberi, pellagra, dental caries, certain types of anaemia and neuropathy. It also opens the gate to infectious diseases, including tuberculosis, the so-called *white pest*. But the diet was not only a factor in the prevention and treatment of certain diseases; it was also related to physical development and, in that respect, public health not only aimed to prevent populations from disease, but also to create a maximum level of wellbeing, with nutrition becoming a central subject.

Under those circumstances, the hygienic control of foodstuffs became a key issue. Public health authorities were concerned about the protection of the public against dangerous contaminated foodstuffs and fraudulent practices in connection with the sale of food and the feeding of population groups in schools, factories, prisons, asylums, naval and military establishments and also in any commercial transaction.[11] In war times, governments had to feed large armies whose physique and morale had to be maintained at all costs, and at the same time responsibility for providing food for the civilian population had to be assumed, a hard challenge to be successfully faced in times of shortage.

As a consequence of the economic crisis, unemployment and poverty had imposed on governments enormous responsibilities in the sphere of public assistance, one of the most urgent being the combat against defective diseases and malnutrition. The emergency situations produced by the war, post-war period and the depression had helped to make clear the importance of public health nutrition work in normal times. In many European countries, concerned governments controlled food availability and the nutritional conditions of the population. State central administrations extended their programmes of action under the influence of public measures and regulations, so that nutrition was paid increasing attention in the field of public health.[12] Governmental involvement was

11 Guillem-Llobat, Perdiguero, 2006, pp. 33-40.

12 Bernabeu-Mestre, J. *et al.*, "La alimentación como problema sanitario: nutrición y salud pública en la España de la primera mitad del siglo XX", *VIII Congreso de la ADEH*, Maó, 2007, 63 p.; Bernabeu-Mestre, J., Galiana, M.E., Esplugues, J.X. and Cid, P. "Overexploitation, malnutrition and stigma in a women's illness: chlorosis in contemporary Spanish medicine (1877-1936)", in Harris, B., Gálvez, L., Machado, E.

easy to understand in a context of emergency, but it was becoming even more systematic for public health and economic reasons. In the 1930s vast numbers of human beings were malnourished or undernourished and, indeed, famine itself had not yet disappeared, remaining a threat.[13] But the situation would only worsen as a consequence of the war, first in Spain and then in most European regions, becoming a sort of social epidemic.

Although the effects of the crisis had not yet been reflected in vital and epidemiological statistics, several indications of increased morbidity among the unemployed and their families suggested a deterioration of their state of nutrition, especially among the social groups badly hit by the crisis. The situation was growing worse, and the resources of the unemployed and assisted persons were so scant in certain regions that they no longer sufficed to procure an adequate diet.[14] A clinical typology of undernourished states and a precise definition of malnutrition were necessary.

The Health Committee of the League of Nations decided to establish contact between the experts responsible for the enquiries at the time, proceeding to reach an agreement on how the state of nutrition could be determined by means of a clinical examination of a standard type to be decided upon. A conference was convened for this purpose in Berlin in December 1932, chaired by Professor E. Gorter, the director of the Children's Clinic of Leyden University (Netherlands).[15] Two possible methods of action were discussed at the conference. One was to study the nature and quantity of foodstuffs consumed by the individuals under examination, discussing records of diet and consumption, and making a decision about whether their diet was adequate or not. The second option was based on clinical examination with a view to determining physical condition by direct exploration. Under such critical circumstances, the second method was regarded as the most reliable to obtain a picture of the situation. Obviously, these medical examinations

---

(eds.), *Gender and wellbeing in Europe: historical and contemporary perspectives*, Ashgate, Hampshire, 2009, pp. 154-171.

13 Burnet, Aykroyd, 1935, pp. 323-474.

14 "The most Suitable Methods of Detecting Malnutrition Due to the Economic Depression, The. Conference held at Berlin from December 5th to 7th, 1932", *League of Nations Quarterly Bulletin of the Health Organisation*, Vol. 1, 1933, pp. 116-129.

15 The Conference was attended by representatives from Austria (E. Nobel), Belgium (D.L.J. Gilbert), United Kingdom (Janet M. Campbell and A.F. Hurst), Denmark (Th. Madsen), France (J. Parisot), Germany (C. Hamel, E. Atzler, G. von Bergmann, W. Bansi, O. Martineck, p. Stefani and H. Zondeck), Italy (C. Gini) and USA (K.D. Blackfan and J.R. Murlin) and several members of the German Reichstag.

had to be applied to a sufficiently large number of people from the various classes of the unemployed and needy groups, comparing data with groups of persons belonging to the same class, whose incomes and living conditions had been unaffected by the crisis[16]

If the number of unemployed individuals was considerable, other tests – anaemia, fatigability, the pulse rate, signs of avitaminoses (xerophtalmia, rickets, oedema) – could also be conducted to a lesser extent. For the organisation of the enquiries, the agencies conducting them were official public health and social hygiene services comprised of doctors, visiting nurses and social workers with the necessary expertise and personal skills to ensure the best results.

Driven by the need to determine nutritional deficiencies according to scientific patterns, a general programme of research into biological measurements and tests for the definition of states of malnutrition was published by H. Laugier in 1936.[17] Notwithstanding the hard methodological difficulties, some interesting points were emphasised in this report in order to make the practical screening of malnutrition possible. If accurate information was available concerning the weight of the person examined before the period of malnutrition, the ratio between the weight at the moment of checking and the previous weight constituted the basic criterion. In the absence of such data, some alternative measures could orient the diagnosis, such as Bouchard's index for adults and Pirquet's index for children. The amount of subcutaneous adipose tissue was also to be ascertained, but always taking into account that some obese individuals do not lose weight even if they eat very little and, conversely, there are thin people who do not put on weight despite their copious food intake.

Research in connection with the physiological effects of fasting might have shown regularities determined by urine analysis, a very valuable way of establishing malnutrition indices. Unfortunately, there was a lack of such investigations and, besides, they had never been applied to determine the state of malnutrition. Some clinical signs could point to deficient nutrition, such as the loss of muscular energy and the capacity for sustained effort – reduced in a state of malnutrition – but they were mainly studied in connection with unusual movements.

All the experimental evidence seemed to prove that an undernourished person reacted to renourishment rapidly and positively.

16 "The most Suitable Methods", 1933, p. 119.

17 Laugier, H., "General Programme of Research into Biological Measurements and Tests for the Definition of States of Malnutrition", *League of Nations Quarterly Bulletin of the Health Organisation*, Vol. 5, No. 3, 1936, pp. 505-530.

Further experiments developed in internment camps and other nutritional experiments on humans confirmed this idea.[18] Weight and the basal metabolism increase, the pulse quickens and the blood pressure rises as motor capacities improve. Moreover, a series of additional tests could be made on a comparative basis before and after this period of feeding. A test consisted of meals rich in proteins. It had been noticed that undernourished persons retained nitrogen, as this element was not found in their urine in sufficient quantities. A glycosemia rate was also considered to be helpful. The general aim was to translate into laboratory indices the biological negative effects of a deficient diet.

The biological supervision of food, especially of its vitamin content, was to become one of the experimental possibilities to modify and improve nutritional qualities through an artificial vitaminisation of foodstuffs.[19] The first technical challenge to solve was the preservation of vitamins, because industrial processes were not free of risks. Some evidence showed that the permanent and excessive ingestion of artificially vitaminised foods had drawbacks over time, and accidents were reported in France, Italy and England. Randoin argued for the strict suppression of advertisements exaggerating the positive effects of vitamins, the expression of vitamin contents in food in international units and the establishment of effective controls over artificial vitaminisation by means of international regulations. Rather than an advantage, some industrial techniques affecting food had become a supplementary risk.

Surveys showed that in the 1930s the problem of nutrition varied widely from one part of the world to another. In some countries, an adequate diet was still probably within the reach of the majority of the population, while in others practically everyone lived just a little above a bare subsistence level. In some countries, food prices were relatively low, but in others they were high in relation to incomes. National surveys were recommended, since local differences implied that nutrition policies varied in different areas, their goal being to ensure that all sections of the population had an adequate diet: sufficient energy-bearing and protective foods for optimum health.[20]

---

18 Nutrition in internment camps and nutritional experiments on the pathological effects of malnutrition in humans will be discussed in a further chapter.

19 Randoin, L., "On the necessity for a biological supervision of food (with Special Reference to its Vitamin Content)", *League of Nations Quarterly Bulletin of the Health Organisation*, Vol. 5, No. 3, 1936, pp. 493-504.

20 *Final report*, 1937, p 32.

Nevertheless, experts reported that food habits were gradually changing in the right direction, and "those communities, on the whole, are now consuming, in addition to the indispensable foods of high energy value, more milk and dairy products, more fruit and more vegetables than a generation ago".[21] Improvement was said to come from the understanding of dietary needs, but the movement towards better nutrition had not gone far enough. Once again, popular culture and tradition clashed with scientific knowledge and, from the nutritionists' point of view, poverty and ignorance were considered to be main obstacles to progress, while the disparity between prices and incomes was a factor that increased difficulties. Indeed, nutrition policy was required to achieve two goals: the consumption of those products recommended as essential by experimental science, but also an improved supply, which required agriculture and commerce to adapt to new demands and cultural patterns derived from scientific knowledge.

Admitting that hunger was a national problem in most countries was the starting point for any solution in nutritional policies. More than ever, politicians became aware of the necessity of bringing together scientists, public health experts, economists, agricultural experts, consumers' representatives, teachers and administrators in some kind of national nutrition committees that recognised the importance of integrating agricultural, educational, health and economic policies.[22] European governments afforded direct relief, especially to the unemployed, and the extension of such social interventions was considered extremely important in order to improve the population's health status, bearing in mind that the problem of malnutrition was urgent. Many governments adopted measures of direct assistance to supplement the diets of the more exposed, especially to prevent malnutrition in childhood by way of giving milk to infants, children, adolescents and expectant and nursing mothers.

From the perspective of social assistance, school meals were to play an important role in a context of dietary policies based on public and private provision of food needs. The crisis forced modern states to become directly committed to intervening in private habits, but also in public and private institutions, shaping a network of community nutrition: school canteens, hospital meals, charitable and benevolent institutions, relief centres, the army and navy, prisons and other state services and institutions. Public and private authorities assumed

21 *Ibidem.*

22 *Ibidem*, p 36-38.

responsibilities for the provision of meals, trying to ensure that all nutrient constituents as defined by experimental science were provided.

In all Western countries, the average diet of the population had become increasingly diversified from the beginning of the 20th century. There had been a tendency for the consumption of dairy produce, eggs, fruit and vegetables to increase; and the great staples, such as cereals and potatoes, had come to constitute a smaller proportion of human foodstuffs. The fact that a larger amount of the total calorie requirements were derived from the highly protective foods represented a great nutritional advance and provided evidence that there was a natural tendency on the part of consumers to become more aware of the importance of rational nutrition as far as economic circumstances permitted. An exception usually mentioned was the increasing consumption of sugar in certain countries.

The most notable trends, apart from the remarkable increase in sugar consumption, were the continuous rise in the consumption of milk, butter and eggs, the steady fall in bread consumption and the post-war decline in the consumption of potatoes. It seemed clear, from the examples given, that the average diet of the urban working classes in Western countries tended to include larger amounts of protective foods. Instead of the general improvements and changes in feeding habits, the diet of a substantial portion of the population remained deficient in essential nutritive elements, giving way to an unquestionable problem of malnutrition, even in countries with the highest standards of living.

The changing content of the diet of Western countries was not an accident; it corresponded to a genuine change both in physiological requirements and in the possibility to satisfy them. Most of the experts believed that the principal factors were the reduction in the expenditure of muscular energy caused by unemployment and increased mechanisation in industry and agriculture. There was also the reduction in the hours of work on the one hand and the rising number of those engaged in commerce, trade, clerical work, administration and other quasi-sedentary occupations on the other. By far, labourers doing heavy manual work spent more energy than machine operators or office workers. Ever a smaller fraction of the population was engaged in the primary industries such as agriculture and forestry, and a constantly increasing proportion was involved in manufacturing, trade, transportation, clerical and professional occupations. Economic facts were also to be kept in mind: the foodstuffs that had tended to feature in the diet were usually more expensive than those they had displaced, and the so-called modern diet became dearer than the diet of previous decades, which had uneven effects upon everyday life in times of crisis.

The effects of deficient nutrition caused by poverty and exclusion was not immediate; it took some time to reach a clinical level, becoming apparent after a long interval. "A child whose diet contains too high a proportion of cheap carbohydrates may retain a *normal* weight for a fairly long time, even though a state of anaemia and debility has already set in. The actual duration of the inadequate nutrition is a very important factor".[23] However, it was widely recognised that even among the very poor, the diet could be influenced by factors other than income, such as maternal efficiency and cultural habits. Nutritional experts suspected some prevalence of hidden undernourishment in all social levels. After the 1930s crisis and World War II relief was necessary as a social tool, but also education in marketing, values, cooking and methods of food preservation. Housewife efficiency was deemed to be a keystone of the problem of nutrition during the economic crisis and it mostly depended upon educating mothers. All instruments had to be put into action to reach this target: campaigns, films, lectures and radio. Mothers became a key player in the process of civilisation. Changing dietary habits was a part of it.

An international food policy, as called for by the international committees, also required the international unification of the technical analysis and control of food quality of foodstuffs, setting up standards of reference and specifications for grading foods of all kinds according to quality. Bearing in mind that each country had previously developed its own regulations and institutions for the control and expertise, coordination of the nutrition work carried out by different authorities was recommended.[24] Based on the collection of records about consumption by families of different occupational groups with different income levels, international comparative records were to become essential in verifying to what extent national dietaries fell short of the new standards. Scientific standards aimed to become references of authority in the process of disciplining both the economy and dietary habits.[25]

During the Depression years it was thought that general incomes would rise sooner or later and therefore special actions had to be taken to improve the nutrition of particular community groups.

A meeting on the *Nutritional state of children* was held in December 1936 following the initiative of the League of Nations Experts'

---

23 Burnet, Aykroyd, 1935, p. 384.

24 Guillem-Llobat, X., *El control de la qualitat dels aliments. El cas valencià en el context internacional (1878-1936)*, Valencia, PUV, 2007.

25 "Report on the physiological bases", 1936, pp. 97-98.

Committee on Nutrition. In their final report, the experts recommended an assessment of the state of nutrition of large numbers of children, and to further develop somatometric, clinical and physiological tests, designed to detect the first signs of malnutrition at the earliest possible moment. Nutritive food requirements in the first year of life were also discussed, paying special attention to breastfeeding and milk supplies as a means to avoid problems in the child's organic development and nutritional deficiencies. In the last meeting, held in November 1937, the technical commission on nutrition endeavoured to show, in the light of recent research, why milk was a foodstuff of such paramount importance, especially during growth in childhood. It also emphasised the need to eliminate the dangers of milk as a vehicle for bacterial infection.[26]

Between June 1938 and April 1939 the work of the Health Organisation Technical Commission on Nutrition concentrated on two main lines. It changed the geographical perspective, previously focused on Western countries and, in pursuance of a recommendation adopted by the General Advisory Health Council in 1937, it was to undertake the study of nutrition in Asia and tropical countries in general. In addition, the Commission was to deal with qualitative and quantitative surveys designed to bring any nutritional deficiencies to light.[27]

With particular regard to the Far East and tropical countries, the Committee considered that fuller information was required on dietary habits, the incidence of diseases connected with dietary deficiencies and the nutritional value of local foods.[28] As a starting point, it reached some general conclusions on national programmes and urged certain adjustments in the sphere of agriculture to increase the production of protective foods. However, more complete dietary surveys were to be made to find food supplies in the rural and urban areas of several countries using statistics on production and consumption as a main tool.

Three types of enquiries into the state of nutrition of populations were suggested. Large-scale demographic investigations were proposed, consisting of a record of the age, sex, physical appearance, height and weight of each subject. They represented a sort of individual chart containing general anthropometric features. A second level of research included more detailed investigations that covered a limited number of

---

26 "Report on the work of the Health Organisation between June 1937 and May 1938, and on its 1938 Programme. 4. Nutrition", *League of Nations Bulletin of the Health Organisation*, Vol. 7, 1938, p. 646.

27 *Ibidem*, pp. 27-32.

28 *Ibidem*, p. 29.

individuals. Among other data suggested were: core features of children's diet; an exhaustive medical examination of individuals; the economic and social position of the family; as well as somatometric records, photographs and tests to detect pre-deficiency conditions. The third level consisted of surveying bio-topological investigations regarding morphological characteristics and biological functions, as well as psychological examination of the population.

During its August session, the attention of the Special Committee was drawn to the fact that, even in Europe, disturbing conditions existed in which the problem was no longer to lay down the bases for a satisfactory diet, but rather to prevent the population from the risk of dying from starvation. This was, more particularly, the position of Spain in 1938, affected by two years of war. To cope with it, the Society of Friends sought guidance in the preparation of an emergency diet for the refugees. The Committee suggested that a diet of this character should be mainly composed of whole wheat, brewer's dried yeast, cod liver oil and various salts. This emergency diet was designed to include vitamins and essential inorganic constituents. At the same time, the Committee pointed out that such a diet was, at most, adequate to sustain life and to prevent the appearance, during a limited period, of the more serious effects of malnutrition. But it was not to be interpreted as a permanent dietary pattern. It could only be looked upon as an emergency diet, to be supplemented at the earliest possible moment by fresh foods.[29] The risk of undernourishment and chronic malnutrition was a real threat and the situation would deteriorate in several European regions in the following years as a consequence of the war.

Looking for Standards of Food Quality

Throughout the 19th century most European countries developed regulations and established local and national institutions to analyse food quality and fight fraud. Experimental procedures in specialised laboratories for analytic chemistry, bacteriology and serology paved the way for stricter control of food quality and for the detection of any sort of adulteration.[30] The increasing process of food industrialisation gave

29 *Ibidem*, p. 32.

30 Guillem-Llobat, *El control de la qualitat*, 2007; Elvbakken, K.T., Lægreid, P., Rykkja, L.H., "Regulation for Safe Food; a Comparison of Five European Countries", *Scandinavian Political Studies*, Vol. 31, No.2, 2008, pp. 125-148; Smith, D.F., Phillips, J. (eds.), *Food, Science, Policy and Regulation in the Twentieth Century. International and Comparative Perspectives*, London, Routledge, 2000.

way to new risks and also led to the search for new solutions. Food quality was the kernel of health and politics.[31]

The establishment of standard values in the composition of each specific foodstuff was one of the main strategies followed by countries to make it easier to control food quality and detect fraud. In most European countries the progressive introduction of a growing amount of standard values for specific foodstuffs increasingly subjected to industrial production resulted from the large-scale issue of food regulations at the turn of the 20th century. Detecting fraud and adulterations when applied to milk, wine, oil, chocolate and other daily products was relatively simple with the new analytical methods. However, the definition of quality standards and the necessity of reaching international homologation in the world food market could be more controversial, giving way to heated debates in some European countries.

In the United Kingdom, the *Society of Public Analysts* campaigned for decades in favour of the establishment of official standard values in the composition of foodstuffs. The issue was also included in some meetings of the FAO committees. Specialised journals such as *The Analyst* and *The British Food Journal* called for an agreement on quality standards. Nevertheless, the social groups influencing the public opinion in favour of the establishment of quality standards were not successful in their campaign, and opposite attitudes that represented the interests of the different groups involved clashed. By the 1930s the issue remained unresolved in Great Britain.[32]

Basically, the need to reach agreements about the composition of certain foodstuffs was linked to the growing industrialisation and internationalisation of the food market. That is why the issue surpassed the national context, reaching the international sphere. In fact, the inter-war period was characterised by intense debate, agreements and negotiations about biological standards, to a great extent promoted by the international agencies, especially the League of Nations. Standardisation was the starting point of any industrial development in key fields such as physiology, serology, bacteriology and the pharmaceutical industry. Obviously, it was also a *sine qua non* condition for the international development of food industries involving quality standards.

---

31 Guillem-Llobat, 2008e, pp. 215-246.

32 Smith, Phillips, 2000.

The establishment of food quality standards was already an old demand in the international conferences of hygiene and demography held in the second half of the 19th century. As a result of this interest, an international commission for the repression of food fraud was created as a permanent conference site under the pressure of some participants calling for the establishment and publication of a code containing the normal composition of foodstuffs in each country. This was likely to be the first step in establishing a global *Codex Alimentarius* some decades later by the FAO. It was approved by international consensus, the only starting point for a practical solution to guarantee the regulation of the increasing industrialisation and internationalisation of the food trade.

Standardisation was also a challenge as far as the methods of food quality analysis were concerned. In the international context, the standardisation of analytic methods was proposed and discussed at international conferences. At the international meeting on applied chemistry held in Berlin in 1903, a resolution was passed on the need to reach an international agreement on the methods of analysis to be used to determine the quality of each foodstuff. In Spain this standardising initiative was pushed for through special governmental requests such as the one addressed to the *Unión Farmacéutica Nacional* [National Pharmaceutical Union] on July 21, 1933.[33] This professional association of pharmacists was commissioned to prepare a list of suitable methods for the analysis of foodstuffs. It was to be the first initiative sent to the *Comisión General de Sanidad* [General Health Board], to be approved and distributed among laboratories, health officers and professionals with responsibilities on food quality control.[34] These initiatives in favour of standardisation – especially those dealing with the composition of foodstuffs – and the request for a more detailed labelling of food merchandise was called for to improve meaningfully the capacity of public administrations to control food quality and prevent adulteration and fraud.

However, these contributions did not always result in effective food quality regulations. Indeed, in some cases these strategies became a way of allowing certain practices that were previously forbidden. The more analytical information established quantitative limits for substances that were not accepted before, considering them simple adulterations.

Another consequence of standardisation was labelling as a means of information to the consumer and a guarantee of publicity about the content and therefore quality control. However, it paved the way for the

33 Guillem-Llobat, 2008e, p. 230.

34 *Ibidem*.

transformation of the composition of foodstuffs. As long as the consumer was informed, the composition could vary within certain limits to a greater extent than before. Labelling opened up a new side to the discussion. Sometimes the capacity of consumers to understand the meaning of the label was put into question by the experts, and some authors even queried the procedure itself, considering the fact that being labelled implicitly meant that foodstuffs had passed quality controls, leading to a non-critical acceptance by the consumer. At the turn of the century attitudes to food regulations varied widely between those defending strict rules and those in favour of more permissive ones.[35]

On the other hand, there was not a uniform trend, and contradictions appeared in the regulations themselves. In the case of the composition of liquors, wines, vinegars and artificial sweeteners, some especially restrictive rules were passed in the late 19th century. But the rules approved during the first decades of the 20th century to regulate the quality of those products were more and more lenient. This example shows that the trend was towards more restrictive regulations to guarantee the quality of certain foodstuffs at the turn of the century and more permissive as time went by. However, the tendency was not the same for every foodstuff and important differences could be found depending upon specific negotiations between the several actors involved. The regulation of each individual product was finally established at a national level only, usually following complex agreements between public health officers, politicians, industrialists and consumer associations. Obviously, depending on the relative strength of the groups involved, the final regulation could be different, which was indeed the case if we look at the European context. Although in the early decades of the 20th century standardising and labelling were at the heart of the legal control of food quality, the process was not exempt of difficulties.

---

35 Frohlich, X.Z., *Accounting for Taste: Regulating Food Labeling in the Affluent Society, 1945-1995*, Cambridge, Ma., Massachussets Institute of Technology, 2011.

CHAPTER 5

Food, Famine and Relief in Wartime

The high hopes on the science of nutrition as the nucleus of social change collapsed under the exceptional economic crisis that hit Europe in the 1930s, the destabilising effects of millions of refugees in Greece, the spread of malnutrition in rural areas, as well as the devastating effects of the Spanish Civil War and World War II. All of these events caused the living conditions of many European citizens to deteriorate, and major concerns grew among national and international organisations regarding food availability and the negative influence of nutritional impairment on the health standards of the population.[1] In the case of Spain, the benefits produced by the social and sanitary reforms introduced by the republican government since 1931 were jeopardised by the 1936 fascist military *coup d'état*.[2]

The Impact of the Civil War on the Spanish Nutritional Condition

At the end of 1936 the League of Nations, following a proposal by the Spanish Republican Government, adopted a resolution to send a group of experts to survey the health situation of the Spanish population after several months of conflict. The evaluation of the nutritional state of the population and the strategy to guarantee food availability was not only a matter that impacted upon the economy and public health, but it was also an essential aspect in military terms. The technical commission sent to Spain by the League of Nations included: Antoine Lasnet, a medical officer and member of the French Academy of Medicine; Jean Laigret, a member of the Pasteur Institute in Tunis; and C. Wroczynski, Chief Medical Adviser to the Ministry of National Education in

1 Biraud, M., "Health in Europe. A Survey of the Epidemic and Nutritional Situation", *League of Nations Bulletin of the Health Organisation*, Vol. 10, 1943-1944, pp. 557-699; Barona, 2007b.

2 Barona, 2006c; Barona, 2007b.

Warsaw. At the beginning of 1937 a report was presented to the Council.[3]

The Commission paid special attention to the dietary condition of refugees as food supply prospects in certain areas were bleak. Its report dealt with four fundamental problems: health organisation, the epidemiological situation, dietary prospects and problems arising from the evacuation of refugees.[4]

During the first year of the war all the available data showed a controlled epidemiological situation without signs of degradation in the level of health. There were no unexpected epidemic outbreaks. The health of the population in the republican zone remained within the usual limits. The stable population had enough supplies, but there were severe shortages among the refugees. This apparent normality came as a surprise to the League of Nations' experts visiting Spain at the beginning of 1937. But the situation began to worsen, as shown by the evolution of the general mortality rates. In the period 1930-35 the rate was 14.5 per thousand, and in 1937 it was only 15.5. But the rate increased gradually during the war, reaching a peak of 19.2 per thousand in 1938. When the Civil War ended, there was a decrease in general mortality for a three-month period, but in 1940 an increase brought the rate up to 16.6 per thousand. 1941 showed a new increase due, in part, to food shortages and high infant mortality subsequent to the spectacular birth rise in 1940.[5]

The excellent system of recording epidemiological data put in place by Marcelino Pascua[6] during the first republican biennium had been profoundly altered by the war and so the collection of data was deficient. Yet it still permitted the identification of the four principal problems that required attention under those circumstances: typhoid fever, spotted fever, smallpox and bacillary dysentery. All of them were expected problems, given the living conditions during the war.[7]

---

3 *Rapport sur la mission sanitaire en Espagne (28 decembre 1936-15 janvier 1937)*, Genève, Société des Nations, 1937.

4 Anguera A., "Servicios sanitarios con motivo de la inmigración durante la guerra", *Revista de Sanidad e Higiene Pública*, Vol. 1, 1938/1939, pp. 25-42; García Luquero, "Aspectos sanitarios de la evacuación de refugiados en Santander", *Revista de Sanidad e Higiene Pública*, Vol. 1, 1938-1939, pp. 68-81.

5 Barona, 2007b.

6 Marcelino Pascua was a former pensionate of the Rockefeller Foundation at the Johns Hopkins School of Public Health and General Director for Health in the socialist government 1931-1933. After the war he went into exile, becoming head of the statistics office of the World Health Organisation.

7 *Rapport sur la mission sanitaire*, 1937, pp. 72-73.

According to the League of Nations' 1937 report, typhoid fever had been an endemic problem in Spain before the war due to poor hygiene in water for human consumption. The number of cases at the start of the 1920s oscillated between 15,000 and 20,000 annually, leading to 3,000 to 4,000 deaths. In 1934-35 the number of cases was strongly reduced. But the situation worsened from the start of the war due to the deterioration of sanitary conditions and the movement of refugees, as shown by the data employed by the expert committee, originally from statistics compiled by the National Hospital of Infectious Diseases. In the second half of 1936 there were 358 cases, 42 of which ended in death. At any rate, the experts expressed their reserve and thought that health services had reorganised and that bacteriological water testing was being carried out on a regular basis. There was no fear of an epidemic, and therefore, an intensification of typhoid vaccination was not recommended.

The whole of the epidemiological survey did not detect the appearance of epidemic or even sporadic outbreaks. The measures adopted by the republican government in this matter consisted of recruiting all the medical professionals of the country, coordinating the actions of the civil and military medical authorities, adopting special measures to ensure the proper functioning of medical aid on the front of battle and developing vaccination campaigns whenever convenient. Typhoid and paratyphoid fever vaccination was administered to the army, and quite widespread paratyphoid fever vaccination was extended among the civilian population. Smallpox vaccination was compulsory, yet vaccination against diphtheria was rare, given that this measure had never been that common with the population. There was no other type of preventive vaccination applied to soldiers, not even against tetanus.

From their direct observations and from the official data compiled, the League of Nations' experts considered the health situation to be satisfactory at the start of 1937, although they feared the spread of typhoid and spotted fevers. They therefore recommended compulsory vaccination and water and food testing. With regard to spotted fever, they laid out recommendations for the improvement of treatment and prevention that included the use of portable de-lousing devices and treatment material, general immunisation against typhus for health workers and improving the availability of vaccines. They thought it necessary to equip municipal and provincial centres with specific areas for the treatment of patients with infectious diseases, provide disinfection devices for health services, these being clearly inadequate. They also isolated contagious patients and improved the system of epidemiological data collection in order to detect any sign of deterioration in the sanitary situation at any time. A central point was the training of doctors specialised in epidemics; these could be specifically assigned to prophylaxis and the fight against infections and be employed in asylums, prisons and other places where large groups of people lived. As a conclusion, let us accept that the international specialists detected neither nutritional problems nor the impairment of health levels in republican Spain.

The report presented by J.A. Palanca to the League of Nations in 1939 on the Francoist side commented on the main health problems in the nationalist sector regarding the army but also the health situation of the civil population.[8] The report was rather unrealistic in trying to show that the actions taken before the war allowed a controlled epidemiological situation during the war in the nationalist zone. The completion of Palanca's report coincided with the end of the war, a time at which the necessary reconstruction of health care for the population was already underway.[9]

The evacuation of refugees fleeing the front to neighbouring areas was a fundamental aspect regarding the health and nutritional state of the population. The report of the League of Nations showed that 250,000 refugees from Extremadura lived in Jaen, Ciudad Real and Toledo; and Catalonia had received a large quantity of refugees from Aragón. The flow of refugees aroused spontaneous solidarity in the families living in the hosting zones, but there was a clear need to set up a National Committee for War Refugees. The provincial and local delegations of this committee were in charge of the evacuation, distribution and fostering of the refugees.[10] The money for their care came from private sources and from the national budget.

The magnitude of the problems posed by the evacuation of the population from the front was enormous. At the end of 1936 they numbered more than one million. Of those, 350,000 were fostered in Catalonia and 250,000 in Valencia.[11] The refugees accounted for 14% of the whole population of the country. The capacity to foster new refugees was on the verge of saturation and food shortages appeared in some areas. The evacuation of the capital, Madrid, which was under siege,

---

8 Palanca y Martínez Fortún, J.A. *Les services sanitaires espagnols pendant la guerre civile*, Genève, Societé de Nations, 1939. Palanca was a conservative hygienist belonging to the group of experts in public health leading reforms in Spain during the previous decade; he was an intern of the Rockefeller Foundation. After the start of the Civil War he became the head of health policies on the nationalist side.

9 *Ibidem*, 1939.

10 *Rapport sur la mission sanitaire*, 1937, pp. 73-74

11 *Ibidem*, p. 86

was extremely hard and the experts predicted the dramatic worsening of the health and nutritional status of the population in this area. In fact, most of the research on the nutritional impairment of the Spanish population regards the dramatic situation of the capital exclusively.[12] However, historians have not taken into consideration the fact that feeding conditions in the principal cities of republican Spain were radically different, as well as access to food. The case of Madrid cannot be absolutely generalised, as unfortunately has been done by a significant part of historiography, simply because medical reports were slanted and focused on a city under siege. Food supplies became a problem affecting more than 1,200,000 inhabitants during the siege of Madrid. It worsened during the first months of the war, with more than 300,000 refugees.

The military front divided the country into two sides. The east was under Republican control and the rebels took the west and the north. The Republican zone produced wheat, rice, vegetables, fruit and wine. The area controlled by Franco's troops produced cereals but mainly for grazing.[13] The experts from the League of Nations predicted that the inhabitants of Madrid would go short of meat and milk. The supply of flour, olive oil, fruit, pulses, and vegetables was guaranteed if the republican authorities were able to defend the transport infrastructure. Although the shortage of milk and meat was alleviated by using other products, shipping difficulties meant serious problems in the distribution of food.[14]

From the second half of 1937 severe food problems hit the Spanish population, comparatively worse than the shortages in central Europe during the First World War.[15] Madrid saw a decrease in the caloric value of its diet as compared with the first winter of the war and this led to nutritional deficiencies and progressive malnutrition in the whole population.[16]

---

12 Del Cura, M.I. del, Huertas, R., *Alimentación y enfermedad en tiempos de hambre. España, 1937-1947*, Madrid, CSIC, 2007; Del Cura, I., Huertas, R., "The siege of Madrid (1937-1939). Nutritional and clinical studies during the Spanish civil war", *Food & History*, Vol. 6, 2008, pp. 193-214; Del Cura, I., Huertas, R., "Estudios nutricionales en Madrid durante la Guerra Civil espanyola", in Bernabeu-Mestre, J., Barona, J.L. (eds.), *Nutrición, salud y Sociedad. España y Europa en los siglos XIX-XX*, Valencia, SEC/PUV, 2011.

13 *Rapport sur la mission sanitaire*, 1937.

14 *Ibidem.*

15 *Ibidem.*

16 Grande Covián, F., *La alimentación en Madrid durante la Guerra. (Estudio de la dieta suministrada a la población civil madrileña durante diecinueve meses de*

The state of war changed the social and political dimension of food availability and nutrition, which now became a military tool. Following international recommendations, the Spanish Government established an *Instituto Nacional de Higiene de la Alimentación* [National Institute for Food Hygiene], where experts in physiology of nutrition aimed to coordinate nutritional policies both for the civil population and the military forces under the direction of José Puche, a Professor of Physiology, Rector of the University of Valencia and an expert on nutrition. The Spanish experts knew about the latest developments in nutrition physiology and the research work discussed and published by the technical committee of the League of Nations.[17] From January 1937 scientific criteria were used to implement a system on the basis of family or personal food rationing and special norms for the sick.[18]

At the beginning of 1937 Spanish health officers advised that the demand for basic products had almost been covered by domestic agricultural production. Nevertheless, in anticipation of future shortages, 120 tons of potatoes were imported from Holland. The main problem, however, was related to transport. In 1937 the food supply had not yet led to critical problems of hunger, deficiency diseases, or malnutrition, but experts expressed their concern: "If we consider the hundreds of thousands of women and children who live in Madrid, we can only conclude that it will be necessary to evacuate them as soon as possible… as food deficiency is a big threat".[19]

Nutrition had become central to the war. In mid-1939 the Technical Commission on Nutrition of the League of Nations presented a report of the work done between June 1938 and April 1939, including a section on the critical situation of the feeding of refugees in Spain and the need to take emergency measures to avoid starvation.

---

guerra: Agosto 1937 a Febrero 1939). Madrid, Publicación de la Revista de Sanidad e Higiene Pública, 1939.

17 The Technical Commission on Nutrition was presided in March 1937 by Edward Mellanby, and composed of 16 members. Teófilo Hernando, a Professor of Pharmacology in Madrid, Enrique Suñer, a Professor of Pediatry and José Murillo, director of the Spanish Institute for Food and Medicines were Spanish representatives.

18 Jiménez García, F., Grande Covián, F., "Sobre los trastornos carenciales observados en Madrid durante la Guerra. I. Los cuadros clínicos presentados con más frecuencia y su clasificación", *Revista Clínica Española*, Vol. 1, 1940a, pp. 313-318; Jiménez García, F., Grande Covián, F., "Algunas observaciones sobre las dietas consumidas por los enfermos carenciales de Madrid", *Revista Clínica Española*, Vol. 1, No. 1, 1940b.

19 *Rapport sur la mission sanitaire*, 1937, p. 89.

From November 1936, as a result of the siege of the city by rebel troops, a period of dietary restrictions started for the population of Madrid, worsening over time and finally affecting the majority of citizens. The City Council introduced a *Family supply card* and placed a ban on the free traffic of foodstuffs. As a consequence, most of the inhabitants were given the same ration for much of the war and Madrid's society was turned into a laboratory to analyse the effects of a prolonged lack of food, since the period of famine and scarcity lasted more than two years. A group of experts from the National Institute of Food Hygiene completed a study of the diet of Madrid's population during the 19-month siege, from August 1937 to February 1939.[20]

The average calorie value of the diets provided in the 19-month period came down to 1,060 calories a day, representing 49.7% of the minimum acceptable level. In the last year of the war the average was 944 calories or 43.3% of the minimum daily intake. The calorie value of the diet dropped steadily, from 1,514 daily calories in August 1937 to 852 in February 1939, a leap downward from 70% to 36% of the minimum diet. From an energy point of view, it was definitely a poor diet; besides, the main foodstuffs were bread, oil, rice, legumes and sugar, with animal products accounting for just 4.7% of the total calorie value. While the approximate protein need was estimated at 60 g per day, the average figure for the 19 months was 34 g, i.e. 56% per cent lower. In fact, the diet on the *Cartilla de Racionamiento* represented an average value of 25 g per day.[21]

The diet was deficient in fats (41% of the minimum diet) and carbohydrates (53 % of the minimum daily intake) but also in minerals and vitamins. Group A and C vitamins were below the minimum threshold, group B vitamins were highly deficient and only the good weather of the city made up for the shortage of vitamin D. All these records placed the population of Madrid in a more negative position than that of Germany in the First World War, whose calorie coefficient ranged between 1,400 and 1,800 calories per person per day. It is worth insisting on the exceptionality of the situation in Madrid, not at all equivalent to that of many other cities and rural areas, which certainly suffered from shortages.

In the study of deficiency diseases associated with malnutrition, the Spanish experts F. Jiménez and F. Grande Covián, who worked at the *Instituto Nacional de Higiene de la Alimentación* during the war, estimated the average caloric value of the diet of the Madrid population

---

20 Grande Covián, 1939.

21 *Ibidem*, pp. 45-46.

to be 2,130 calories daily before the conflict. In August 1937 that figure had been halved.[22] The feeding of the population reached a critical point in October 1938 when only 150 g of bread per person could be allocated and the daily diet of a great deal of people was limited to a cup of Malta coffee with or without sugar for breakfast, a plate of lentil soup with a little bread for lunch and some rice with a little bread for dinner. That type of diet only provided between 800 and 1,000 calories and caused a very significant loss in body weight. Surveys developed by nutritionists at the end of the war indicated that the average loss of weight of the population in Madrid as a result of deficiency diseases represented approximately 30% of their weight before the war.[23]

The Spanish group of experts began to detect simple, non-specific malnutrition signs and several deficiency diseases, which attracted the attention of physiologists, nutritionists and clinicians. There were neither reliable nor comprehensive statistics. Only data on mortality in the first year of the war were available, but they were inaccurate due to an inefficient system of recording epidemiological data. From the research published by nutritional experts we know that the main deficiency illnesses in Madrid were pellagra – the so-called *pellagra sine pellagra* – neuropathies associated with nutritional deficiencies, optic and acoustic neuritis, simple glossitis and hunger oedema.[24] Most of these conditions were associated with avitaminoses or with a deficiency of proteins. The situation worsened in the post-war period.[25]

In the early 1940s Jiménez García and Grande Covián published a series of research articles in the *Revista Clínica Española*, including plenty of records on the deficiency illnesses suffered by the inhabitants of Madrid during the war and the early post-war period.[26] Notwithstanding the dramatic nutritional status of the population, avitaminoses A, C and D were very infrequent, exceptionally causing

22 Jiménez García, Grande Covián, 1940a, 313-318; Jiménez García, Grande Covián, "Algunas observaciones sobre las dietas consumidas por los enfermos carenciales de Madrid", 1940b.

23 *Ibidem*.

24 For a broader analysis see Barona, 2010, pp. 105-118; Barona, Perdiguero, 2007, pp. 115-122; Huertas, R., Del Cura, I., "Deficiency Neuropathy in Wartime: The "Paraesthetic-Causalgic Syndrome" described by Manuel Peraita during the Spanish Civil War", *Journal of the History of the Neurosciences*, No. 19, 2010, 173-181; Del Cura, M.I. del, Huertas, R., *Alimentación y enfermedad en tiempos de hambre*, 2007.

25 García-Albea Ristol E., "Las neuropatías carenciales en Madrid durante la Guerra Civil", *Neurología*, Vol. 14, 1999, pp. 122-9.

26 This research has been partially analysed by Del Cura, Huertas García-Alejo, 2006, pp. 50-89; Barona, 2007b, pp. 31-34; Garcia-Albea Ristol, 1999, pp. 122-129.

haemeralopia, scurvy and rickets. In 1943 and 1944 deficiency illnesses similar to the ones described in Madrid began to appear in some European countries as a consequence of the Second World War.[27]

The situation of the Spanish population hardly improved in the first years after the conflict. In fact, in several ways, the nutritional status of the Spaniards worsened during the post-war period, as reflected in 1943 by Yves Biraud, an expert form the League of Nations, in his assessment of nutrition in Europe.[28]

Famine and Nutritional Deficiencies during World War II

Between 1942 and 1946 a series of studies devoted to assessing the negative effects of World War II on the nutritional situation of the European population were published. Some of them were direct contributions from the experts of the League of Nations.[29] John Lindberg played a main role as the coordinator of a number of surveys discussed in the Financial Section and Economic Intelligence Service of the League of Nations. When the third volume of the Lindberg reports went to press in 1946, the President of the United States, Herbert Hoover, had already warned in Chicago (May 17, 1946) that: "Hunger hangs over the homes of more than 800,000,000 people, over one third of the people of the earth". Consumption and rationing had a strong economic dimension and therefore several issues of the *World Economic Survey* published by economy experts of the League of Nations and FAO dealt with this matter.

---

27 Barona, 2007b.

28 Biraud, 1943-1944.

29 Bourne, G.H., *Starvation in Europe*, Allen & Unwin, London, 1943; FAO, *Standing advisory comité on nutrition. First report to the director-general. Nutrition Division*, Copenhague 23-31 August, 1946, FAO, Washington, 1946; *Food Rationing and Supply, 1943/44*, Geneva, League of Nations, 1942; [Lindberg, J.] *Wartime rationing and consumption*, Geneva, League of Nations Financial Section and Economic Intelligence Service, 1942; *Malnutrition and starvation in Western Netherlands, September 1944-July 1945*, The Hague, 1948; [Lindberg, J.] *Food rationing and supply 1942/43*, Geneva, League of Nations Financial Section and Economic Intelligence Service, 1943; [Lindberg, J.] *Food, Famine and Relief, 1940-1946*. Geneva, League of Nations Financial Section and Economic Intelligence Service, 1946; Muehel, W., "Ill effects of food restrictions in Europe, 1940-1944", *League of Nations Bulletin of the Health Organisation*, 1945-1946, Vol. 12; Orr, J.B., *The role of food in post-war reconstruction*, International Labour Organisation, Geneva, 1943; Puche Alvarez, J., "El hambre en Europa", *Ciencia (México)*, Vol. 1, 1940, 6 p.; *Rationement alimentaire et ravitaillement 1943-1944*, Société des Nations, Genève, 1944; Rosen, J., *Wartime food developments in Switzerland*, Stanford, Cal., Stanford University, 1947.

Shortly after the start of the international conflict, José Puche, the aforementioned Spanish physiologist, specialist in nutrition and head of the Spanish *Instituto de Higiene de la Alimentación* during the Civil War, wrote a survey about hunger in Europe and its influence on the evolution of the war. This was written just after he went into exile in Mexico.[30] In February 1939 the German Institute for Commercial Research had published data about self-sufficiency in the provision of food, but the records were immediately altered by the negative effects of the war. According to Puche's calculations, Germany and the invaded countries were to suffer strong shortages in wheat and corn, quantified as being between seven million and 8.5 million tonnes, reaching ten million tonnes if the deficit on rice were added and multiplied considering the lack of fertilizers, fuel and other goods. His forecast was for a strong shortage in many European countries such as Poland, Belgium, the Netherlands, France, Denmark, Norway, Spain, Austria, Italy, Czechoslovakia, Albany and Germany. He drew a very negative picture just as the World War broke out.

From the beginning of the conflict an evaluation of the nutritional problems in Europe was required, but a complete and accurate survey was not possible until some time after the end of the hostilities. But the health authorities and relief organisations needed some type of helpful information to be able to overcome the harsh wartime situation regarding both nutrition and epidemics. The League of Nations' Health Organisation made two principal reports public in 1943. One of them was published under the title "Health in Europe" by Yves M. Biraud, the Head of the Service of Epidemiological Intelligence and Public Health Statistics of the League of Nations.[31] The second one was a technical report on "Famine disease and its treatment in internment camps". Both painted an appalling picture of the health and nutritional situation in Europe in the early 1940s.

Biraud's report was preceded by a series of articles in the medical literature pointing out "the shortcomings of rationing, losses of weight of children and adults; increase in the incidence of certain communicable diseases; changes in the prevalence and character of tuberculosis; the increase in both infant and general death rates".[32] Notwithstanding the usefulness of those partial approaches, no comprehensive study had been published based on a large body of statistical records and therefore his aim was to furnish a first approach to

30 Puche Alvarez, 1940.

31 Biraud, 1943-1944.

32 *Ibidem*, p. 559.

a series of materials collected from many reports at the Service of Epidemiological Intelligence and Public Health Statistics of the League of Nations in Geneva. Biraud was aware of the limitations of those records: they did not adequately cover countries like Poland or Greece, which were suffering from severe nutritional deficiencies and famine in those days. The makeup and size of populations and cities in many European countries were deeply altered by conscription, refugee migration, deportation, attraction towards war industries and evacuation, thus making it difficult for any sort of epidemiological rates to be satisfactory.

But Biraud's memorandum was accurate enough to give a general picture of the dimensions of health impairment and nutritional problems in Europe in 1943. Divergence in the trends of general mortality in different countries, for instance, gave a measure of the influence of insufficient feeding. Although his main target was to report on the consequences of the war on the health situation, Biraud aimed to "give a measure of the influence of insufficient feeding".[33] To estimate the food situation in Europe, he made use of computations concerning the normal consumption of staple foods in European countries. These were based on documents issued by the Economic Intelligence Service of the League of Nations, including documents on wartime rationing and consumption, and a series of monographs published in 1939 for the European Conference on Rural life, which covered the agricultural situation in European countries. He also collected data on food restrictions, taken from the daily press, medical periodicals, private studies and reports from national health administrations and relief organisations, both official and private.[34]

Notwithstanding the methodological limitations caused by the exceptional circumstances of the war and the scarcity of reliable records, Biraud offered a convincing landscape of the nutritional situation in most European countries. According to his memorandum, food availability in Poland varied enormously depending on the location and social circumstances, ranging from practical sufficiency in some agricultural areas to acute shortages in cities and famine in ghettos. The effects on health were different: from mere deficiency diseases such as rickets to mass starvation. In 1943 relief efforts had been greatly reduced, due to the opposition of the German occupation forces, and they chiefly concentrated on children.

33 *Ibidem*, p. 561.

34 *Ibidem*, pp. 561-562.

In the Balkan area there were also considerable local differences in terms of the effects of the food shortage, which was something fairly general in the south west of the region. In the absence of reliable vital statistics, the situation for the USSR was no better, especially considering the negative effects of the German seizure of a large part of its most fertile agricultural land.[35] The situation of the besieged population of Leningrad was dramatic and millions of refugees had been evacuated from the war zone. According to Biraud, "[...] The hugeness of the food stores sent to the USSR under lend-lease agreements is an indication of the extent of the need".[36]

Special reference was made to the food shortage in post-war Spain: "Food shortage was severe during the civil war in a large part of the country, indeed acute for two winters in Madrid and among the large number of prisoners. The economic and social consequences of the civil war were prolonged and aggravated by the European war, so that in 1941 the serious nature of the nutritional situation of the country appeared to be second only to that of Greece".[37]

In the early 1940s actual famine and subsequent starvation hit many population groups across Europe: inmates in internment camps, prisoners of war camps, Jews in ghettos, civilians and soldiers of besieged cities, patients in hospitals and prisoners. A considerable loss of weight and deficiency diseases had been detected in great numbers of people in the cities of occupied countries, but the lack of food had been nowhere as intense and general on a nation-wide scale as it had been in Greece. Even in the peacetime period before the war, only a small portion of the staple foods needed to meet the population's dietary requirements were grown, according to official records.[38] Famine affected the towns first and then extended to the countryside. The situation became much worse in 1943-44 due to the negative effects of inflation. In addition, the limited relief supplies that were allowed to enter the country were insufficient and could hardly transform the extended famine condition into a situation of chronic and severe shortage.

In its milder but chronic form, food insufficiency was considered to have caused a definite increase in tuberculosis mortality and in the general mortality rates of several countries. It was the main cause of many deaths, but also an effective contributory cause in a much greater

35 *Ibidem*, p. 694.

36 *Ibidem*.

37 *Ibidem*.

38 *Ibidem*, p. 695.

number, particularly among elderly people and certain population groups living under exceptional circumstances.

As far as mortality is concerned, rates indicated that infants had been spared, generally speaking, although they suffered from many forms of non-fatal malnutrition, as many adults did. On the other hand, food shortage and malnutrition prevailed far more severely in cities than in rural areas, a fact that showed the capital importance of planning food relief. Prospects were uncertain for prompt and adequate relief which – if followed by rapid economic improvement – would result in a comparatively rapid physical rehabilitation of population groups suffering from malnutrition, with a quick fall in tuberculosis mortality rates. Experience gained in the aftermath of the First World War reinforced this perspective.

But the health situation at the end of World War II was not optimistic. Increased contacts due to community life and migrations resulted in a fairly marked rise in diphtheria, scarlet fever and meningitis in Central, Northern and Western Europe. A similar effect was caused by typhus fever in Eastern and South-Eastern Europe. Destitution in terms of lack of food, soap, home and body linen, had contributed to the increase in typhus fever in endemic areas and among prisoners and inmates of relief institutions. However, those epidemics did not influence the incidence or severity of traditional and other epidemic diseases at the end of the war. Typhus fever was probably a threat, since its prevalence in eastern and southeastern countries of Europe could be the origin of a breakdown that was eventually extended to other regions by troops coming from those areas, as well as from North Africa.

Biraud tried to fight exaggerated fears among the public and medical professionals regarding the spread of epidemic diseases during and after the war. The diseases with the heaviest toll in the past had been mostly controlled: typhus fever, smallpox, enteric fever and malaria. After the Great War rural populations in Russia had a low degree of acquired immunity to common infectious diseases and migration contributed to the spread of contagion and epidemics. According to this, the danger of dissemination of infection under the circumstances in 1945 was infinitely smaller than in 1919. The United Nations' Relief and Rehabilitation Administration had benefited from the pioneer work of the Inter-Allied Relief Committees in London, as well as that of national health administrations, to prepare plans for the repatriation of refugees and prisoners. National Red Cross Societies were also prepared for emergencies, and the collaborative commitment of health and statistical authorities from different countries with the Epidemiological Intelligence Service of the League of Nations was expected to tackle epidemic diseases and keep health administrations and relief organisations informed.

Food Rationing Systems during World War II

Food rationing policies were introduced in most European countries as an early measure, even before scarcity had time to develop. Rationing systems were designed to secure an equitable distribution of the available supplies of essential food to the entire population, regardless of their level of income. They were a strategy for preventing the waste of essential foodstuffs by means of the control of foreign exchange, shipping facilities and manpower. In addition, food rationing sought to supplement and reinforce measures of price control and production planning, something necessary for managing the economy of war. Without effective coordination between the various phases of social and economic policies, and more particularly between the availability of supplies, an organised system of distribution, and price control, food rationing could not have worked smoothly. In this case, thanks to the experience gained with the Great War and the Spanish Civil War, on the basis of the latest developments in the experimental science of nutrition, European governments were in general remarkably successful in managing their rationing policies, a central aspect of the political economy in war time.

Two main models of rationing were applied during World War II, conceived by the experts according to their suitability to the economic situation of the country involved. One was the *German-type*, also called *Continental*, and the other one the *Anglo-American-type*.[39] The German system represented an improvement on the rationing schemes that were applied during the Great War. This system was adopted all over the European continent with some particular modifications. It was conceived according to a supply situation that was more stringent than in the Anglo-Saxon countries. Food imports to Europe accounted for 10 per cent of the supplies before the world conflict, but due to the exceptional situation of the war period they were entirely cut off, whilst the production of domestic crops contracted to approximately 80 per cent of the normal standards by the end of the war.[40] Therefore, the problem in continental Europe was the capacity to satisfy the nutritional requirements of the whole population, the total food consumption, according to nutritional requirements. The solution of this challenge was sought by introducing a reduction in livestock, particularly pigs and

---

[39] [Lindberg, J.], 1942.

[40] [Lindberg, J.], 1946.

poultry, transferring to human consumption a greater part of the crops released from animal feeding. This policy resulted in a lower animal-vegetal ratio in the human diet, with a higher proportion of vegetable calories being consumed.

However, in considering the nutritive value of the diet, it was extremely important not to excessively reduce the proportion of animal proteins and calories, since some of them – such as milk for children – were deemed to be essential for health, to maintain organic defences, avoid undernourishment and secure the adequate organic development of infants and children. Indeed, economies of scale were required in the distribution not only of animal foodstuffs, but also of vegetable foods. Under the German or continental rationing system any important foodstuffs or groups of foodstuffs were particularly rationed in amounts per person, per day, per week or per month. Rationing was the system applied by nutritionists to guarantee both the quantity and quality of diets. It must be kept in mind that the logic of markets in times of scarcity tended to increase prices and produce maladjustments. As a counterbalance strategy, rationing tried to avoid foodstuffs becoming too expensive and diets too low in daily calorie intake.

A plurality of factors had to be considered in order to adjust rationing to the needs of the population groups. Physiological needs for food varied in a significant degree according to sex, age and occupation. Attempts were therefore made to make rationing differential in order to minimise inequalities. To do so, consumers were divided into several broad categories, each one receiving rations in proportion to previously calculated physiological needs. But the number of categories was limited for practical and administrative reasons, and the system did not fully eradicate inequalities, at least in terms of calorie needs. The system was considered to be "cumbersome, inelastic and altogether devoid – at least in theory – of a free consumer's choice".[41]

Experts were aware of the negative social attitudes towards rationing. Therefore, to be successful, rationing required a highly efficient administrative apparatus and also the support of public opinion. When those fundamentals were missing – and this applies especially to the procurement of food from farmers – an increasing proportion of the total food supplies were shifted to the more attractive and more lucrative black markets. The smaller and less popular the official rations, the greater the alternative paths. When they were accepted by public opinion, this was an incentive to use and supply black markets as a normal practice. Economists and public health experts associated the

[41] *Ibidem*, p. 2.

failure of rationing systems in guaranteeing an adequate diet with the spread of black markets.

The efficiency of rationing was directly proportional to the amount of calories that the rations afforded: the bigger the rations, the less important the black market. Qualitative or cultural elements (the prestige or bad reputation of certain foodstuffs associated with consumption by upper or lower social groups) were not taken into consideration. On the whole, rationing proved efficient throughout the war in Germany, Czechoslovakia, Denmark, Sweden and Switzerland, and also in the Netherlands for most of the time, but it was less successful in countries such as Belgium, France and Norway. On the contrary, in southern and eastern European countries, rationing collapsed altogether at the end of the war. Official records about actual consumption were hard to collect, since under conditions of extreme scarcity, as was the case with Greece in 1943, black-market supplies entered the scene.[42]

The situation was quite different in the United Kingdom, and rationing was never stopped during the war. Although access to overseas supplies was seriously threatened, rationing was chiefly introduced in order complement the scarce shipping space and foreign trade. The domestic output was directed towards the production of bulky or perishable foods, such as wheat, vegetables and milk, whilst food imports were primarily directed towards providing concentrated animal products, such as fats, meat and other dairy products. Throughout World War II no absolute limitation on the supply of total calories took place in Britain. The consumption of bread and most vegetables remained free, operating as a sort of *budget regulator* and permitting consumers to purchase as many calories and foodstuffs as they required if they could afford them. On the other hand, rationing was designed to distribute scarce foodstuffs, animal products, sugar and fats equitably.[43] It was devised so as to meet the average needs for all the main nutrients and it was considered that there was no need for differential calorie rationing (the Continental rationing style), with basic rations being based on an equal *per caput* allocation.

Some specific population groups required quality foodstuffs. This was taken into account by special distribution schemes, complementary but separate to the general rationing system. In this respect, reference must be made to special rations of milk and protective foods for children, nursing and pregnant women, to communal feeding and

42 For more detailed information, see the Appendix "Legal Food Rations by Countries, 1940-1945", [Lindberg, J.], 1946, pp. 121-159.

43 *Ibidem*, p. 3.

industrial canteens. Additional, non-essential rations were also supplied by the so-called *point-rationing* system. This method ensured a fairly wide consumer's choice between different commodities. Indeed, the Anglo-American system remained more flexible than the German or continental system throughout the war and, therefore, it was better adjusted to individual choices and family habits. On the whole, rationing was limited to animal foodstuffs, mainly to prevent the uneconomic expansion of animal farming products, while providing for a sufficient amount of export, lend-lease and military needs.[44] In the USA, the British system was adapted to a separate rationing of meat, fats and canned goods, with little restriction to consumer's choice.

Food Consumption Levels during the War

The surveys conducted by the Economic and Financial Department of the League of Nations indicate that an adequate consumption of foodstuffs – just as satisfactory in calories and quality as before the war – was maintained in the Americas, the British Dominions, the United Kingdom, Ireland, Denmark, Sweden and Switzerland until the end of the war. In other countries, such as Bulgaria, Rumania and Hungary, even the pre-war intake, though adequate calorie-wise, was of lower nutritional quality, and was maintained during most of the war. In the rest of Europe, critical local shortages were identified, mostly affecting urban areas and population groups that were too poor to access the black market. Even in those cases, farmers were little affected by food rationing and apparently managed to maintain their pre-war consumption level, except in areas directly exposed to warfare. But the critical situation of many rural areas in Europe in the years previous to World War II must not be overlooked: their marginality, famine, underdevelopment and exclusion, especially as a consequence of the economic crisis that hit the rural districts in the 1930s.

In Germany and the Protectorate of Bohemia and Moravia, calorie consumption in urban areas was slightly lower than before the war, but not much shorter than 3,000 calories per day and consumption unit. In Belgium, Finland, the Netherlands and Norway, rations varied from 2,300 to 2,800 calories per consumption unit a day approximately, although the intake per consumer was a bit lower, in some cases 20 per cent lower than before the war.[45] These figures did not point to a truly critical deficiency of calories, but local shortages became more severe at times.

44 *Ibidem*, p. 4

45 *Ibidem*.

A total of between 1,500 to 2,300 calories per consumption unit was the level found in the Baltic States, Slovakia, France and Italy, although the experts thought it convenient to include substantial additions coming from the black market, especially in France and Italy.[46] The situation was much more critical in other European countries. In Poland, Greece, and some areas of Yugoslavia and Albania, food distribution was not regular, and consumption fell for shorter or longer periods to levels of semi-starvation or outright famine.

Generally speaking, milk consumption in Europe was relatively well maintained during the war, but the proportion of most foodstuffs of animal origin, particularly meat and eggs, decreased; fats were scarce, whilst the consumption of vegetables increased both in absolute and relative terms. The nutritional composition of the diet, especially regarding vitamins and minerals, was not much worse than before the war, and in some exceptional cases it even improved. However, absolute deficiencies of specific nutrients became more frequent as the calorie intake dropped below safe levels, with malnutrition appearing as a consequence. Calorie rations in the Soviet Union were about 1,800 calories per head per day, a figure apparently similar to that in Germany, but the diet included almost no milk and dairy products, fats and eggs, and very little meat. Severe local, temporary shortages arose in the low-consumption areas in the Far East. Some parts of India suffered a famine in 1943, as well as several regions of China, and rations were reduced in Japan during the war, which led to a dramatic food situation at the end of the Pacific war.

The European feeding situation, food availability and the efficiency of the rationing policies varied enormously across countries and between social groups within the same country. Therefore, drawing general conclusions may involve a risk of misinterpretation and an oversimplification of a plural reality. While it was true that peasants, farmers and other country dwellers were less affected by nutritional problems, it must also be noted that living conditions and nutritional health were considerably worse in many rural areas of Europe than in the cities. The most evident critical food shortages arose mainly in urban areas, proportionally taking a greater part of the fall in national food supplies. The average level of food consumption depended on the size of the official rations, but also on the extent to which these rations were made available and on the purchasing power of incomes that could obtain additional food from other non-rationed sources, including the black market. All those factors were very difficult to assess by the

46 *Ibidem*, p. 5

experts, who estimated that contributions to food consumption from the black market generally exceeded deficiencies derived from low incomes and hindered access.

The urban populations suffered shortages in varying degrees in the different countries. The League of Nations reported that the calorie level was maintained at 3,000 calories as the daily consumption unit or slightly below in Denmark, Germany, Bulgaria, Czechoslovakia, Rumania and Hungary. This level was in general slightly lower than in the pre-war period, but it was not physiologically deficient. In Belgium, Finland, the Netherlands and Norway rations were lower than before the war, representing 2,300 to 2,800 calories per consumption unit a day, as much as 20 per cent below normal calculated requirements.

Severe partial shortages affected the lower income groups in urban populations, those who were too poor to patronise the black market. In the Baltic States, Slovakia, France and Italy, rations shrank, ranging from 1,500 to 2,300 calories, to which those obtained in the black market were added. "Where such additions were not forthcoming in any significant amount, however, the rations were too low to permit full working capacity and health".[47] In Poland, Greece, some parts of Yugoslavia and Albania, distribution was very irregular, and consumption levels fell for shorter or longer periods, even in agricultural regions, to levels of semi-starvation. In some regions and during certain periods, especially in Greece in 1942, famine prevailed.

There was an absence of official, statistically measurable calorie deficiencies, which does not imply that the diet was adequate and balanced in any respect. In wartime, the struggle to have access to foodstuffs and to obtain enough calories to prevent starvation sometimes overshadowed the composition of the diet, its balance and proportion of elements to maintain optimum health and the best efficiency. If we take into consideration not only calorie contribution, rationing diets in wartime did not satisfy the accepted standards of physiological requirements regarding a balanced composition and proportion of nutrients. Even in peacetime, balanced diets were the exception rather than the rule in many areas of Europe.

The official reports of the League of Nations identified fully adequate diets only in certain Scandinavian and North and Western regions. Considering the situation of the continent as a whole, it would appear that the deterioration in the balanced composition of the diet was less marked than what it was often assumed. The National Institutes of

47 *Ibidem*, p. 54.

Food and other similar agencies had been quite efficient in benefiting from the teachings of modern nutritional science and the experience of other countries circulated among experts, who were able to avoid the many mistakes made during the Great War.

In most of the countries that maintained their calorie intake, the composition of the diet was increasingly vegetarian. But since milk consumption was fairly well maintained, the nutritional efficiency of the diet was not impaired. However, the experts stressed the fact that, generally speaking, the diet was impoverished by the waning presence of fat, meat and eggs, and consequently a smaller variety of foodstuffs was available and palatability reduced. This gave rise to some discomfort among the population, but there was no evidence that the war-rationed diet had become much poorer in essential minerals and vitamins than before the war. Indeed, owing to the increase in the consumption of vegetables, the intake of these nutrients probably rose in some cases.

In the group of countries that reduced the calorie intake, the quality of the diet was not too different from the one previously mentioned, but as the number of calories available per consumer was lower, and distribution usually less uniform, a number of shortages were identified, not only in the amount of calories but also in that of proteins, minerals and vitamins. Regarding food shortages, a social division became evident, under-nutrition being on the whole limited to the poorer sections of the urban population.

Finally, in the third group of countries, mainly those in eastern and southern Europe, the problem with quality was almost completely subordinated to that of quantity. The diet was virtually composed of vegetables, and the calorie intake was so low that absolute deficiencies of almost all essential nutrients were common. In this case, deficiency was not only associated with calorie intake but to the poor composition and variety of the diet, which was a source of malnutrition, deficiency diseases and other clinical problems.

At the end of World War II, rationing records comparable to those discussed above were still unavailable in relation to the situation in the Soviet Union. It is well known that the German invasion resulted in a severe shortage of Russian crop production. Indeed, the occupied territories comprised some of the richest agricultural districts that usually supplied agriculture and farm products to the rest of the country. In addition, in 1941 and 1942 the country lost its best winter wheat-producing areas, its principal sugar beet regions, and much of its oil seed land.[48] It was estimated that, on a *per caput* basis, grains harvested in 1943 did not exceed 80 per cent of the normal pre-war production.[49] Such a deficit could not be overcome by a mere reduction in the grains used for animal feeding, in spite of a great reduction in livestock numbers, including: seven million horses out of a total 12 million in the invaded territory; 17 million cattle out of 34 million; 20 million hogs, 27 million sheep and goats, and 110 million head of poultry.[50] The situation severely affected diets, as it was estimated that normally at least 75 per cent of the calories for human consumption were derived from cereals. Neither pre-war stocks nor lend-lease imports were sufficient to make up for the deficiencies of home-produced supplies.[51]

The decrease in the supplies of crops and animal products in the free portion of the Soviet Union was in part compensated by potatoes and vegetable products, the supply of which, according to the information published in *Bolshevik*,[52] was larger than usual. Therefore, the majority of people survived chiefly on a diet based on black bread, boiled potatoes and cabbage.[53] The League of Nations reports stated that the system of distribution was less egalitarian in the Soviet Union than in most European countries. Rationing covered the staple foods and the rations were sold at fixed prices that were within reach of ordinary wage earners. In addition, there existed a legal free market in which privileged groups able to afford the high prices could benefit from their superior purchasing power in acquiring extra necessities and luxuries. Those food supplies in the open market were derived from the share received by collective farmers after the division of the harvest. Prices were 800 to 15,000 per cent above the ration prices.[54]

Ordinary rationed consumers were divided into four categories: manual workers, office workers, dependent adults and children under 13, receiving a different amount of bread, cereals, meat, potatoes, sugar, vegetables and cheese. According to the estimations, the calorie intake *per caput* was about 1,800 a day, being higher for workers and lower for children and dependent adults. Other calculations indicated 1,600 calories. Although these rations were apparently as high as in Germany

48 *World Food Situation*, Geneva, League of Nations, 1946, p. 103.

49 Farnsworth, H.C., Timoshenko, V.P., "The Food Situation in Soviet Russia, 1943/45", *World Grain Review and Outlook*, 1945.

50 *World Food Situation*, 1946.

51 [Lindberg, J.], 1946, p. 56.

52 *Bolshevik*, March, 1944, num. 5.

53 [Lindberg, J.], 1946, p. 56.

54 *Ibidem*, pp. 56-57.

for the same year, they were of an inferior nutritional quality, containing almost no milk, dairy products, fats and eggs, and insignificant amounts of meat.[55]

Throughout the war, the nutritional situation in the United Kingdom and in the neutral European countries was more favourable than in the rest of continental Europe and the Soviet Union. Greater availability and a more flexible supply were reflected in the rationing systems. In the United Kingdom, rationing emerged out of the necessity of husbanding shipping space for war imports and as a result of restrictions on the supply of foreign currency.[56] Nevertheless, the food supply remained adequate throughout the war and stable rations were ensured. The British rationing system had greater adaptability to individual needs; it maintained an unlimited total consumption of calories of vegetable origin, though some vegetables and fruit were scarce and other imported stuffs were almost unobtainable. But all consumers could buy as much bread and potatoes as they liked. Rationing was chiefly intended to maintain a balanced diet in nutrients and not just to guarantee a minimum calorie intake.

As it usually happens in times of war, the agricultural strategy focused on reducing the consumption of foods that required a lot of shipping, land and labour. The policy stimulated the home production of bulky foodstuffs, such as cereals, potatoes, vegetables and milk, using the shipping space for imports of concentrated foods, such as fats and meat. Indeed, milk consumption increased by about 28 per cent in 1943, compared with pre-war levels. Wheat-growing land rose by 82 per cent, and all cereal crops by 86 per cent. Potato crops increased by 116 per cent.[57] Rationing included protein foods, milk and fats. Since the need for quality foods varied less than for energy foods between different social groups, a uniform basic ration per head was adopted for meat, bacon, cheese, fats, sugar and jam. These rations, together with the free foods, were adequate to meet average physiological requirements. The introduction of whole bread and the supplement of margarine with vitamins A and D contributed to safeguarding the nutritional adequacy of the ordinary diet.

Obviously, this system did not satisfy all the requirements of groups with special needs and therefore several additional schemes of *communal feeding* were implemented. While in continental Europe workers engaged in heavy work received additional rations, Great

---

55 *Ibidem*, p. 57.

56 *Ibidem*.

57 *Ibidem*, p. 58.

Britain adopted the policy of supplementing useful additions out of the ration. Communal feeding adopted three main forms: industrial canteens in factories, mines and docks; school canteens for children; and *British restaurants* for the public. Industrial canteens were introduced early in the war. Employers of more than 250 workers and sometimes smaller ones were required to operate canteens, pooling resources together with other factories to operate a single canteen. School canteens also expanded during the war to supply school children with one well-balanced meal a day. The Board of Education paid between 70 and 95 per cent of the cost to local authorities. Sponsored by the Ministry of Food, and with the assistance of local authorities, the so-called *British restaurants* were initially conceived as an element of the emergency programme, but they became part of wartime living and by the end of the war more than 2,000 were in operation, serving about 600,000 meals a day on average.[58] The government encouraged their establishment in areas where there were many small factories without independent canteens. The canteens were classified in two categories, the first catering to heavy workers and the second to ordinary workers.

Preschool children, nursing and pregnant women did not generally benefit from the communal feeding schemes. These special groups demanded diets rich in first-class proteins, minerals and vitamins, and therefore they received a special rationing card that entitled them to extra quantities of protective foods, such as milk, eggs and fruit. Vitamins were also supplied for free or at a very low cost, and children under one year had a priority right to two pints of milk a day, while nursing and expectant mothers and two to five-year-old children received one pint a day. Milk was supplied free if the parents' income fell below a minimum. Schoolchildren received milk under the *milk-in-school* scheme inaugurated before the war.

A third measure called the *point-rationing scheme* was introduced in 1941, to distribute commodities whose supplies were too small to permit specific rationing. Each consumer received a card containing a set number of points and the commodities were priced not only in ordinary currency but also in points. This system allowed certain foods to be included, giving the consumer a much greater choice. Economic and financial calculations proved that such a rationing system would have been useless if part of the population had not possessed the income needed to purchase the legal rations. Certainly, the British system, and its aim of establishing a healthy minimum diet for all, required close coordination between price policy and social policy.

---

58 *Ibidem*, p. 59.

In addition to the previously mentioned initiatives, the Ministry of Food had almost monopolistic power over the distribution of all imported and most homegrown foodstuffs. It fixed the price of essential foods to the consumer based on social policy considerations. Prices were stabilised at low levels and the difference between the cost of production and the cost of import was contributed by the Treasury, sometimes from subsidies, sometimes from the profit made from the sale of other products. When the policy of price stabilisation was introduced at the beginning of the war, subsidies were already being paid at a rate of about 50 million pounds a year. At the end of March 1945 they were running at a yearly rate of 225 million.[59]

As a consequence of this social rationing scheme, the average consumption of milk, potatoes, vegetables and bread increased, while that of sugar, animal products other than milk, fats and imported fruit declined. Official figures indicated an estimated daily supply of 2,900 calories per caput per day, which was considered to be sufficient. Generally speaking, the nutritional level of the civilian population was deemed to be even better than before the war. The chief shortcoming of the nutritionally improved national wartime diet in Great Britain was monotony and the lack of palatability. But the general improvement in public health, even though the country was at war, testifies to the success of the British food distribution and rationing systems.[60]

Sweden was almost self-sufficient in food before the war, enjoying a high level of consumption, and did not suffer any serious food shortages during the war. Milk, potatoes, meat and fish were not rationed most of the time and they operated as budget regulators, permitting the population to satisfy their total needs for calories in a balanced manner. The proportion of animal and vegetable foods consumed did not really change. The foods rationed followed the German-Continental pattern, although a point-rationing system similar to the British one was intended to safeguard the consumer's free choice.

The situation in Switzerland was a bit tighter than in Sweden, as the country was more dependent upon imported food. Bread was rationed and only potatoes remained free. The rationing system was gradually rendered more and more flexible by the introduction of certain adaptations and modifications of the German model. In 1943 lower income groups could not always afford to buy the full ration of the more expensive foods. Consumers were given a choice between two rationing plans at different prices but with equally nutritive calculations. In

59 *Ibidem*, p. 61.

60 *Ibidem*, p. 63.

addition, coupons for certain foods could be legally substituted, at specific rates of exchange, for coupons of other food items. These modifications gave the Swiss rationing system with some flexibility, limiting a differentiation by consumer's category.[61]

Conditions in Ireland did not require rationing of more than a few imported foodstuffs, and in Portugal domestic food production before the war rendered the country 90 per cent self-sufficient in cereals and 100 per cent in fats. Figures remained like that until 1943, when serious droughts reduced crops and forced the country to ration bread. By the end of the war, consumption was about 95 per cent compared to what it was before the war, but inadequate administrative control caused city dwellers to suffer all the impact of a decreased supply.

Spain was almost self-sufficient in food before the Civil War, although the standards of consumption were slightly low. As a consequence of the war, technical reports showed that the situation had impaired drastically, the amount of area sown and productivity were decreased to such an extent that Spain became dependent upon the importation of staple foods. By the end of the war, the total supplies, according to the estimates of the Department of Agriculture of the United States, provided some 2,300 calories per person a day, as compared to 2,650 before the Civil War. The reduction was unequally distributed, heavily hitting the lower classes in cities. Their official rations – less than 1,200 calories per head – were not always available. But non-rationed food, such as meat, fruit and vegetables, and additions from the black market perhaps, permitted an urban consumption of about 2,000 calories, this being valid, obviously, for those groups that were able to purchase these relatively expensive foods.[62]

Starvation, Malnutrition and Experimental Research in the Camps

Internment camps worked as large detention centres to confine selected groups of the population. In Germany, the Nazi regime established concentration camps after reaching power in 1933, and during World War II camps increased in size and number in many areas of Europe. Inmates came from every occupied country and others were transported from different areas. Early in 1942 the *Wirtschafts-Verwaltungshauptamt*, the Central Office for Economy and Administration of the SS, took control of the camps, and inmates were

61 *Ibidem*, pp. 63-64.

62 *Ibidem*, p. 64.

frequently worked to death as forced labourers in industrial production. They were also used for medical experimentation.[63]

The German population grew rapidly in the 1920s and 1930s, as agricultural innovations led to increased food supplies, and medical progress together with better nutrition contributed to extending life expectancy and reducing mortality. During the Nazi rule, the German medical profession acted as an extension of the regime and the concept of *Rassenhygiene*, which was coined by Alfred Ploetz in 1895, became widespread with the new genetic theories, giving supposedly scientific support to the application of genetic laws and the natural selection of humans.

The *racial hygiene* programme was deployed once Hitler arrived in power on January 30, 1933. The *Deutsche Ärztevereinsbund* and the *Hartmannbund* were placed under the control of the *Reichärzteführer*.[64] Gerhardt Wagner was appointed to the post; he was already head of the Reich's Physicians Chamber, the Association of German Health Insurance Physicians, the Office of Public Health, the National Socialist Physician's League, the Office of Racial Policy, the Expert Committee for Public Health and the Office for Genealogical Research.[65] A significant portion of German physicians participated in the racial hygiene programme, with 45 per cent of professionals joining the Nazi Party and becoming accessories to Nazism even before they began assisting in the camps' experiments.[66] From the early days, the Nazis set in motion a programme of medical intervention, including compulsive sterilisation that was made legal through the "Law for the Prevention of Genetically Diseased Offspring" (July, 1933). An individual could be sterilised if a genetic health court determined that he or she suffered from what was considered to be a genetic illness, such as schizophrenia, manic-depressive psychosis, syphilis or alcoholism. In May 1934 the former Bureau of Education for Population Policy and Racial Hygiene became the Office of Racial Policy, charged with bringing all education and training on population and race matters into line with Nazi ideology. In 1934 a total of 181 genetic health courts were established in

63 Weindling, P., *Nazi Medicine and the Nuremberg Trials: From Medical War Crimes to Informed Consent*, New York, Palgrave Macmillan, 2004

64 Pasternak, A., *Inhuman Research. Medical Experiments in German Concentration Camps*, Budapest, HUN Akadémiai Kiadí, 2006, p. 16.

65 *Ibidem*, p. 16.

66 *Ibidem*, p. 17.

Germany, operating as part of the civil justice administration, composed of one lawyer and two doctors.[67]

> The results of the sterilisation programme reveal the degree to which physicians participated from the very beginning in Nazi programmes. An estimated 400,000 persons were sterilised, 95 per cent before the outbreak of World War II. The majority of these sterilisations were done by surgical means, vasectomies for men and tubal ligations for women. In some instances experimental means such as chemical injections or radiation were used. Persons chosen for sterilisation had the right to appeal but almost all appeals were rejected. The so called feebleminded were almost frequently targeted (42.5% of the total number of procedures).[68]

After 1939 the sterilisation practices slowed down, with the euthanasia programme becoming one of the new priorities. It was grounded on two main assumptions: first, that human beings were not biologically equal; and second, that this inequality relieved the State of the duty to protect all citizens equally, so that the weak could be simply abandoned or sacrificed. Assisted death could be justified on medical and legal grounds, and also on utilitarian ones, freeing state and society from the burdens associated with caring for the incurable, the mentally ill, the feebleminded, the retarded, and the deformed.

The idea that the state should place a greater value on the healthy than on the sick was commonly accepted. Although the euthanasia programme was to be clandestine, its implementation required extensive cooperation from medical professionals. Doctors and midwives were put under pressure to report degenerative diseases, contributing to this medicalised form of killing.[69] A Committee for the Scientific Treatment of Severe, Genetically Determined Illness started to administer an adult euthanasia programme in 1939. The war provided a smokescreen behind which the murders could take place. The euthanasia programme was named T4 and managed by a bureaucratic body consisting of 50 volunteer physicians headquartered in Berlin.[70]

> The Working Committee for Hospital Care was the name that appeared on letterhead for official correspondence; The Charitable Foundation for Institutional Care, or Central Clearinghouse for Mental Hospitals, handled fiscal affairs; and the Non-Profit Transport Corporation and the Common

67 *Ibidem*, p. 18.

68 *Ibidem*, pp. 18-19.

69 Lifton, R.J., *The Nazi Doctors. Medical killing and the psychology of genocide*, New York, Basic Books, 1986.

70 Pasternak, 2006, p. 23.

> Welfare Ambulance Service, Limited, moved patients from their care facilities to extermination centres.[71]

The programme involved most of the German psychiatric asylums, and questionnaires about the presence of *genetic disease* (schizophrenia, Down's syndrome, Huntington's chorea, and others) were sent to hospitals and homes for the chronically ill. Adults hospitalised for five or more years were checked as well. The first murders were carried out in Poland in January 1940, where 4,400 incurable mentally ill patients were shot.[72] Injection was initially envisioned as the preferred means but it was soon substituted by carbon monoxide administered in special tiled gas chambers designed to resemble a shower room, complemented by crematoria ovens for burning the bodies. Initially six hospitals were chosen and outfitted with special gas chambers and crematoria. By August 1941 a total of 70,273 individuals had been murdered. The extermination camps were the end point in a graduated series of institutions designed to serve the goals of the Nazi programme of racial hygiene. The system of prison camps, which included forced-labour camps, prisoner-of-war camps, transit camps, concentration camps and extermination camps, thus completed the work begun in the ghettos and mental institutions.

> One of the first concentration camps was Dachau, opened in 1933, just outside Munich. At first Dachau held only political opponents, such as Communists and Social Democrats, or those who had been sentenced in a court of law. But its population soon expanded to include Jews, homosexuals, Jehovah's Witnesses, Gypsies, clergy and others who were denounced for making negative comments about the regime. The other concentration camps filled quickly as well. Meanwhile, the conquest of the East was bringing ever greater numbers of Jews and other "undesirables" into the boundaries of an expanding Reich.[73]

As this sort of medicalised killing was accepted and extended, the Nazi Reich faced new strains. Six extermination camps were constructed in Poland: Auschwitz-Birkenau, Treblinka, Belzec, Sobibor, Majdanek and Chelmno, all being operational since 1942.

"On 12 August 1942 Himmler instructed Oswald Pohl, Director of the SS *Wirtschafts-Verwaltungshauptamp* (WVHA), to organize experiments on nutrition in the concentration camps. The goal was to identify the cheapest method of supplying the minimal nutrition needed

---

[71] *Ibidem*.

[72] *Ibidem*, p. 24.

[73] *Ibidem*, p. 28.

by active labourers in the camps".[74] Several diets, with and without nutritional supplements, were tested. The physician and chemist Ernst-Günther Schenck was appointed Nutrition Inspector and commissioned to assess the status of nutrition in the camps. Schenk spent the period of November 1942 to January 1943 visiting eight concentration and penal camps. He reported that the quality of food was good, including excellent vegetables, but that 20-30 per cent of the prisoners seemed, nevertheless, to be suffering from malnutrition.

Some dietary supplement, cheap and readily available was needed. Schenk suggested brewer's yeast, which could be provided without taxing the civilian food supply. However, the WVHA favoured the implementation of another supplement, a mold-infused egg white available under the trade name *Biosyn*. In 1943 *Biosyn* was incorporated into a vegetable sausage that resembled common *liverwurst* in smell and taste, and the product was sent to the camps for initial tests on 100 prisoners. The sausages were alleged to have come from the cellulose and paper factory in Lenz, but camp rumours said they were actually made out of sewage sludge. The undernourished experimental subjects suffered from intestinal problems after eating the sausages, and 70 to 80 per cent of them became seriously ill. These dire results did not stop Pohl from continuing the experiments. He actually expanded their scope for three months between January to March 1944, including 100,000 prisoners in Dachau, Buchenwald and Sachsenhausen.[75]

The results of these tests were among the reports presented in1944 at a conference held in Berlin, with the participation of experts in nutrition. The participants included the 1938 Nobel Prize winner for chemistry Richard Kuhn, Otto Flossner, Director of the Nutrition Physiology Department of the Reich's Health Department, and Wilhelm Nonnenbruch, Professor of Medicine, among others. The vote was unanimous in favour of continuing the experiments.[76]

Between December 1, 1943 and March 31, 1944, a series of experiments on nutrition were conducted in the Infirmary at Mathausen Concentration Camp. The objective of the experiments was to find the most beneficial form of nutrition for concentration camp inmates. For comparison purposes, three basic types of diet were established: type A, the so-called "eastern diet"; type B, a normal diet plus nutritive yeast; and type C, normal diet.

---

74 *Ibidem*, p. 230.

75 *Ibidem*, pp. 230- 231

76 *Ibidem*.

Type A or eastern diet consisted of vegetables and farinaceous food, served exclusively in the form of a thick soup without any meat or bread. Type B was the normal diet at the concentration camp, without any hard-labour rations but with an added 30 g of nutritive yeast per person, evenly mixed into the midday diet.[77] The majority of the prisoners sought out for experiments consisted of invalids, cripples and those over 55 years of age. Only 30 per cent were strong, young individuals. Weakness was a common characteristic, which made the prisoners more susceptible to different types of illnesses. They worked in the weaving mill, located near the infirmary block. Their work was done while seated most of the time and was in general less exhausting, and so their caloric need was much lower than that needed by those doing hard work.

The clinical and laboratory experiments conducted in conjunction with nutrition tests were expected to give a picture of the influence of the respective forms of diet on the human body, especially on haematopoiesis or blood cell production, and on the circulatory and excretory systems. The experiments were also expected to cover the pathological changes that occurred. In addition, they were also expected to differentiate between the changes that could be attributed to the diet and those that were associated with pathogenic causes. Nevertheless, many practical difficulties arose: the emergence of acute enterocolitis and oedema, both affecting the weight curve in a different way. Other problems were related to haematological analysis, furunculosis and infections influencing the blood leukocyte formula.

The tests were conducted during three periods. The nutrition experiments started on December 1, 1943 and completely ended on May 31, 1944. Further comparative experiments were performed until July 31, 1944, at which time a normal diet was prescribed to all prisoners. The numbers initially selected for the experiments were:[78] group A, eastern diet, supplied to 150 prisoners; group B, normal diet plus yeast, supplied to 110 prisoners, and group C, normal diet, supplied to 110 prisoners. The total amount of inmates involved in the experiment was 370 prisoners.

By the end of the experimentation period – July 31, 1944 – the death toll came to 116 (31.35 per cent), the causes of death being diagnosed as follows:

---

77 *Ibidem.*

78 *Ibidem.*

Colitis 62
Myodegeneratio cordis...................... 19
Tuberculosis 12
Pneumonia.. 8
Cachexia universalis 3
Septicopyaemia 2
Erysipelas 2
Phlegmona gangrenosa...................... 2
Exudative pleurisy 1
Glomerulonephritis 1
Uremia.. 1
Septicaemia 1
Epidemic meningitis 1
Hepatic carcinoma............................ 1

The percentages of survivors were:
67% in group B
54% in group A
48% in group C

Through the clinical examinations and the hematologic, electrocardiographic and clinical evidence obtained while conducting the experiments, it was concluded that the most suitable diet was the normal diet plus yeast, and the most unsuitable the normal diet given to all prisoners in the concentration camps.

In general, the nutritional situation of inmates in internment camps during the war was a descent to hell. A report about the health condition of inmates in those institutions was published in the *League of Nations Bulletin of the Health Organisation* in 1944.[79] The memorandum was received for publication in August 1943 and showed the clinical research completed over one year. According to the figures in the memorandum, internment camps investigated in the south of France harboured some 20,000 adolescents and adult internees in 1943. The published report focused on medical aspects related to the state of health of the confined population, excluding any reference to living conditions, human rights or internal rules that could incriminate authorities. The research was published as an *anonymous* report. The work done was justified for the scientific interest and experimental value of the observations, and the practical application of the results in communities suffering from famine. The names of the doctors participating in the research were suppressed, as well as those of the internees and any geographical references of the camps.

---

[79] "Famine Disease and its Treatment in Internment Camps", *League of Nations Bulletin of the Health Organisation*, Vol. 10, 1943-1944, pp. 722-772

Between 1940 and 1943 the internment camps received a big influx of inmates, the number and composition of whom were variable. Internees showed amazing physical and moral resilience to the very negative health and nutritional conditions to which they were submitted. The situation changed completely 12 to 16 months after the internment of about 20,000 inmates. A first outbreak of famine disease had already occurred in spring 1941, but famine invaded the camps from August 1942 onwards.

The death rate continually increased, revealing, after a period of resistance, the deep exhaustion and extreme physiological destitution of the weakened organisms of the inmates. Men appeared to be much less resistant than women, teenagers and children. Private relief organisations drew up a plan of action, which found strong obstacles to its implementation, but was finally deployed with the help of large relief organisations and the goodwill of administrative authorities in the camps.

The plan comprised five main aspects: the examination of all internees from the point of view of their state of health and nutrition in order to spot inmates suffering from famine disease; the hospitalisation of famine patients in special huts for observation and treatment; the establishment of special dietetic kitchens under the joint responsibility of the relief organisations; emergency medical treatment consisting of dietetic products, vitamins, minerals and tonics, and segregation of threatened patients in a centre for prophylactic treatment separate from the camp. This medical relief intervention started in February 1942.

Internment camps became a large laboratory for clinical research on malnutrition and physical exhaustion under extreme circumstances. The medical programme included the screening all inmates in order to select those patients showing nutritional deficiency syndrome. A clinical and therapeutic study of the sick hospitalised in the quarters for cachectic patients followed. The food situation was analysed, all activities of the relief organisations coordinated, doctors gave medical instructions to be followed and finally a critical examination of the results took place.

In the course of a preliminary examination, all internees were weighed and measured, their pulse-rate and blood pressure recorded, as well as the main facts of their personal medical history. Patients were submitted to a simple medical examination and the results recorded on individual cards. A classification of the examined persons took place according to the following data: weight in relation to height; condition of the skin and subcutaneous tissue; muscular tone; station; cardiovascular system; oedema; and blood counts. Patients were divided into three main categories: cachectic, pre-cachectic and threatened.

Special infirmaries called cachectic quarters received those patients who suffered from extreme skeleton-like emaciation.

Many adults of medium height only weighed about 40 kg. Their physical condition was extremely impaired: dry skin, subicteric pallor, signs of cyanosis or haemolytic process and anaemia. Pre-cachectic patients displayed the same symptoms but to a lesser degree, and their general condition was not so seriously damaged. Threatened cases were in better shape, with a tendency to show symptoms of hunger oedema, some emaciation and weakness. Most of these patients were convalescing from typhoid fever, gastric or duodenal ulcer, tuberculosis and chronic uncompensated cardiac disease. Based on the quantitative results for a camp with a population of about 11,000 internees, of whom 9,000 were examined, 331 were classified as cachectic, 839 as pre-cachectic and about 4,000 were under the label of threatened cases.

"These proportions, however, were not static. *Famine disease*, which developed like a virulent epidemic, constantly progressed in the camps. Every week systematic investigation discovered new pre-cachectic and threatened cases, as though the virulence of the pathogenic agent were far from spent".[80] From the first results of the screening work, it appeared that more than half the inmates were threatened by symptoms of famine disease. This research on camp inmates allowed the definition of clinical forms of famine:

> *Humid famine*: the principal form being hunger oedema.
>
> *Dry famine:* characterised by the absence of oedema; it was most common among Spaniards and Italians, showing dry and scaly skin.
>
> *Anaemic famine:* blood examination and neurological symptoms "of considerable pathogenic and therapeutic interest".
>
> *Circulatory famine:* unstable blood pressure, hypotension, bradycardia showing heart suffering.
>
> *Neurological famine:* ataxia, paresthesia, polyneuritis symptoms, mixture of Parkinsonian and ataxic symptoms.
>
> *Mental famine:* patients showed a "fixed, lifeless and apathetic gaze", confusion, prostration and extreme weakness.

The famine categories found in internment camps, with their physical and physiological symptoms, were carefully detailed in the published report. The determination of these clinical categories

80 *Ibidem*, p. 730.

contributed to medical knowledge; they were also useful for prognosis and for the orientation of the treatment.

The genesis and evolution of the physical and mental impairment associated with the famine syndrome were followed carefully after the arrival of new internees in a normal state of nourishment. Those inmates were abruptly subjected to the camp fare. The deterioration of the general food supply and the growing destitution of the internees led to the appearance of the first symptoms of malnutrition at the end of 1942 "after a certain time-lag". Careful clinical observation of the internees revealed that once signs of nutritional deficiency appeared they followed each other in a particular order. During the first three months of a deficient dietary, a heavy loss of weight took place, from eight to 15 kg per month. After that initial period the weight loss would decrease gradually from month to month. A gradual disappearance of the fatty tissue was observed and inguinal hernia was frequent. A general feeling of fatigue followed, accompanied by irritability and a change of the bodily complexion, which turned straw-coloured, lemon-yellow, or white; dry skin and fugitive oedema in the mornings, sometimes lasting for about ten minutes.

The headaches appeared later, sometimes accompanied by mental disorders, depression or excitement, excited reflexes, static disturbances and amenorrhea in women. Finally, giddiness and ankle-cramps appeared, oedema became permanent, showing a tendency to generalisation, and cardiac arrhythmia appeared. At this point impairment was so deep and global that if actions were not immediately taken, the outcome of famine disease was inevitably death. Malnutrition was not the only cause; restrictions on freedom of movement, the cold weather, unfavourable hygienic conditions, moral depression, in other words, the appalling living conditions could "only hasten this fatal development".[81]

The medical research programme did not finish with the death of the patient; it also included a careful and detailed observation of the conditions under which the death had happened, something considered by the medical experts "very instructive from the pathogenic point of view". The permanent impairment of physiological conditions finally led to a state of coma, which was followed after a more or less short interval, by death. Sometimes, patients were suddenly struck down and collapsed while walking, sometimes they died in their sleep.

---

[81] *Ibidem*, p. 735.

Some patients passed away slowly, showing signs of progressive asthenia, or died from pre-existing or inter-current diseases. An autopsy was performed, which did not usually reveal anything macroscopically relevant, "apart from the occasional presence of cerebral oedema".[82]

The medical research programme was developed in two internment camps; mortality in January and February 1942 was:

	January	February
Internment camp holding 400 people	45	49
Internment camp holding 2,800 people	59	38

Internment camps were equipped with technology to carry out clinical exploration: fluoroscopic examination, X-ray screening and blood analysis were applied to almost all of the inmates. Cases of pulmonary tuberculosis were detected, as well as cardiovascular disturbances such as heart enlargement and broncho-vascular inflammation, and the bones were extremely decalcified and demineralised, all such observations being typical of a deficiency condition. Clinical and X-ray screening detected endocrine disorders. Hyperthyroidism cases were rare but goitre was frequent; puberty was delayed in girls and a great deal of women over 15 and under 45 had amenorrhea. Adrenal alterations led to hypotension, hypoglycaemia and asthenia. Men suffered from alterations of spermatogenesis. Dysfunctions of the genital endocrine glands suggested pituitary disturbances. On the contrary, diabetic patients seemed to benefit from a deficient diet, as well as rheumatic and metabolic diseases.

Considered by medical researchers as an epidemic situation, the evolutionary curve showed, in a first phase, a progressive increase in morbidity, "consequent upon contamination, till it reaches a high level or a peak, and then falls again when a sufficiently large proportion of the population has acquired immunity, or when active measures effectively prevent the spread of the disease".[83] When the medical research was brought to an end, famine disease had not yet reached its peak in the camps. Every week the screening of the patients revealed new pre-cachectic and threatened cases, for the causes of the famine were far from disappearing.

---

82 *Ibidem*, p. 736.

83 *Ibidem*, p. 738.

The gender divide showed important features. Compared with men, women were affected after a time lag of ten months. Keeping this fact in mind, the increasing number of women affected by the deficiency syndrome in July 1942 was a clear expression of the general impairment of the overall situation. The medical experts did not take into consideration any external or social aspects such as the intensity of physical work, which could contribute to explaining this situation. On the contrary, they argued that "[…] the fact that the calorie requirements of women are 20% lower than those of men, and the slowing-up of metabolism due to amenorrhea, explain in part why they have been more resistant to famine than men. It appears that in the end their resistance broke down in its turn, and that the prognosis in the case of women became less favourable than it had previously been".[84]

On the other hand, climate conditions seemed to have a strong influence over evolution and survival. The chances of saving a patient were greater during milder seasons than in wintertime. The cold weather had a weakening influence because calorie losses and existing vascular and nervous disorders were aggravated. Patients who died in winter did so as much from the cold as from famine. On the contrary, a warm temperature had positive effects over oedema. The medical report found that those patients suffering from neurological and mental forms of famine had the most negative prognosis, as well as the appearance of abundant diarrhoea, which is a cause of dehydration, demineralisation and bad assimilation of nutrients and vitamins.

Some signs indicated a fatal prognosis. The inability of patients to stand on their feet for a few minutes was most serious. Medical experts found it indispensable to prescribe strict and complete rest if those patients were to be protected from sudden death. Also, pronounced atrophy and extreme emaciation accompanied cachexia, and, a as a general rule, patients already suffering from other diseases got worse due to famine.

The medical research experts responded to famine disease as if it were not a social problem provoked by living conditions at the internment camps but a sort of epidemic with a purely medical and scientific perspective. The possibilities of cure depended upon age, the season of the year, the early establishment of treatment and the extent of the therapeutic action undertaken. They were explicit; "[…] an incurable condition (apart from terminal coma) does not exist. Notwithstanding a remarkable loss of weight, profound asthenia and a very serious general condition, it was found possible, through *persevering an energetic*

[84] *Ibidem*, p. 739.

treatment, to save individuals considered to be irrevocably lost".[85] With treatment being based on a substantial diet rich in fats and proteins and on hypertonic injections of glucose, the medical research found that patients who had been considered hopeless cases were saved. They had been suffering from generalised oedema, ascites, pleural effusion, myocarditis, hemorrhagic purpura and losing as much as 55% of their physiological weight. Segregation of severe cases was considered to be an indispensable therapeutic factor, especially for those suffering from mental disorders.

One of the experimental targets of the research project was to assess the exact role played by vitamin deficiency in famine disease. However, the exact participation of it in clinical signs and physical deterioration was impossible to ascertain. Obviously, the experts discovered the consequences of a deficient calorie intake easily – emaciation, loss of weight and disappearance of fat – but clinical examination did not enable them to assess specific signs resulting from the lack of any definite vitamin. "Moreover, the vitamin requirements of the human body can vary and be subject at the same time to individual factors and to endogenous influences, which govern the absorption and utilisation of the vitamins consumed".[86] They talked about clinical symptoms related to vitamins C, D, A, nicotinamide and decalcification.

Indeed, it was obvious that the appalling physical condition of the internees was due to the inadequacy of their diet, both from the viewpoint of quantity and quality. A simple comparison between the indispensable elements of a normal diet and the one served to the inmates of the camps provided blatant conclusions. Famine disease was considered the consequence of a chronic quantitative and qualitative deficiency in the diet.[87]

The experts calculated that about 15 to 20% of the theoretical energy value of nutrients in the diet was in reality lost, and therefore the actual value of the daily ration per person was not 1,188 calories but around 950 calories a day on average. As we analysed in previous chapters, in 1942 a great deal of experimental and clinical research on nutrition had established solid patterns regarding the necessary intake of calories for health. In addition, numerous technical reports and articles were available about the consequences of shortages and malnutrition during the Great War, from 1914 to 1918. The situation was considered to be

85 *Ibidem*, p. 740.

86 *Ibidem*, p. 741.

87 More details about the daily rations in Barona, 2010, pp. 130 passim.

critical when the daily protein intake fell to 40-50 g per day, the fats intake to 20-30 g, and the daily calorie value between 1,400 and 1,800.

The daily protein ration in the internment camps was no more than 30 to 40 g of foodstuffs that were almost exclusively of vegetal origin and the fats intake was 8 to 10 g a day, which in no case allowed the protein balance to be maintained. When the protein ration and the calorie intake fell simultaneously below the physiological minimum, it was not only the nitrogen balance that was disrupted; the elimination of proteins was also abnormally increased. Cachexia cannot be overcome, even by giving large amounts of fats and carbohydrates, and the weight cannot rise if the minimum requirement of proteins is not supplied. Instead of one gramme of protein per kilo of body weight, defined as necessary by nutritionists, the diet only provided 48 g of vegetal protein. A continual nitrogen deficit followed, which, even though it amounted to only 9 g a day, represented for these internees 3,300 g of protein in the course of a year, a serious impairment of the muscles and other organs being the consequence. The same vegetables were served for weeks on end. Besides, they were badly cooked and inadequately stored for too long. A significant number of inmates suffered from intestinal disorders, and defective absorption was yet another factor of vitamin deficiency, even though the intake was adequate.

Medical researchers then made a comparison with the food situation of a large industrial town near the camps, in collaboration with the Nutrition Section of the Regional Hygiene Institute. Quantitative data for February 1941 showed that the average for different social groups was 1,737 calories for adults and 1,565 calories for teenagers. The lowest figures accepted by physiologists were 1,600 calories for male adults, 1,400 for women and 1,400 for adolescents. At the end of 1941 figures were similar: for the least favoured group, 1,764 calories per male adult, 1,509 per female adult and 1,614 per teenager.

Based on these figures, the experts compared the food situation in the town to that of other German towns in 1917. As for the food situation in the camps, the ration average was not unlike that in Madrid towards the end of the siege, during the civil war, when the ration was 852 calories (it was 1,514 calories at the beginning of the siege).[88] From the comparative study, medical experts concluded that the ration supplied to the internees in the camps was 40% to 50% lower than that of the civilian population of the nearby industrial town, which was itself seriously affected by a food shortage. They predicted that the *epidemic of famine disease* would persist in the camps and that the efforts of the

[88] "Famine Disease", 1943-1944, p. 750; Grande Covián, 1939, p. 22.

organisations to combat the situation by supplying additional nourishment and intensive drug therapy would remain ineffective under the existing conditions. It was urgent to raise the ration in all the camps to the level of the civilian population.

Relief organisations made considerable efforts by sending supplementary foodstuffs to the camps but, according to the medical report, failure was due to the insufficient food rations given to the internees. When the relief organisations discovered that famine disease was spreading in the internment camps, they intensified their efforts; several kitchens were installed especially designed to feed cachectic patients, who received a daily ration of between 2,200 to 2,500 calories, with an appreciable improvement in the quality. Relief organisations sought to procure a nourishing diet, scientifically calculated and adapted to patients in a state of advanced cachexia. On the other hand, to stop the *famine epidemic*, they supplied an ever-growing number of *threatened* patients with food supplements in the form of pea or rice soups, pasta, pearl barley or dried or fresh fruit, accounting for 250 to 400 calories.

> It is impossible in the present study to give an adequate idea of the immense effort exerted by the organisations engaged in relief work, the flexibility of their action and the spirit of cooperation animating them. Some inkling of it may be given by the fact that in less than a week there were numerous developments: the kitchens were installed; a detailed card-index was prepared and kept up-to-date containing the follow-up observations concerning patients cared for by each organisation; most of the necessary foodstuffs were purchased in the Balkans, Turkey, Portugal and Spain, and others were dispatched from the two Americas; storehouses were built; and a great deal of work was done in connection with the handling and storing of the supplies. When we add that, in addition to these material arrangements, many necessary negotiations were undertaken with the authorities on behalf of the internees either in general or in individual cases, a fair idea is given of the impressive work carried out jointly on behalf of the internees by a dozen international and national relief organisations.[89]

The work of the organisations covered between 65 and 70% of the internees in the camp. In June 1942 a total of 1,958 rations a day were distributed among 2,750 inmates in one large camp. Specific actions were taken in the maternity section, where the weight of the newborn infants shifted from an average of 2.1 to 2.5 kg in 1941, and from 2.9 to 3.1 kg in 1942 and 1943. No infant mortality rates appeared in the medical report.

---

[89] "Famine Disease", 1943-1944, p. 753.

Some sort of drug therapy was also implemented, depending on the various clinical forms of famine. Patients suffering from *dry famine* were supplemented with tonics, drugs containing amino-acids, stimulants, vitamins and phosphorus-containing products. In those affected by *humid famine*, diuretics were added to the above, and for patients suffering *neurological and mental famine*, brewers' yeast, glucose and aneurin were added. In cases of anaemia, iron extracts and vitamins were administered. The effects of a wide range of drugs was evaluated: brewers' yeast, calcium, glucose, iron, insulin, coramin, vitamins A, B, C, D and E, nicotinamide, hepatogastric extract, wheat germ, ortedrin, pervitin, and sulphonamides. The medical treatment was accompanied by rest, and there was segregation for permanent care and systematic supervision in the case of cachectic and pre-cachectic patients.

According to the evaluation of the medical experts, dietary and drug treatment had completely changed the appearance and condition of the patients. There was a rapid decline in mortality once relief had been well organised. During the last two weeks of April 1942 an increase in weight was recorded in 32 out of 100 cachectic patients in one camp, 20 patients remained in a stable condition, there was weight loss owing to a decrease in fluid (oedema) in 40 cases, and a real loss of weight in eight patients. In the first two weeks of May the number of cachectic patients who gained weight was 60.4%. But after the medical programme of intervention and the two months of therapeutic experience, the cachectic and pre-cachectic patients who returned to everyday life at the camp relapsed because they were still exposed to the same pathogenic factor: famine. According to the experts working on the relief programme:

> The inadequacy and the irregularities of the rations effectively supplied to the inmates by the administrative authorities of the camps made it definitely impossible to save them. Those who were saved from the consequences of famine, at the cost of great effort on the part of the relief organisations in supplying supplements of food, would thus still have a suspended sentence of death, unless the camp authorities supplied them with a more or less adequate basic ration, this basic ratio remaining the prime factor in the problem of saving famine-disease patients. When all is said and done, the obligation to solve this problem rested with the authorities responsible for the internment of the inmates of the camps.[90]

At the end of the medical report, a postscript was added. The changes in the military and political situation in Europe, characterised by the advance of allied troops and the consequent Nazi retreat, enabled

---

[90] *Ibidem*, p. 761.

the humanitarian experts' group to lift the veil of anonymity, giving some information about the camps. The "Health Commission" of the "Co-ordination Committee for Relief in Camps" consisted of: Rene Zimmer, representing the Unitarian Service Committee of the United States; Maurice Dubois, member of the Swiss Red Cross and Children's Relief (*Secours aux Infants*); and Joseph Weill, of the O.S.E. Union (Jewish health organisation). The camps in which the observations were recorded were situated in the south of France and, more particularly, in the Eastern Pyrenees. They were set up in 1939 and 1940, first of all to accommodate Spanish refugees, under the name of *Centres d'hebergement*, and then, during the first part of the world war, to receive "enemy aliens". From July 1940 these camps were mainly filled with Jews of various nationalities. During the second half of 1942 tens of thousands of them were deportees from camps in Poland. The camps designated by the letters "G" and "R" in the medical report were those at Gurs and Rivesaltes. The town and its food rations have been indicated for purposes of comparison with those of camps in Marseille. The charitable organisations that took part in the provision of relief for the internees were: *Aide aux Emigrés*, the Swiss section of the International Migration Service, Geneva; The Confederation of Swiss Jewish Communities; The Joint Relief Committee of the International Red Cross; The Ecumenical Council, Geneva; The *O.S.E. Union* (Jewish Health organisation), Geneva; *Schweizerischer Aerzte verein* (Swiss medical union), Zurich; *Secours Suisse aux enfants*, Geneva; The Society of Friends, United States; The Swiss Red Cross; and The Unitarian Service Committee, United States. Consignments of medicines were supplied free of charge by the following manufacturers of pharmaceutical products in Basle: C. Boehringer & Co., C.I.B.A., Geigy; and Sandoz.[91]

Following the pattern of internment camps and the excellent conditions they offered to investigate the effects of malnutrition on human health, at the beginning of 1945 the American physiologist Ancel Keys, head of the Laboratory for Physiological Hygiene at Minnesota University, initiated a series of experiments on starvation with a group of volunteers.[92] The experiments were implemented by a research group headed by Keys and composed of doctors Henry Longstreet Taylor, Josef Brozek, Austin Henschel and Harold Guetzkow. As a previous

91 *Ibidem*, p. 772.

92 The general results were published some time later: Keys, A. *et al.*, *The biology of human starvation*, Minneapolis, 1950; Tucker, T., *The Great Starvation Experiment: Ancel Keys and the Men Who Starved for Science*, Minneapolis, University of Minnesota Press, 2007.

stage, researchers travelled around the country in order to choose a significant group of volunteers for the human research experiment on nutrition deprivation. They interviewed a long series of volunteers, performed a medical examination and asked the men about their health, taking as a key factor their psychological balance. They also reviewed the Selective Service health record of each candidate. Men whose weight varied greatly from the norm were dismissed, as well as husbands. Keys considered that married life interfered with the maintenance of control conditions in the experiment.

Main requirements were enjoying good physical and mental health, measured according to a clinical tool: the Minnesota Multiphasic Personality Inventory (MMPI), published in 1943. Keys' goal was to analyse scientifically the effects of prolonged hunger on the impairment of health and bodily functions. He originally wanted 40 men in the study, but could only select 36 volunteers who met the minimum requirements. The loss of a man would represent an almost three per cent loss in the study's total data, something which would also reduce the statistical reliability of every test ran because of the small sample size. J. Brozek acted as the psychotherapist. Volunteers received extensive information about the experiment: they were instructed about body functions, changes to be expected both in organic and psychological aspects, patterns of behaviour, living conditions and the organisation and length of the research programme. Under difficult circumstances, the participants took frequent advantage of the rule that allowed them black coffee and water in unlimited quantities, an opportunity to put something in their mouths and stomachs.

They were submitted to frequent and systematic medical exploration. Increasing the intake of water resulted in polyuria of transparent colourless urine per day, as coffee and water consumption soared. If patients experienced any exceptional or unexpected changes, they were to inform the research team. Obviously, as the time went on, the reactions among the guinea pig group were plural. One of the participants waited weeks before telling any of the scientists that his urine appeared to be changing colour. As the days passed, his urine darkened and he was eventually obliged to report the problem to the staff: he was actually urinating blood. Keys wrote that the problem was "of obscure aetiology". It was the 18th week of starvation and Keys was forced to drop another man from the experiment. The affected man stayed to help in the kitchen until the end of the experiment. Like other guinea pigs, within a few days of normal meals, all symptoms, mental and physical, disappeared, but Keys thought the blood in urine somehow represented a personal failure, not a direct result from starvation.[93]

During the experiment, body temperatures decreased from the normal 98.6°F to an average of 95.8°F and in one of the more striking changes, the average heart rate slowed from an average of 55 beats per minute in control to 35 beats per minute, the bodies trying to conserve every calorie. The lowest recorded pulse rate was a startling 28 beats per minute. Participants saw their weight loss begin to stabilise around the 20th week of starvation. Unlike a couple of them, their stalled weight losses were entirely explicable and did not put them under suspicion of cheating. A few of them were suffering from oedema. Keys considered this the chief *stigmata* of starvation.[94] Oedema was caused by retained water and occurred chiefly in the ankles and knees, but also in the face; some cases adopted extreme forms.

While oedema had traditionally been linked to famine, the causes were obscure, as it was a conspicuous symptom of starvation. Keys devoted a chapter to oedema in his final study, where he analysed different explanations. One theory considered it as a cause of increased pressure inside the capillary vessels, pushing fluid from the blood vessels into the interstitial space between cells. Another explanation attributed it to increased permeability in the capillaries. Oedema complicated weight calculations due to the water retention.

In the 20th week of the experiment, on June 22, 1945, the guinea pigs received the visit of a young army sergeant, whose testimony translated the starvation experiment to the German concentration camps.

> I was captured in December during the Jerry breakthrough in Belgium. I weighed 190 pounds when they captured us. I was fat, friends! Anyway, the first thing the Krauts did was take our boots and our socks – I do not know if this was to keep us from escaping, or because they needed the boots and socks. Probably both. Then they marched us for four days in just our galoshes. That was entirely without food. Finally, they gave us a loaf of bread for every four men. I wanted to save a little piece of mine for later, but I couldn't. I ate all of my share right then and there. Then they loaded us into boxcars, and we took another four-day trip locked up like cattle. At the end of that, we hiked three miles up a mountain to Bad Orb Prison Camp. There we got our first hot meal- a bowl of grass soup. Most days after that, a smudge of margarine, and some kind of tea. That was it. I was there a hundred days and lost fifty pounds. So, I guess the reason I'm telling you all this is that I also used to hide food under my pillow and stare at pictures of

[93] Tucker, 2007, p. 132.

[94] *Ibidem*, p. 140.

> bread like they were pinups of Betty Grable – I recognize your deviant behaviour. So how about it – are you fellows ready to eat? You'll have to forgive my table manners, though. I've been a guest of the Nazis – the bastards.[95]

On July 20, 1945, the final week of starvation, a military visitor and Army major visited Keys' Laboratory of physiological hygiene. He was Marvin Corlette, a doctor who had seen first-hand the starving victims of the Nazi concentration camps. He was also the chief of the Civilian Nutrition Branch of the Army's Medical Corps, owing all the credentials and the experience to rigorously evaluate the starvation experiment.

> Keys showed Major Corlette the barracks… and their array of testing equipment. Corlette was more eager to get to the men. Keys watched from across the room as the major talked to them, took notes, and examined their swollen ankles. Key's wasn't about to ask this young major his opinion, but he listened closely to the major's questions and comments in an attempt to discern his frame of mind. Did he think that Keys had accurately recreated concentration camp-style famine? Or did he think the whole experiment was a circus, a dangerous, indulgent exercise in scientific showmanship? Major Corlette was civil and cheerful, but he left the laboratory without sharing his conclusions.[96]

Keys got a letter from the major dated August 18, summarising his visit to the lab. After describing the clinical symptoms of the guinea pig group he concluded: "Except for the absence of filth and secondary skin infections in the experimental subjects, it appears that the fundamental clinical pattern of partial starvation as we observed in Europe has been duplicated".[97]

A specific aspect of the experiment was the assessment of the influence of hunger on sensorial perception. Hungry people were said to be more sensitive, but Keys found it difficult to believe that hunger really improved hearing and sight; he therefore devised a series of laboratory tests to examine sensorial perception and reactions. The most meaningful results were those regarding hearing improvement by a full standard deviation that apparently demonstrated that hunger sharpened hearing. On the other hand, the intellectual capacity of the men in the study was largely unaffected by hunger.

July 28, 1945, had been announced from the beginning of the experiment as the last day of the starvation phase:

---

95 *Ibidem*, pp. 141-143.

96 *Ibidem*, pp. 144-145.

97 *Ibidem*, p. 145.

The thirty-two men who made it to the rehabilitation phase were in many ways different than the men who had shown up at Memorial Stadium in November of 1944. They were smaller – they had dropped from an average of 152.7 pounds to 115.6 pounds, an average weight loss of 24.29 per cent. They were shorter too – the average man had lost about a third of a centimetre in height. Their total blood volume had been reduced by almost 500 cubic centimetres. The heart that pumped that blood had shrink by 17 per cent. More significant, and more difficult for Keys to measure, their world had shrunk. The men had come to Minnesota to be part of a global mission to help all of humanity. Now they didn't care about starving refugees… Now their world consisted only of the South Tower of Memorial Stadium and the food line at Shevlin Hall.[98]

[98] *Ibidem*, p. 161.

CHAPTER 6

The Post-war Food Crisis and the Impairment of Health Conditions

While the war was still in progress, political and military authorities believed that once hostilities ceased, trade would recover previous standards, food would flow abundantly from the surplus countries to the deficit areas and food habits would soon revert to a normal situation. However, their expectations were not fulfilled and, as backed by historical experience, the aftermath of war is often almost as difficult as war itself. World War II proved not to be an exception. The food situation worsened markedly over wide areas towards the end of the war and subsequently continued to deteriorate at an accelerated pace until, in the spring of 1946, famine conditions prevailed in several parts of Europe. The post-war food crisis cannot be fully understood without some reference to the wider aspects of the food problem, since its intensity was due in part to adverse natural factors such as droughts, and to the upheavals of the closing phases of the war, but fundamentally it reflected the dangerous unbalance of world agriculture and food trade systems.[1]

Even before the war, the international organisations had had great difficulty in compiling reliable statistics on world food production, basic estimates usually being simple approximations subject to a margin of error. The accuracy of the records did not improve during the war and in many countries the disorganisation of the civil administration rendered reliable statistics almost impossible. Especially in those countries where food shortages and inflation were most critical, farmers and producers had perfected the devices of withholding supplies from their governments. In addition, in competing for the scant post-war supplies, deficit countries tended to exaggerate the hard domestic situation of their crops and their capacity for food production.[2]

1 [Lindberg, J.], 1946

2 *Ibidem*, p. 72.

According to the estimates of a report by the United States Department of Agriculture,[3] the calorie value of the world food production had declined at the beginning of 1946 by about five per cent of the global average just before the war. The American experts expressed that if allowance were made for population increase, the *per caput* production would have declined by about 12 per cent during the war. The decrease was unevenly distributed across the world. Data suggested a similar production or even a slight increase in food production in Asia, Australia, South Africa and New Zealand, and an approximate 20 per cent decrease in continental Europe and North Africa, contrasting with a striking increase in the British Islands, which normally, however, produce only about one per cent of the world's total. North America was the only major producing area that showed a significant increase, accounting for about 30 per cent compared with pre-war figures.

To gain an insight into the seriousness of the food shortage confronting the world in 1946, the amount of production and also the many difficult problems of national and international distribution must be considered. Under those circumstances, it would have been necessary to increase the supply of cereals for human consumption to maintain the calorie intake, by reducing livestock numbers, not only in Europe, where a substantial reduction was in fact brought about during the war, but also in the other parts of the world. From the experts' point of view, wheat and rice were truly the "stuff of life" of mankind. As regards wheat, practically the whole exportable surplus came from the four chief exporters: the United States, Canada, Australia and Argentina. Production in these countries averaged about 40 million tons for the period 1935-39, versus a little more than 46 million tons in 1945-46. The pre-war production of rice amounted to about 200 million tons, of which about 96 per cent was grown in Asia, and the crop in 1945-46 fell to about 168 million tons, 15 per cent below pre-war levels due to disorganisation that was a consequence of the war. India and China suffered from droughts and great deficits were noted in Japan and former Japan-occupied areas.[4]

However, most of the countries that produced a surplus of cereals increased the feeding of them to their livestock population, in some cases substantially increasing their number during the war. When the war came to an end, most of these countries liberalised or abolished

3 *World Food Situation 1946*, Washington, US Department of Agriculture, February, 1946.

4 [Lindberg, J.], 1946, p. 74.

rationing. As a result, it proved impossible for important food exporting countries to meet more than a part of the import requirements of deficit areas. Although it was impossible to obtain exact estimates of export surplus and import requirements, and absolute quantities that depended on variable circumstances such as the standard of consumption adopted, international experts' boards estimated a world deficit of nine to 10 million tons, especially considering that wheat demands rose as a consequence of the fall in the Asiatic rice crop. Exportable supplies amounted to less than 60 per cent of the stated requirements.

In 1946 a report of the Economic and Financial Department of the League of Nations pointed out the following:

> In spite of belated efforts to meet these requirements, it is, at the moment of writing, clear that famine cannot altogether be averted. The Emergency Committee for Europe has estimated that approximately 100 million people in Europe will receive less than 1,500 calories a day, and of these many, particularly in Germany, Austria and Hungary, are already receiving 1,000 or less. In India, the cereal crop is short by about 8 million tons, and a large part of the city population is existing on rations of 1,000 calories a day or less. With recent allocation of wheat it is possible that further widespread deterioration will be avoided. In China, acute local famines are reported, but transport obstacles make adequate relief extremely difficult. In Japan, as well, famine conditions will develop unless large imports materialize.[5]

The serious sharpening of the food crisis at the beginning of 1946 was partly due to unforeseeable circumstances and partly to overconsumption in the first half of the crop year based on optimistic prospects. The war had left behind a serious disequilibrium between supply and demand, which could have been overcome only by a strict application of an economy of food controls, something dropped by most countries wishing to go back to *normality* after the war. Crops were by and large divided between human and animal consumption. However, a number of crop calories were used to feed animals and only a part of them was returned in the form of animal foodstuffs fit for human consumption. Hence, when total crops decreased, human consumption could be maintained within certain limits by diverting feed grain from animals to humans. In that case, a reduction in livestock was needed and a more vegetarian diet implemented. In many Asian countries, but also in eastern and southern European countries, during the post-war period, the diet was completely vegetarian and the deficit could not be made up for other than through increased imports. While consumption levels

5 *Ibidem*, p. 6.

were barely maintained or declined in Eastern Europe, Germany and Italy, food consumption increased in Western Europe.

On the other hand, international food relief to the liberated areas had been severely hit by the food crisis. The Fourth session of the UNRRA Council (Atlantic City, March 1946) recommended that where livestock numbers had been drastically reduced efforts should be made to rehabilitate livestock herds, in spite of shortages of human food. A series of recommendations were passed, such as: the elimination of any avoidable food waste; the diversion of maximum quantities of grain to direct human consumption and the consequent reduction in livestock numbers; the raising of the rates of extraction in the milling of cereals; and the diversion of fats from industrial use to food use. In addition, the experts in nutrition recommended more efficiency in the procurement of foods from farmers and a continuation of rationing policies as a positive way to regulate food production and distribution, regulating prices and consumption. According to John Lindberg's report for the League of Nations, such measures were feasible in the surplus areas, but they were not likely to yield appreciable results in the deficit regions, where waste was rare, inflation rampant and the administration structure not efficient in the managing of the situation.[6]

Farmers demanded an increasing supply of consumers' goods as an inducement to part with their food. In the spring of 1946 the rate of extraction in the milling of cereals had been generally increased to levels similar to those prevailing during the war, or even higher. Sweden, in addition to food exports of about 400,000 tons between 1944-46, had voluntarily given up import contracts for about 100,000 tons of wheat and rye. But it was in the United Kingdom, the greatest importer of food in the world, that the conservation policy had been most energetically pursued. Controls of food production and distribution continued after the war and in some cases rations were lowered. Moreover, import requirements were scaled down, with a reduction of nearly 30 per cent. From the summer of 1945 the United Kingdom exported 80,000 tons of cereals to continental Europe, drastically reducing the bulk stocks held by the Ministry of Food.[7] A nation-wide campaign to save still non-rationed bread and the milling extraction rates was implemented, and feed rations to animals stood at a sixth of the pre-war average levels.

In France, bread was once again rationed in January 1946, and the extraction rate of cereals was raised to 90 per cent. According to experts

6 *Ibidem*, p. 77.

7 *Ibidem*.

on the political economy of food, the deciding factor in the world food balance was rather to be found in the surplus countries, particularly in the United States, and their capacity to fulfill their export commitments, let alone surpass them. Except for Argentina, most surplus countries had introduced the rationing of animal food produce during the war, which resulted in the evaluation of the expansion of animal production. After the war, when the world's heavy needs for wheat and quality foods had become apparent, the eating by animals of the scarce cereal supplies continued at an accelerated rate. Rationing of food, except sugar, was rapidly lifted in the USA, and the consumption of animal food continued above wartime levels. At the beginning of 1946 it had become evident that the rate of grain consumption by livestock would render it almost impossible for the USA to meet its export commitments.[8] In order to achieve the goals, a Famine Emergency Committee was created, under the Chairmanship of former President Hoover, to plan and implement the steps to reduce domestic food consumption. In other supply countries, such as Canada and Australia, measures to prevent the expansion of domestic consumption of animal products were to be taken too. The Canadian government introduced food saving campaigns as well as meat rationing in October 1945.

Globally considered, the situation in the surplus countries in 1946 was very pessimistic with regard to their commitments on food production and exports. The situation was so serious that is was virtually impossible to make a forecast of the coming crops. There was no reason or evidence to believe that the productivity of European agriculture was going to recover and increase rapidly. "The disorganization of transport and administration and the lack of fertilizers, machinery and draught power are cumulative in effect".[9] A serious crop failure, in the absence of any reserve stocks, would have been catastrophic and, to prevent this threat, the experts recommended conservation measures.

From May 20 to 27, 1946, an international conference called by the United Nations Food and Agriculture Organization met in Washington DC to discuss global measures to tackle the most urgent food problems. The emergency programme for food conservation was based on the following recommendations: 1) Raising the extraction of wheat flour to a minimum of 85 per cent where lower rates were applied; 2) Stretching the supply of wheat flour by at least five per cent admixture of flour from other grains or from potatoes; 3) Limiting the use of grain for

8 United States Department of Agriculture, Production and Marketing Administration Press Release, March 16th, 1946.

9 [Lindberg, J.], 1946, p. 80.

alcoholic beverages and "other non essential purposes"; 4) Maximum diversion of grain and potatoes from feed use to human consumption, while giving priority to milk herds and draught animals in whatever feeding of coarse grains that may be necessary; 5) Reduction of grain-absorbing and quality-meat production; 6) Reduction of food waste; 7) Reduction of Government stocks of food; 8) Taking steps to render it possible to put direct rationing of bread into effect at short notice, whenever this proved to be necessary. The Conference also recommended the setting up of an international research and information service to survey and report quarterly on the world food situation. It also proposed the creation of the International Emergency Food Council to carry on the work of the Combined Food Board, to be initially composed of representatives of those 20 nations with a presence on the Board.

Levels of Food Consumption in 1946

The Emergency Economic Committee for Europe advanced the first estimations on the impact of the shortage at the end of the war.[10] Its reports showed, on the one hand, *normal consumer* rations in December 1945 and, on the other, weighted average rations of all consumer groups, plus estimated additions from non-rationed sources. It attempted to show the total diet of non-farmers, as well as the predicted average diet of non-farm consumers, offering a range of countries ordered by their levels of consumption.

Just after the war a first group of countries made up of Denmark, the United Kingdom, Sweden and Switzerland had a level of calorie consumption that was not significantly below their high pre-wartime averages. Notwithstanding the changes in the composition of their diets during the war, there was no reason to assume that the real nutritional situation of the population was much inferior to that of the pre-war diets. The Committee stressed that, owing to a more equitable distribution of the available supplies, the lower social groups of the population were better nourished than before.

A second group of countries that included Belgium, France, Luxemburg, the Netherlands, Norway and Czechoslovakia had an average consumption that amounted to about 2,500 calories per head in the autumn of 1945.[11] A net allowance of this order would equal more than 3,000 calories per consumption unit, since an efficient system of

---

[10] Emergency Economic Committee for Europe, *The Winter Food Position in Europe*. Report by the Sub-Committee on Food and Agriculture, London, 1946.

[11] This estimation was made by the United States Department of Agriculture.

distribution could achieve an equitable sharing of available resources. In France, farmers were consuming more or less at a normal rate, while the city population was much less well off. The normal consumer in Paris had rations worth 1,400 to 1,500 calories, to which free foods and eventual black market purchases were added.[12]

The same variation in consumption was observed in Bohemia and Moravia, provinces of Czechoslovakia, where farmers' consumption was similar to that of the pre-war years, while the urban population consumed about 1,840 calories per day in February 1946. The differences between the urban and rural diets were less evident in Belgium, the Netherlands and Norway, where at the end of 1945 average consumption was about 2,500 calories per day. While the composition of the diet had deteriorated as a consequence of the war, particularly regarding animal foodstuffs, the levels were considered acceptable to maintain health and efficiency. When serious shortages occurred, the international reports attributed them to the result of inefficient distribution rather than to overall supply shortages.[13] Some cutbacks were inevitable, although a truly critical situation was not expected in these countries, with the possible exception of Czechoslovakia and urban France.

A third group of countries including Greece, Finland, Portugal and Spain hovered, at the end of 1945, on the critical level between just enough and starvation. The average consumption of the total population was rather less than 2,000 calories a day. Consumption among the non-farm population in Greece was down to about 1,700 calories a day in January 1946 and depended upon UNRRA assistance. The normal consumer ration was down to little more than 1,100 calories, something indicative of the critical position of the urban population where extra food was not obtained from the black market. In Spain, owing to the lingering effects of the Civil War, the disorganisation of transport and the lack of fertilisers, and owing, in addition, to drought in 1945, food production remained at a low level, perhaps 70 per cent of the average for the period 1931-35. The low rations were irregularly available and the prospects were not optimistic. The situation in Portugal was probably less precarious, but the maintenance of rations depended upon imports.[14]

The situation in the Balkans and the countries of Eastern Europe was more difficult to assess, being, by all indications, exceedingly serious,

12 [Lindberg, J.], 1946, p. 83.

13 *Ibidem*, p. 85.

14 *Ibidem*, p. 86.

and starvation or semi-starvation a common threat. The Danubian countries were normally food-surplus areas and production was relatively well maintained in the war years, but was drastically reduced in 1945. As these countries were predominantly agricultural, the reduction in the total supply affected the city populations heavily. In Bulgaria, the situation was critical and the level of consumption less than 1,500 calories a day. In Romania, the official ration supplied 600 calories only and there was a threat that official food stocks would run out by the spring of 1946. In Hungary, starvation appeared to be common and runaway inflation complicated the problem of food procurement and distribution. The city food rations amounted to no more than 500 to 1,000 calories a day. In Poland, domestic supplies allowed a ration of some 1,300 calories a day for the urban population. Shortages were so serious that urban populations in certain areas and social groups were dependent upon UNRRA help and other imports for additions.

No information was available in 1946 for the Baltic States and the Soviet Union. In the latter, grain exports in 1946 suggested an improvement in the food crisis: official rations were more filling, sugar and bread rations for children increased and prices in the free market were reduced.[15]

The German situation was exceptional because Germany was occupied in 1946 in four zones. In the occupation zones of the Allies, domestic supplies were estimated to be sufficient for an average consumption of 1,500 calories and 1,100 for the non-farm population at the end of 1945.

> Until November 1945 normal consumer rations in all occupation zones remained below the 1,500 calorie level, which the Combined Nutrition Committee (composed of experts from the United States, the United Kingdom and France) considered insufficient for the maintenance of health for more than a short period. The rations were highest (1,550 in December 1945) in the British zone, followed by the American zone (1,500 calories). The rations (not always honoured) were considerably lower in the French and Russian zones, where distribution also was rendered more uneven by transport and storage difficulties. The normal consumer rations varied between 800 and 1,200 calories a day.[16]

The situation in Austria was also critical, although it was difficult to obtain a picture of the general conditions in the country. In autumn 1945 normal consumer rations amounted to 800 calories in the Soviet zone,

---

15 *Ibidem*, p. 87.

16 *Ibidem*, pp. 87-88.

1,490 in the American, 1,425 in the British and 1,445 in the French. For the countryside, non-farm consumption, including black market additions, was estimated to be less than 1,800 calories a person, a level only possible to maintain with large imports. From 1946 the situation deteriorated and rations in Vienna were no higher than 800 calories. The total non-farm consumption in Italy at the beginning of 1946 was less than 1,550 calories a day on average, and "normal consumer" rations supplied 820 calories a day, depending largely on imports of wheat.

The Emergency Economic Committee for Europe summarised the situation in January 1946: "After taking into account all home-grown and imported food supplies available or in sight, 140 million people will have to continue to live on a diet which provides an average of less than 1,500 calories.[17] The remaining 40 million may be expected to receive 1,500/2,000 calories.[18] These estimates excluded Albania, Turkey and the Soviet Union".[19]

Diets between 2,000 and 2,500 calories were recommended for the non-farmers in Belgium, Bulgaria, the Netherlands, Norway and some parts of Yugoslavia, amounting to some 21 million people. Average diets above 2,500 calories were available to non-farmers in Sweden, the United Kingdom, Denmark and Switzerland. About 150 million Europeans were threatened with famine or semi-starvation, not far from 40 per cent of Europe's population of just over 400 million, excluding the Soviet Union. The situation was hard to handle, politically and economically untenable, and a source of social conflict.

Post-war Food Relief

In August 1940 Prime Minister Churchill promised in a speech in the House of Commons that "after the defeat of the enemy" Europe would receive food and relief from abroad. A few months later Great Britain set up a Committee of Surpluses with the purpose of acquiring stocks of relief goods. As early as September 1941 an Inter-Allied Committee on Post-War Requirements was set up in London. In the following year and a half, the Committee compiled detailed schedules of the post-war import requirements of the occupied areas in Europe. Also in 1941 a

17 The non-farm populations of Austria, Eastern Slovakia, Finland, Germany, Hungary, Italy, Romania, and possibly Spain. Further, the farm population in the tobacco-growing districts of Bulgaria, and German residents in Czechoslovakia.

18 The non-farm populations of France, Bohemia, Moravia and Western Slovakia, Greece, and certain districts of Yugoslavia. A bare 2000 calorie diet may be in store for non-farmers in Luxembourg and possibly Portugal.

19 [Lindberg, J.], 1946, p. 88.

Middle East Relief and Refugee Administration with headquarters in Cairo was set up in order to care for the Polish and Greek refugees who had escaped from the Germans. As we know, their activities were later taken over by the UNRRA. Meanwhile, various interdepartmental committees in the United States had been actively studying post-war needs and, after Pearl Harbour, all these activities were centralised in a special Office of Foreign Relief and Rehabilitation Operations under the Department of State. Operations were carried out in 1943 in Tunisia, where feeding programmes were launched, refugee camps established and health services provided.

But as a consequence of the invasion of Europe, the need for large-scale international action and coordinated efforts became more apparent and necessary. After consultations between the American and British governments, the aforementioned institutions presented a draft agreement for a Relief Organisation to the United Nations. The proposal was adopted by representatives of 44 states from United and Associated Nations of the UN on November 9, 1943, in favour of the creation of a United Nations Relief and Rehabilitation Administration (UNRRA). Its member states were later increased to 48. The purposes of the new organisation were broad and sweeping, as stated in Article 1 of the Foundational Agreement:

> (a) To plan, coordinate, administer or arrange for the administration of measures for the relief of victims of war in any area under the control of any of the United Nations through the provision of food, fuel, clothing, shelter and other basic necessities, medical and other essential services; and to facilitate in such areas, so far as necessary to the adequate provision of relief, the production and transportation of these articles and the furnishing of these services.
>
> (b) To formulate and recommend measures for individual or joint action by... member governments... for the purpose of achieving an equitable distribution of available supplies.
>
> (c) To study, formulate and recommend... measures with respect to such related matters... as may be proposed by any of the member governments...[20]

The UNRRA Council, which was made up of one representative of each member state, was the central policy-determining body. Decisions were made by a simple majority vote. A Central Committee composed of representatives of the USA, the United Kingdom, the USSR and China made policy decisions of an emergency nature between sessions,

---

[20] *Ibidem*, p. 92.

although they were subject to reconsideration by the full Council. Two Regional Committees were created, one for Europe and another for the Far East, made up of representatives of the member governments in each area. They were competent to make recommendations to the Council for their own area. A number of technical committees advised the Council on specific questions, such as supply, agriculture, displaced persons and health. A Director General was the executive authority responsible for the carrying out of the directives given by the Council. Headquarters were established in Washington DC and the European Regional Office was located in London.

In the years between its creation and 1946 numerous regional offices and country missions had been established, comprising a staff of almost 17,000 officials. A great number of the staff were involved in relief work, with the activities supposed to finish at the end of 1946 in Europe.[21] The UNRRA was financed by the governments of its member countries and initial contributions fixed in Atlantic City totalled approximately one per cent of the national income for the year ending June 30, 1943. In August 1945 the Council recommended a second contribution from each such country on the same basis, the total funds of the organisation being estimated to reach 3.77 billion U.S. dollars.[22]

In practical terms, large as these sums were, they proved small when compared with the enormous needs, and therefore assistance, that had to be arranged in a highly selective way. Relief was limited to such liberated areas that lacked the foreign exchange needed to pay for their own imports. Only health and welfare services could be provided to all liberated areas under the authority of the Director General. Indeed, the UNRRA's activities came to be restricted to a relatively small group of liberated countries, with limited relief programmes authorised later for some ex-enemy countries, notably Italy, Austria and Finland.[23] Requirements were determined in practice on the basis of estimates submitted by claimant governments. The regional committees for Europe and the Far East first determined the needs of different commodities for their own geographic area and, since national relief budgets began to emerge, funds could be translated into real programmes of operation, eliminating less urgent requirements and placing increasing emphasis on food.

---

21 *Ibidem*, p. 93.

22 *Ibidem*.

23 *Ibidem*.

The estimated quantities and value of supplies by main groups shipped by the UNRRA from all sources to liberated areas up to the end of 1945:

	Total	Food	Clothing, textiles, footwear	Agricultural rehabilitation goods	Industrial rehabilitation goods	Medical and sanitation goods
Tonnage shipped (1000s)	3,959	2,663	188	346	738	25
Value (1000s US Dollar)	681,553	316,777	173,325	46,505	116,073	28,873

Source: [John Lindberg], *Food, Famine and Relief*, p. 94.

An *ad hoc* Sub-Committee for Europe drew up the theoretical scales of nutritional relief requirements for Europe after the war. This Committee met on May 5, 1944, under the chairmanship of Karl Evang, a Norwegian physician who was active in the Norwegian Support Committee for Spain. It also included representatives from Australia, Belgium, Brazil, Czechoslovakia, the French Committee of National Liberation, Greece, Iceland, Luxembourg, the Netherlands, Norway, Poland, the United Kingdom, the USA, the USSR and Yugoslavia.[24] The standards considered were declared to be in the nature of "minimum requirements, which, if possible, should be introduced as soon as territories have been liberated". As a general basis for determining such minimum requirements, the Committee recommended "the use of an average level of consumption of the total population of each of the countries concerned of 2,650 calories per head per day for essential relief needs for the period under consideration".[25]

Regarding the composition of the diet, the experts' commission included sufficient amounts of milk and eggs for special groups of the population: pregnant and nursing women, children aged up to seven and sick individuals. All in all, the average diet had to contain a daily allowance of 75 g of fat and 60 g of protein, of which about half was of animal origin. The committee looked forward to excluding bread from rationing policies in liberated areas as soon as possible. Although these scales were lower than the recommended allowances for optimum health

---

24 *Ibidem*, p. 94.

25 *Ibidem*.

and efficiency, the experts estimated that family budgets could contribute some extra food purchased from the retailers. The *ad hoc* sub-committee for food regarded these requirements as "inadequate in respect to total protein and animal protein" for populations whose health had been seriously undermined by prolonged existence barely above the starvation level. A higher protein intake of around 80 g – of which no less than 30 g was to be of animal origin – was the recommendation of the experts in those cases. However, the determination of needs was separated from the procurement of supplies to meet the requirements, as supply allocation was not handled by the UNRRA but by the Combined Food Board, which was made up of representatives of the USA, Canada and the United Kingdom. The various commodity committees were composed of representatives of the main exporting and importing countries for each commodity.

After the UNRRA had explored national requirements and brought the relief budgets of the receiving countries into line with real resources, it presented the claims on food for the liberated areas to the Combined Board, trying to match legitimate claims with available supplies. Having its own service of official information, the Combined Board was not bound to accept the UNRRA claims as they were proposed.

In April 1945 the UNRRA began to deploy large-scale activities, and by the end of February 1946 it had shipped 3.8 million tons of food to 12 nations. Also in April 1945 the Allied military authorities entrusted the organisation with the responsibility of relief in several liberated countries, and throughout the year assistance was given to 12 countries, although substantial supplies began to reach the Far East only in the last part of the year. The UNRRA's food requirements in the second half of 1945 were about 2.9 tons. Although at the time some foods, especially wheat, were not under allocation, by the beginning of 1946 it had actually shipped 1.8 million tons, which meant roughly 62 per cent of the actual requirements.[26] But with the need for meat amounting to 304,817 tons, allocations were only 63,000 tons, which represented 20 per cent. It was only in terms of wheat, milk, cheese and some minor items that shipments almost reached requirements. At the top of the list: Greece received 1.3 million tons, about 35 per cent of the total; Italy received 381,000 tons; 279,000 tons went to China; other countries received a total of 14,000; while 0.7 million tons went to the rest. Food relief after the Great War – when the needs, according to the experts, were smaller – amounted to 6.2 million tons, of which not less than 4.8

26 *A statement by the Director General on the War Food Crisis*, Council IV, Document 50, C(46) 30, 18 March, 1946.

million were shipped during the first eight months of 1919. In 1946 deliveries continued to fall short of scheduled operations.

The 3.8 million tons of food shipped up until the end of February 1946 were composed of cereals, enough to feed about 12 million people during one year. The total relief deliveries of food after World War I amounted to 6.2 million tons, including large quantities of lard.[27] Although total UNRRA shipments increased in March 1946 to 1.5 million gross tons, shipments of food fell below this schedule.

Negative Effects of Famine upon the Public Health of the European Population

After a long period of negative living conditions under the influence of a plurality of negative factors associated with the economic crisis, political tensions and the war, changes in morbidity and mortality were expected to occur. Average life expectancy was probably the more direct and simple long-range index of public health. Under the effect of malnutrition and poor living conditions, resistance and immunity were gradually lowered, morbidity increased, although it took time for individuals to complete the whole cycle of exhaustion and sickness, ending in a deterioration of health standards and in death rates. The cumulative effect of all of the negative factors was estimated to appear relatively slowly, and several years were needed before the damage to health could be estimated in full.

As a consequence of food shortages and the subsequent reduction of calorie and nutrients intake, public health was affected. Food is not the only factor determining the health status of the population, but it is remarkable that during the war most of the determinant variables upon which health depended developed in a negative direction. Most cities had been destroyed by bombing and land warfare, residential construction had come to a practical standstill in belligerent countries and the housing shortage became a general problem. Many families were forced to share narrow quarters, and in many bombed-out areas, the population lived in improvised shelters or in cellars of ruined buildings. The impairment in housing conditions influenced health negatively. Overcrowding had become a generalised problem at the end of the war, even more acute where whole population groups evicted from their home regions had been moved to areas scarcely equipped to receive large numbers of refugees, destitute people, or where the military had requisitioned civilian buildings. The lack of housing

27 *Relief Deliveries and Relief Loans*, Geneva, League of Nations, 1943.

affected health in particular, considering the fact that feeding was deficient all over Europe and general hygiene conditions, clothing, bedding and safe water had become scarce resources.

In general, the meagre supplies of pre-war textiles and shoes were used up, and replaced, to some extent, by articles of less quality.

> The lack of soap, the almost complete absence of hot water, and the difficulty of finding decent privacy have naturally affected the habits of personal cleanliness. On top of all this, the efficiency of public health services has lessened in many cases owing to the destruction of hospitals or their requisitioning, the mobilization of doctors and nurses for military service, and the gradual exhaustion of the supplies of medicines, drugs and medical equipment.[28]

In this dramatic sentence, John Lindberg summarised the harsh living conditions of most of the European population in the 1940s. In addition to the general degradation of both diet and living conditions, increasing pressure was exerted upon people. Working hours were generally longer and household duties became harder for housewives. Overwork, fatigue, lack of sleep and stress – as well as the psychological pressure that comes with uncertainty, instability and the disruption of previous lives – aroused a negative perception about people's quality of life. All these factors, moreover, damaged health, influencing bodily wellbeing, organic defences and immunity. Risks to life posed by aerial bombardments, as well as the presence of enemy soldiers in occupied areas, exposed the population to intense nervous and physical strain. During the war and post-war years, civilians were submitted to high levels of anxiety and had to face an uncertain future. Although the real impact of the deterioration of living conditions and the psychological impairment of the health situation were difficult to assess, it seemed evident that all those factors, together with an insufficient diet, did have a negative effect.

Statistical measures on the evolution of public health were mainly based on scarce epidemiological records, principally morbidity and mortality rates, as there existed no direct measures of health, the previously mentioned ones being indirect negative indices pointing to a waning health situation. Neither anthropometric series of records nor clinical data were collected or made available. Even in the case of morbidity and mortality records, it is important to note that the national epidemiologic services were not always reliable to the same extent – this was particularly important for morbidity statistics. Under extraordinary circumstances, such as the war and post-war, they basically included

---

28 [Lindberg, J.], 1946, p. 92.

cases of serious diseases, excluding other conditions, and they often related to deaths rather than to incidence or prevalence figures. Reports and surveys on the state of health of the European population at the end of the war could not draw far-reaching conclusions because the available records were partial, unreliable or unrealistic. The overall picture of the evolution of health that those reports showed was expressive enough, but they were short on specific details. Reports usually referred to urban areas, hardly comparable with total national records. In addition, both morbidity and mortality statistics were likely to be less reliable in countries where health was badly deteriorated and the administration disorganised by war or civil strife.

Traditionally, wars were followed by health crises and disastrous epidemics. After World War I the repercussions of war on health were partly stopped due to improved methods of epidemic control. The international quarantine diseases, plague, cholera, yellow fever, smallpox, typhus and relapsing fever, still affected certain geographically circumscribed areas of the planet endemically, but they could still spread with great violence under exceptionally negative health conditions. All these diseases had been stirred up by the war, yet the new outbreaks had been successfully localised. Since some of these epidemics were transmitted to humans by animal vectors, the war had favoured their breeding and spread to such an extent that they continued to constitute a source of potential outbreaks and risks for human health.[29]

Cholera was endemic in India, Burma and China and had gained little ground outside these areas. A minor smallpox epidemic hit Naples in Italy in the spring of 1944, persisting until 1945. Plague and yellow fever did not affect European countries. There had been outbreaks of typhus in Eastern Europe, Italy and in Germany at the end of the war. A few cases had also occurred in Northern and in Western Europe, transmitted by displaced persons. Typhus was initially controlled "due largely to the efficiency of modern delousing techniques, and, after the liberation of Europe, to the liberal use of the new powerful insecticide, DDT".[30] However, the dangerous consequences of the use of DDT were not evident.

---

29 *Ibidem*, p. 104.

30 *Ibidem*, pp. 104-105. The main surveys on epidemiologic records of the European population during and after WWII come from the *Weekly Epidemiological Record of the Bulletin of the Health Organisation.* The 4th issue of volume 10 was devoted to "Health in Europe".

Since the introduction of vaccinations, typhoid fever was no longer the typical war disease, affecting soldiers and the army, but due to the destruction of cities and sanitation systems, and the uprooting of populations, the disease spread to civilians. The destruction of public health care services, together with polluted drinking water and the worsening of the health conditions of the population, were among the main factors of the serious spread of epidemic diseases.

> A quite serious epidemic occurred in September 1939 in Warsaw, after the bombardment of the city, and its spread has since been determined by the progress of bombing; it appeared in the United Kingdom in 1940 and 1941, in Germany after 1942, and epidemically in Japan in 1945. But considering Europe alone, reported cases before the end of the war rarely exceeded twice the normal number. In Germany the incidence in 1943 – the peak war year – was 2.3 times normal, as was also true in France. The incidence was low in Scandinavia, the United Kingdom, the Netherlands, Belgium, Switzerland and northern France, increasing progressively as one moved east and south from this area. But with the end of the war, and the upheaval of life in central Europe, the situation rapidly deteriorated, until typhoid fever came to outweigh diphtheria (previously the chief wartime epidemic) both in frequency and severity.[31]

Typhoid fever cases increased in Switzerland, the Scandinavian countries and in the United Kingdom, although absolute figures remained low. But since the summer of 1944 new heavily infected areas extended from the Baltic Sea and the North Sea to the Danubian countries, becoming one of the main sanitary threats in the geography of disease at the end of the war.

While medical controls contributed to keeping pestilential diseases supervised, certain other epidemics had increased – although influenza, the great killer after the Great War, had not been severe in the months following the end of the conflict. Some epidemic outbreaks were widespread in the winter of 1943, 1944 and 1945, both in Europe and America, but mortality rates remained low. Emerging as a new serious threat, poliomyelitis showed a growing incidence in many European countries, including France, Switzerland, Norway, Sweden and the Netherlands. Meningitis also became more frequent in Europe and Japan.

Diphtheria was the disease that showed a greater increase during the war. It was almost controlled in Sweden, Denmark, Switzerland and the United Kingdom, although it became an increasing problem in Germany from the late 1930s. Total records registered on the European continent

---

31 [Lindberg, J.], 1946, p. 105.

rose during the war: there were 173,000 cases registered in 1941; 283,000 in 1943; and the figures grew even more in 1944, all within the pre-Munich territory. Mortality rates were high and the epidemic spread from Germany to the occupied countries. Incidence was greatest in those countries where the level had previously been the lowest. The situation in Norway and the Netherlands became worse than in Germany itself, since incidence increased 112 times in Norway and 40 times in the Netherlands.[32]

> The number of cases in France rose from two thousand in 1939 to 16 thousand in 1943. In all some 630 thousand diphtheria cases were reported in 1943 in such European countries as maintained tolerably efficient registration. Considering non-reported cases, Knud Stowman, chief of the Epidemiological Information Service of the UNRRA, estimates that there were about one million cases in 1943 in Europe (excluding the USSR), and that the figure was at least as high in 1944. This disease involved about 50,000 deaths in 1943, mostly of children. It is reported that in 1945 diphtheria had become the leading epidemic disease in Japan, with a case mortality much higher than that encountered in Europe.[33]

The war also had very negative consequences in terms of the emergence and spread of several skin diseases linked to very unsatisfactory hygienic conditions. Scabies increased spectacularly all over Europe; official figures showed that in Norway it was seven times as prevalent in 1943 as in 1938 and in Amsterdam 75 times. In some devastated towns of central Italy, such as Aquila province, 85 per cent of the population was infected, and similar tendencies were described in the case of other skin diseases such as impetigo.[34]

The fight against the spread of tuberculosis was one of the most important sanitary challenges after the war. As has been generally recognised, the expansion of tuberculosis was particularly susceptible to the impairment of social and economic conditions and above all to the state of nutrition, the excess of working and bad hygienic living standards. In the war and post-war period the systems recording disease incidence and prevalence were heterogeneous and incomplete, and therefore mortality figures were the most reliable index for assessing the spread of the disease among the weakened population. From a policy perspective, however, mortality rates offered a slower and delayed perspective of the evolution of the disease and the impact of the changing situations.

---

32 *Ibidem*, p. 106.

33 *Ibidem*, pp. 106-107.

34 *Ibidem*, p. 107.

In spite of being one of the main social diseases and a core epidemiological problem, the number of tuberculosis cases had started to fall in most European countries in the Inter-war Period. However, this tendency was reversed by the war, when the disease became more severe, producing an unusual number of acute cases, accompanied and sometimes described as interstitial pneumonia and tuberculous broncho-pneumonia.[35]

> Increases in mortality are noted over most of the Continent, and were marked in Belgium, France and the Netherlands, and also in Eastern Europe, Yugoslavia and Greece. It is significant that in France, for instance, mortality from tuberculosis per 100,000 inhabitants in the Department of the Seine increased from 172 in 1939 to 234 in 1941, falling to 191 in 1943, whilst in Brittany (where food was plentiful) it continued to fall, being, in the Department of Côtes-du-Nord, 257 in 1938 and 148 in 1943. The most seriously threatened areas were Paris, Marseille, Lyon and the cities of the Riviera. In Greece the death rate from tuberculosis in 1942 was 456 per 100,000 inhabitants. The increase in active cases has been accompanied by a large increase of pre-tubercular conditions and latent tuberculosis. Where food conditions remained reasonably good, tuberculosis has on the whole either been fairly stable or has continued to fall. It should be noted, however, that owing to intensified industrial activity the rate has tended to go up in industrial centres, even in the United Kingdom and the United States.[36]

Similarly, malaria had become more severe in war-stricken areas. In Greece, malaria mortality was usually high, affecting 40 out of every 100,000 inhabitants in 1939, but in the autumn of 1942 an evident increase was developing. In addition to favourable climatic conditions for the reproduction of the carrier of the microbe, the anopheles mosquito, the outbreak was also associated with the displacement of populations, refugees, low resistance and poor immunity in the weakened population due to famine and bad living conditions, as well as the lack of medicine such as quinine and other drugs. Malaria was essentially concentrated in poor rural districts, where people seldom required medical care, and therefore statistics were neither complete nor reliable.

On the other hand, wartime generally resulted in a sharp increase in venereal diseases, not only in war-involved countries but also in neutral ones. The situation was particularly acute in internment camps and occupied regions. Only Scandinavian countries reported specific figures

---

35 *Ibidem.*

36 *Ibidem.* pp. 107-108.

about the increment of syphilis cases. For the war period 1941-44, cases increased 7.7 times in Denmark, 6.13 times in Norway and 3.9 times in Sweden.

> Fragmentary evidence indicates that, as might be expected, the situation is even less favourable on the Continent. Syphilis was made notifiable in Belgium in 1942, and the incomplete returns show a 70% increase between 1942 and 1944. Records of dispensaries in France indicate a doubling of cases between 1941 and 1942, and again between 1942 and 1943. Unofficial reports from other countries indicate similar developments.[37]

At the end of World War II the prevalence of specific nutritional deficiency diseases was almost impossible to measure statistically. A generalised loss of body weight had been reported in adults all over Europe and cases of delayed growth amongst children and adolescents were frequent. This evident loss of body weight could be partially attributed to stress, psychological strain and greater physical activity. But it was mainly due to the fact that diets were widely rationed and, even in those cases in which calorie amounts were adequate, rations were uniformly dull and the lack of appetite became a limiting factor. It had been noticed that newborn babies were generally underweight in areas with food shortages. A portion of adolescents and adults also suffered from serious deficiency diseases such as rickets, scurvy, as well as gastro-intestinal problems due to the lack of vitamin B, pellagra, hunger oedema, and other consequences of undernourishment. In any case, reliable statistics were always scarce.

In general terms, the health situation in the United States, the British Commonwealth, Sweden, Switzerland and Denmark was considered to be improving despite the war. In the Netherlands, Norway and Czechoslovakia, and during part of the period in Finland, a serious deterioration in the state of health of the population was averted. In Germany, France and Italy, the situation was less favourable, according to the experts' reports. Those countries made the political decision of registering mortality increases. The situation in other countries such as Bulgaria, Hungary and Romania did not seem to have deteriorated in a significant manner, something quite different to what was going on in Poland, Yugoslavia and Greece, where the severe impairment of the nutritional condition and the state of health of the population had intensified mortality, infectious diseases and epidemic outbreaks. It is true that the end of hostilities was followed by some improvement in the health indicators in most Western countries, but the positive tendency

37 *Ibidem*, p. 108.

experienced a drastic retrogression afterwards in Germany, Italy, Austria, Hungary, Romania and Japan.

From a mortality perspective, the death rate continued its pre-war downward trend in a significant number of European countries: Denmark, Sweden, the United Kingdom, Switzerland (except in 1944), Ireland and Bulgaria, in the last country until 1943. This tendency persisted probably until the end of the war, except in the case of Bulgaria. The lowest death rate was that of the Netherlands in 1938, amounting to only 8.5 per cent, an indicator that increased to 11.5 per cent in 1944. A similar trend was noticed in Norway, Germany, Italy, France and most other European countries. If birth rates were on the decline, absolute numbers of infant deaths would also fall, reducing the general death rate as a consequence. However, birth rates went up in the Netherlands, Norway, Czechoslovakia and Finland and, due to this widespread increase in the birth rate, the population did not generally drop in the European context; only Belgium and France were the exception.

Infant mortality remained on a considerably lower level during World War II compared with the Great War. Most countries succeeded in safeguarding the nutritional intake of children, although a difficult challenge was to protect children from the negative impact of displacement and the breakdown of public services. In Sweden, Switzerland, the United Kingdom and Denmark, infant mortality continued to fall, reaching new record lows, notwithstanding the impairment of the nutritional problems. The situation was similar to the pre-war period in Czechoslovakia, Bulgaria and Norway, and also for Finland, except during specific acute warfare and aggressive moments. In the Netherlands, infant mortality rates rose but were still very low when compared with other European countries; something similar happened in Belgium and France, a sharp increase between 1938 and 1940 was followed by a recovery.

At the end of the war, infant mortality rates were less favourable than in the preceding war years and nutritional deficiencies were considered to be one of the contributing factors. "The deterioration was partly connected with the sweeping land warfare, the heavy aerial bombardments and the consequent breakdown of public services, communications and administration, as well as the displacement of populations; but it reflects also, no doubt, the further deterioration in the supply situation over wide areas".[38]

[38] *Ibidem*, p 117.

At the end of the war official reports regarding the health situation of the European population by the League of Nations, the Food and Agriculture Organisation and the World Health Organisation indicated that it was methodologically convenient to analyse the war years and the period after the end of the conflict separately. During the war period the health status and the nutritional condition of the population became widely diversified. The United Kingdom, Sweden, Switzerland and Denmark succeeded to a great extent in preventing the deterioration of health, even improving their pre-war health and nutritional standards. Other countries, such as the Netherlands, Norway and Czechoslovakia, and also Finland during certain periods, succeeded in avoiding serious impairment, although pre-war gains were partially lost or at least not improved upon. In Germany, France and Italy, the situation was more serious, as morbidity and infant mortality went up and large groups of the population had lived under such negative conditions that it would have lasting effects on their future health. On the other hand, Eastern and Southern European countries formed an area ordinarily characterised by high mortality rates and low life expectancy, although general conditions did not deteriorate greatly during the war in countries such as Bulgaria, Hungary and Romania, and it would even improve in others. For Poland, Yugoslavia and the Soviet Union the international agencies did not have statistics, although in some regions in these countries the health and nutritional conditions were as bad as in Greece during the famine of 1942. In Greece, all indices of morbidity and mortality indicated a serious deterioration of health and high rates of mortality. The situation was considered to be a sanitary emergency.

In 1946 the world health situation as a whole, apart from the specific areas of deep crisis already mentioned, was better than expected. This was largely due to the absence of serious epidemics of the type occurring after the Great War, but also, without doubt, to the relative success of the rationing systems and distribution schemes. The experts emphasised that the full effects of malnutrition, starvation and a deficient diet would take a long time to become evident. But the situation in the early post-war years was extremely fragile and uncertain and a general assessment of the impact of the war and rationing over public health could not be undertaken in a consistent way.

CHAPTER 7

The Global Politics of Food and Hunger

From the International Institute of Agriculture (IIA) to the Food and Agriculture Organisation (FAO)

The Origins of the International Institute of Agriculture

The International Institute of Agriculture, the forerunner of the Food and Agriculture Organisation (FAO), was created in 1905 following the initiative of David Lubin (1849-1919). With support from King Vittorio Emmanuele III of Italy, his dream of an international agricultural organisation to bring some order to agricultural production and trade organisation all over the world became reality. The work of the IIA over a 40-year period proved to be useful for the establishment of an international transdisciplinary referent of technical work around food, agriculture and nutrition, especially in critical periods.

David Lubin was born in Klodowa, Poland, on June 10, 1849. He was a merchant and agriculturalist, who possessed exceptional entrepreneurship to run ambitious projects. Like many other Polish citizens, his family emigrated first to England in 1853 and then to the USA when he was only six years old, living in New York initially and then in Sacramento, California. It was in Sacramento that he started a prosperous career with his cousin Harris Weinstock, setting up a successful *One Price Store* known as the Weinstock-Lubin Company. While in Sacramento, he bought a fruit ranch and land for wheat cultivation. He felt drawn to agriculture and immediately understood its huge importance for the global economy and future of humankind. His interest in agriculture prompted him to get involved in the foundation of a farmers' union called *California Fruit Grower's Union.* He also helped in the settlement of Eastern European Jewish refugees who worked on various farms in California, and in 1891 he became the head of the *International Society for the Colonization of Russian Jews*. The aforementioned details point to the profile of an active man, a global thinker full of ambitious initiatives.

Absolutely involved in farming, agricultural production and trade, he was very active in campaigning for subsidies and protection for farmers, not only on a local scale in California, but also on an international level. He soon developed a proposal for an international chamber of agriculture and, following the same project, in 1896 he travelled to Europe for the first time with the aim of establishing contacts to implement the idea of an international agriculture organisation. According to his project, this institution was to act as an international research and technical organisation and an intergovernmental consulting body. It was also to provide farmers across the globe with a means to improve productivity, innovative technology, new methods of cultivation and helping to control the fluctuations of the prices. His proposal established a cooperative system of rural credit, exerting some control over the marketing and trade of agricultural products. In 1904 he travelled to Italy and had an interview with King Vittorio Emmanuele III about his idea. The Italian king was keen on the initiative and set the wheels in motion by bringing the idea to the attention of the Italian government.

One year later an International Conference in Rome (May, 1905) decided on the foundation of the International Institute of Agriculture (IIA), with sponsorship from the Italian King Vittorio Emmanuele III. Forty states confirmed they would engage with the new international agency and David Lubin became the USA's permanent delegate to the organisation in 1906. He died in 1919, shortly after the end of World War I, and in 1946 the IIA was dissolved and its functions and assets transferred to the newly founded FAO, under the umbrella of the recently set up United Nations.[1] In the meantime, the IIA developed a great deal of technical work, sometimes in collaboration with other international organisations such as the League of Nations and the International Labor Organization, and influence on agricultural policies characterised the IIA activities in the inter-war period.

At the end of World War II the defeat of the Axis and the victory of the Allies gave way to a new period characterised not only by the end of the international conflicts and catastrophic wars, but also by the start of a new international order. Priority was given to the idea of founding a new order in the world, in accordance with the political ideology of the victor forces, free of war and the economic, social chaos and inequality that marked the big crisis in the 1930s. Already during the war, the Declaration of St. James's Palace in 1941, the United Nations Declaration of 1942 and the Dumbarton Oaks Conference of 1944 were international agreements preceding the formation of the United Nations in San Francisco in 1945. Held in 1944, the Breton Woods Conference prepared the ground for a post-war economic order through the creation

---

[1] Hobson, A., *The International Institute of Agriculture*, Berkeley, University of California Press, 1931.

of an International Monetary Fund (IMF) and an International Bank for Reconstruction and Development (IBRD-World Bank) in 1945, and later for the International Trade Organization, a portion of which emerged in 1947 as the General Agreement on Tariffs and Trade (GATT). In 1943 a total of 44 governments committed themselves to creating a permanent global organisation for food and agriculture in Hot Springs, Virginia.

At least three major issues dominated the post World War II landscape. The first and more urgent necessity of the international community was *post-war reconstruction and reestablishment of global order*. There were major concerns about rebuilding destroyed infrastructures and restoring agricultural production from a global perspective, but especially in the regions most badly affected by the consequences of the war in Europe and Asia. A second challenge was *creating a global mechanism to promote peace*, an international space of political negotiation and agreement to overcome disputes, prevent war, create international public goods, improve health and promote an exchange of technical expertise. The third major concern regarded the creation of a *functioning and effective international economic system*, avoiding fluctuations and big crises, which recognised national sovereignty over economic policy but also became the referent of an international framework promoting international cooperation, facilitating trade through a managed exchange rate regime, working for the reduction of trade barriers and facilitating long-term capital transfers.[2]

The authorities shared serious worries about post-war food shortages, famine and rural poverty becoming extremely high. The main causes identified were the destruction of the productive capacity of many societies, the damage to a transport system at national and international scales, and the loss of technical capacity for many countries in agriculture, including their access to basic seeds and other necessary inputs. Shortages and famine immediately became a serious problem. Food security debates, as well, were dominated by concerns about inadequate production. Thus, the creation of the FAO, which occurred early in the aforementioned process, first focused on assessing the food situation, projecting what would be needed to stave off starvation and recommending how the necessary increase in the world food production could come about.

---

2 McCalla, A.F., *FAO in the Changing Global Landscape. Working Paper No. 07-006*, Davis University of California, Department of Agricultural and Resource Economics, 2007.

First Steps for the Foundation of the FAO

In May 1943, just in the midst of the critical situation of a world economy conditioned by World War II and particularly by the obstacles to food trade, availability and rationing, the United States President, Franklin D. Roosevelt, invited representatives of 44 countries to meet in Hot Springs, Virginia, to discuss post-war plans for rebuilding and meeting the challenges of a world in need. One of the most important issues on the agenda was the idea of a serious improvement of food and agriculture, or in the words of the conference delegates, "a secure, adequate, and suitable supply of food for every man". The Hot Spring delegates created a working group commissioned to draft a proposal for the creation of a permanent international organisation that would deal not only with food and agriculture but also with forestry and fisheries. Once the project was accepted within the framework of the UN organisations, the International Institute of Agriculture ceased its operations in 1945, at the end of the war.[3]

On October 16, 1945, representatives of 34 nations signed the charter of the Food and Agriculture Organization of the United Nations (FAO). Sir John Boyd Orr, a man with experience in the political management of scientific knowledge on nutrition, was then appointed the first FAO Director General. Boyd Orr (1880-1971) had been a Carnegie research fellow in physiology and in 1914 arrived in Aberdeen to take the lead of a new Institute on Nutrition. During World War I he served as a physician that challenged the reality of malnutrition and poverty, evident in the poor physical condition of many of the army's recruits. Upon his return to Aberdeen, Boyd Orr was determined to complete the institute and investigate the role of nutrients, minerals and vitamins in animal health. In 1925, interested in the diets of farm animals and humans in other parts of the world, he embarked on journeys to Africa, the Middle East, New Zealand, Australia and India. He later discovered that milk added to the diets of children in Scotland and England led to gains in height and weight, becoming increasingly concerned with British food and agriculture policy. His research culminated in the publication of *Food, Health and Income*, an unprecedented and very influential introduction to food policy, inspiring directly the British food-rationing system during World War II.

---

[3] The Library of the FAO was named the David Lubin Memorial Library in honor of the founder of the IIA. It keeps the personal archives of Lubin and the documents, technical reports and publications of the IIA. The Western Jewish History Centre of the Judah L. Magnes Museum in Berkeley (California) has a large collection of papers, correspondence, publications and pictures of David Lubin.

In 1931 he founded the journal *Nutrition Abstracts and Reviews*, becoming chief editor of the publication. Notwithstanding that his duties were time consuming, he was still able to direct fundamental research in nutrition, primarily in animal nutrition in the early days of the Rowett Institute in Aberdeen. His influential *Minerals in Pastures and Their Relation to Animal Nutrition* (1929) was published in this period. In the 1930s, however, after extensive experiments with milk in the diet of mothers, children and the lower social groups of the population, and after large-scale surveys of nutritional problems in many nations all over the world, Boyd Orr's interests swung to human nutrition, not only as an experimental physiologist but also as an active worker for the instruction on healthy diets for people everywhere. His aforementioned report, *Food, Health and Income* (1936) revealed the "appalling amount of malnutrition" among the population of England, regardless of economic status. His surveys and criticism about the negative effects of deficient nutrition on human development and health conditions became the basis for British policy on food during World War II, which he helped to formulate as a member of Churchill's Scientific Committee on Food Policy, a successful programme that has been discussed in a previous chapter. At the end of the war, Boyd Orr, aged 65, and already retired from the Rowett Institute, accepted three new positions: he was appointed Chancellor of Glasgow University for a three-year period; he also occupied a seat in the Commons representing the Scottish universities; and he was also appointed to the post of Director-General of the Food and Agriculture Organization of the United Nations when it was founded.

Boyd Orr and the Failed World Food Board

Notwithstanding Boyd Orr's long experience in the field of nutritional policies, his time as the first FAO Director-General was very short. Both practical and political reasons made him resign just a few months after his appointment. In 1946, under the aegis of the FAO, an International Emergency Food Council was founded in Copenhagen, representing 34 member nations and commissioned to address the post-war food crisis and discuss the global programme. The central issue was the creation of a World Food Board, a technical commission to oversee the purchase of surplus food from food-exporting countries and the delivery of the surplus to countries in need, which would then pay back the food loan through various agricultural activities. He travelled extensively throughout the world trying to get support for a comprehensive food plan and was bitterly disappointed when his proposal for the establishment of a World Food Board failed in 1947, when neither Great Britain nor the United States voted for it. Boyd Orr became convinced that the FAO could not, at that point, become a spearhead for a movement to achieve world unity and peace without the support of the global powers, and therefore resolved to resign as Director-General.

In 1949 he was awarded the Nobel Prize for Peace, and the principal merit stated was his efforts to eliminate hunger in the world. However, he donated the prize money to the National Peace Council, the World Movement for World Federal Government and various other philanthropic organisations. In the years following the Second World War Boyd Orr was associated with virtually every organisation, acting for world government, in many cases devoting his efforts, skills and influence to the cause.

In the years preceding World War II as much as a third of the population of the United Kingdom suffered from poverty-induced malnutrition, a factor influencing poor health. Nutritionists saw the insufficient consumption of milk and fresh fruit as the main cause. Taking this hard reality for a modern and rich country as a starting point, John Boyd Orr came to advocate the establishment of an agricultural economy of abundance, described in his 1936 publication, *Food, Health and Income.* Orr's investigation on the interactions between food, health and income constituted a major contribution to the field of the political economy of nutrition. The study attracted the attention of world leaders in terms of their responsibility to satisfy food production needs on the global level.

On July 5, 1946, the FAO Conference met in Washington and approved a document presented by Director General J. Boyd Orr, containing the proposals for the creation of a World Food Board (WFB). The proposal had to be submitted to the Second Session of the Conference of the Food and Agriculture Organization, to be held in Copenhagen on September 2, 1946. The document was a schematic analysis of the critical situation of food and nutrition, consisting of 12 pages where the long-term problems of nutrition and agriculture, the inter-relationship of nutrition and agriculture with industry and trade and the economic advantages of a world food policy based on human needs were discussed. According to Boyd Orr's analysis, to reach this goal, purchasing power had to be generated. In the context of the existing inter-governmental organisations – commodity organisations for producers and United Nations organisations – a WFB could coordinate actions. The document summarised the structure, operations and actions for short-term and long-term perspectives.[4]

When the FAO was founded in 1945 it was generally assumed that with the policy of cooperation and mutual aid of the temporary international organisations dealing with food, the European nations would be able to cope with emergency situations and the critical circumstances arising after the war. Reasonable agreements between the governments involved would allow the FAO to implement a global food policy. In February 1946 the United Nations' General Assembly called on the governments and international agencies concerned with food and agriculture policies to *make special efforts* in this direction. Under logical expectations to coordinate international policies on food, considering the positive call from the UN, in May 1946, the FAO convened the aforementioned *Special Meeting on Urgent Food Problems*, which was held in Washington. The special meeting requested Sir John Boyd Orr, Director General, to prepare a set of proposals for dealing with long-term issues. Immediate problems of emergency food supplies were the first concern at that critical moment, but the meeting also called for the analysis of long-term issues related to the production, distribution and consumption of food and agricultural products, including the risk of surplus build-ups.[5]

The technical report prepared by Boyd Orr started by recognising that there had never been enough food in the world to satisfy human necessities. Before the war there were 1,000 million people consuming less than 2,250 calories.[6] At the lower levels of intake, the food mainly consisted of cereals, which were the cheapest satisfiers of hunger in most areas of the world, but a balanced diet had to contain a large proportion of animal products, fruit and vegetables. Since food consumption depends on people's purchasing power, as family income rises, the consumption of more expensive foodstuffs increases. Before the war the diet of about the poorest third of the population in the United States was estimated to be below the levels of a healthy diet owing to insufficient consumption of animal products, fruit and vegetables. Full employment and high wages during the war increased the consumption of these foodstuffs, particularly of eggs and milk, whose consumption increased by 30 per cent.In the United Kingdom, in spite of the national food shortage, the consumption of certain foods of special value for

4 *Proposals for a world food board and world food survey. World Food Program, 1946*, Washington, FAO, World Food Program. 1946.

5 *Report of the special meeting on urgent food problems*, Washington, FAO, 1946.

6 World Food Survey, Washington, FAO, 1946.

health rose substantially.[7] As food consumption is directly correlated with health, as the diet deteriorates, health and physical abilities decline, as well as life expectancy. The remarkable betterment in health following improvement in the diet showed that inadequate food was one of the main causes behind preventable diseases, misery and premature death.

The general situation after the war was the great opportunity for Boyd Orr to realise the dreams he had mentioned in his address at the first FAO Conference in Quebec just after his election as the FAO Director-General. The central point was the constitution of a *World Food Board*, a proposal that Orr submitted to the FAO conference at its second session, the one previously mentioned, held in Copenhagen in September 1946. The proposal aimed to prevent the impact of the deep interwar crisis, the negative effects of the war and post-war shortages: the dramatic fall of agricultural prices and incomes, the general economic slump and the fast rise of large-scale unemployment, as a source of widespread depression and massive poverty. Boyd Orr was convinced that food was something more than merely a commodity, and the World Food Board was not only to be an international trade regulator. Its vocation was mostly to end hunger through a three-pronged system: one part dealing with credit given to nations to increase food production; another to regulate prices of agricultural products with buffer stocks of key commodities; and a third one to distribute famine relief. Boyd Orr's logic was clear and evident: "There is no measure which would contribute more to human welfare than the application of a food policy based on human needs…"[8] With food and nutrition being essential human rights, as well as an element for political and social stability, he was convinced of the moral obligation to provide food for the hungry poor. If nations were not able to agree on a food programme affecting such a basic right, he was very pessimistic about the hope of the international community to reach agreement on anything else. As fate had it, his worst presages came true.

International reports and technical surveys during the war and in the early post-war years on nutrition and health suggested that the more income increased, the more morbidity and mortality decreased, children development was easier, adult stature got higher and general health and social indicators improved. Hunger and health raised important economic and political questions. The political dimension of hunger and

---

7 *Proposals*, 1946, p. 2.

8 Orr, J.B., *Food: The Foundation of World Unity*, London, National Peace Council, 1948.

health came across the contradiction that there was not a single national agency or government department. The politics of hunger and the political management of the new knowledge on nutrition were considered by Orr to be essential for the improvement of the health and welfare of the nation, but also a fundamental factor for the politics of justice and the practical implementation of human rights.

The plan for a World Food Board included several dimensions regarding the political economy of food, nutrition and hunger. The first major problem was producing sufficient food not only to feed the expanding world population, but also to feed people according to new scientific patterns of healthy diet, and this implied changing dietary habits and traditional patterns. Advances in agricultural technologies had helped increase the world production of foodstuffs. However, the fast population growth in some regions gave rise to a tough political challenge: ensuring an adequate production and distribution. Scientific knowledge and farming technologies could improve production and give a boost to an increasing industrialisation of food, but distribution was really the main economic and political challenge. Other collateral effects such as the lack of regulations for food quality and systems to fight adulteration had to be avoided as well. But at the end of World War II the idea that industrialisation could be a tool to compensate for unemployment, and particularly underemployment in agriculture, was widely accepted.

The production of foodstuffs led to different types of problems depending on the agricultural pattern. In most developing countries, food was produced on very small holdings and traditional farming techniques were followed. The kernel of political action in these cases consisted of providing peasants with jobs in other industries and educating them in modern methods of cultivation and equipment for technical modernisation. On the contrary, in countries where modern technologies were already applied, the main problem was finding stability for the market and guaranteeing remunerative prices. This had become a problem in the 1920s, appallingly expressed in wartime, when rising prices had to be controlled to avoid maladjustments and cyclical oscillation. Uncontrolled fluctuations in prices hindered agreement on a common price for agricultural products on the world market. This phenomenon resulted in the necessity to ensure a world market for exportable surpluses at stable prices to protect availability for the lower income sectors of the population or for the poor countries. Price variation was not unfair but also an economic problem, as the low purchasing power of food producers was a constricting factor for the development of a market for industrial products. Conversely, reducing industrial prosperity and the purchasing capacity of industrial producers limited the markets for agricultural products.

The volume of trade was also considered to be a core factor for the future of human nutrition and the prosperity of agriculture.[9] A long-term policy on nutrition, health, food production and agriculture was most challenging, as the interests of agriculture, trade and public health in the post-war years had to be reconciled. Food was considered to be a tradable commodity, but it was also an essential element of human rights and life itself. Therefore, the establishment of a World Food Board spelled out the economic advantages of a world food policy based on human needs: if any governments assumed the responsibility to improve the level of nutrition of its nationals up to the scientific standards of a healthy diet, an expansion of food supplies would take place even in the richest countries. This was, certainly, what member nations agreed to do when accepting the FAO's constitution, adjusting agricultural policies to that end. To reach this ambitious goal, the additional food production required was so great that it could only be implemented if production were progressively coordinated on a worldwide scale. Global coordination involved farming diversification, concentrating on the more perishable foods owing to their special value for human nutrition and health, such as wheat and sugar, which could be grown in areas where they were best adapted for production, since they were easily stored and transported.

Rhetorical arguments in favour of a World Food Board were evident and unquestionable. The expansion of agriculture would accelerate the development of mechanisation and would expand the market for agricultural equipment of all kinds, for fertilisers, and for facilities linked to food storage and shipment. In poor countries, the need for technological improvement was urgent in agricultural techniques, irrigation, food control and quality regulation, drainage systems and land reclamation. The capital requirements for the great expansion needed for the global development of agriculture would help to sustain industrialisation and contribute to employment. Prosperity in agriculture would also increase demands in consumption among agricultural producers. A world food policy, based on and dimensioned for the fulfilment of human needs, would provide a programme for agriculture and trade, contribute prosperity and be the point of departure in achieving the humanitarian goals proclaimed by the leading authorities of the United Nations.

---

9 *Proposals*, 1946, p. 6.

The scientific knowledge on nutrition, the innovative technologies in agriculture and the demographic conditions to set off the global economic expansion were already available, but consumption was only possible if people's purchasing power was increased in the same measure as food production. In many developed countries governments had taken steps to bridge the gap between the price of food integrating an optimum diet and the purchasing capacity of the population. However, poor countries and other regions devastated by the war were unable, in practical terms, to give access to a healthy diet to the most damaged sectors of the population. Some financial arrangements, such as supplying capital equipment involving deferred payments and long-term credits to the countries concerned, would lead to the development of natural resources. This world food policy was to be applied according to the proposal put forward by the League of Nations' Committee on Economic Depression. It was not only credit for development purposes that had to be given, but a solidarity fund also had to be allocated to countries in great nutritional need and suffering from shortages and malnutrition. This was required if they wanted to purchase the agricultural surpluses of other nations on special terms and conditions.

Once the need for a World Food Board and its field of operation was accepted, a question remained unanswered: what were the terms of operation of the new institution? Was there to be a new international board or could existing international organisations for specific products such as sugar, rubber, tea, minerals and others be pooled together? Such existing organisations were born as a consequence of the depression and lacked an overall agency coordinating all the strategies for the expansion of an inclusive worldwide perspective. The initiatives had been mostly plural. Further developments during World War II were the creation of an Inter-American Coffee Agreement (1940) and the creation of the International Wheat Council (1942), composed of Argentina, Australia, Canada, the United Kingdom and the United States.[10] Other countries were also invited to participate in an international agreement for submission to an international conference. On the other hand, the governments of Australia, New Zealand, South Africa and the United Kingdom had set up a Joint Organisation in 1946 to undertake the marketing of accumulated wool surpluses; other initiatives were linked to cotton production and trade.

> All existing and projected commodity councils suffer from two important defects, both due the same cause – the need for a more comprehensive

10 Shaw, J., *World Food Security. A History since 1945*, Hampshire, Palgrave Macmillan, 2007, pp. 22-23.

> organization. First, when each commodity is considered in isolation it is impossible to contemplate certain remedies and opportunities, which are feasible when commodities are considered jointly. Secondly, when commodity councils are not part of a larger organization, they lack the financial resources, which would enable them to hold stocks, bring stability to existing markets, and develop new ones.[11]

During the war the United Nations prepared to set up a number of international bodies, establishing the FAO for studies and recommendations on developments in the field of food and agriculture, forestry and fisheries. Its technical advisory services were concerned with a wide range of scientific, technical, economic and statistical problems involved in the improvement of production and distribution. As we already know, an International Bank was established by the United Nations to assist in providing funds for the large investment needed for agricultural and industrial development, a concept including health, education, working conditions, funding and trade. From this perspective, UNESCO, the WHO, the ILO, the IMF and the ITO [International Trade Organization], were among many international agencies created. The Economic and Social Council was internationally responsible, and again the ILO was specifically concerned with improving wages and assisting in alleviating the balance of payment difficulties of member countries, which in itself was considered to be a major contribution toward mitigating international trade obstacles. In addition to this, there were proposals for the creation of an International Trade Organization, which contemplated international machinery for encouraging a progressive reduction in trade barriers, the elimination of restrictive business practices and actions in the field of commodity policy.[12] Apart from the World Bank and the International Monetary Fund, which were designed to facilitate the solution of financial problems on an international level, the functions of the international organisations were limited to the accumulation and interpretation of facts, the production of technical reports, the summary of information and surveys and the issuing of recommendations. No single organisation or combination of them had the capacity to take measures and transform recommendations into action, since they had neither authority nor funds for taking coordinated international action.

In addition to the FAO and the proposal of a World Food Board, a series of temporary organisations were created to deal with the food scarcity caused by the war. As mentioned, the International Emergency

---

11 *Ibidem*, p. 23.

12 *Ibidem*.

Food Council, working through commodity committees, encouraged the stabilisation of prices by reaching agreement on price schedules and by promoting unified buying, recommending the allocation of export surpluses according to the needs of different countries. The UNRRA also managed funds to provide food and agricultural implements, fertilisers and other supplies for the rehabilitation of war-devastated countries. The proposal of a permanent World Food Board was more ambitious and established a permanent executive agency.

> A continuation of this international cooperation is needed because if these temporary organizations bring the world out of the present food emergency, there will still remain the great scarcity of food that existed before the war and at the same time the agricultural problems of fluctuation in prices and the accumulation of unmarketable "surpluses".[13]

In order to solve the lack of coordination, the World Food Board had to be given the necessary authority and funds to confront the long-term problems of world food security. Whether as a new agency or integrated into the FAO structure, it would be appointed by the FAO Conference that included representatives of all countries. Commodity committees were to be the operating bodies. Since the World Food Board was to face great problems relating to the world economy and finance, it was thought necessary to include representatives of other international organisations.

The project presented by J. Boyd Orr to the FAO Copenhagen Assembly attributed four main functions to the WFB:

> 1. The stabilization of the prices of agricultural commodities in the world markets, allowing for the necessary funds for stabilising operations.
>
> 2. The establishment of a world food reserve, adequate for any emergency that might arise through crop failure in any part of the world.
>
> 3. The provision of funds for financing the disposal of surplus agricultural products on special terms to countries where the need for them is most urgent.
>
> 4. The cooperation with other organisations concerned with international credits for industrial and agricultural development, and with trade and commodity policy, in order to facilitate that their common ends might be more quickly and effectively achieved.[14]

For the stabilisation of prices, the WFB would operate through its committees to hold stocks of the most important commodities. The

---

13 *Proposals*, 1946, p. 10.

14 *Ibidem*, p. 11.

Board would announce a maximum and minimum price and would undertake to buy into its stock when the world price fell below the declared minimum and sell from its stock when the world price exceeded the maximum. Price stabilisation appeared to be one of the main aspects of its policy. A revolving fund to operate such a policy would be needed, although since the agency would normally buy at its minimum price and sell at its maximum price, it was expected to earn enough to cover the cost of storage. The most general and important objective of the strategies of the World Food Board would be to ensure that sufficient food was produced and distributed to bring the consumption of all populations in the world up to a health dietary standard. Technical reports showed that the need for additional food was so great that if human requirements could be translated into economic demand, there would be no surpluses of the basic products. The fundamental problem in 1946 was to increase the purchasing power of the population unable to obtain sufficient food to satisfy their needs, with the main duty of the Board being to divert surpluses to these consumers and arrange for financing for the cost of selling at prices that the consumers were able to afford.[15]

The need for immediate action was recognised in the creation of the WFB, a call for action summarised in the FAO approved *Proposals* with the following words: "There are only two alternatives for the nations today: either cooperation for mutual benefit in a world policy, or a drift back to nationalistic policies leading to economic conflict which may well be the prelude to a third world war that will end our civilization".[16] Consequently, the WFB was presented as the main instrument for global stabilisation.

But the Copenhagen Conference did not follow up on any of John Boyd Orr's substantive recommendations in a truly effective manner, and the proposal for a World Food Board slowly disintegrated and disappeared off the agenda in favour of national interest. Orr was acutely disappointed at what he regarded as the failure of his attempt to establish a world authority of global governance with full competence to embark on the path that would ensure that all people of the world were adequately fed. Soon after this failure he resigned as the FAO Director-General. Orr had given the FAO an ambitious start, and as its beneficial work in the task of improving world agriculture and nutrition became more widely realised, some of his proposals that were previously rejected were eventually incorporated into the organisation's programme.

---

15 *Ibidem*, p. 12.

16 *Ibidem*.

Nevertheless, despite a later attempt made by others in 1949, the project of a World Food Board was never resuscitated. However, he continued to believe until his death that the plan would have to be taken up again.

In 1948 John Boyd Orr made a clear statement that spelled out his ideas about the political dimension of hunger and food. He made a global assessment of the problem in a lecture that was followed by an interview and summarised in a newspaper for the general public:

> Not more than 20 to 25 percent of the population of the world enjoy food, shelter, and clothing on a health standard and have the environment needed to promote intellectual and cultural development. Today the masses who have never enjoyed the environmental conditions necessary for a full life are realizing more and more that the poverty which has cramped their existence is no longer necessary; it was not ordained by God that they should be born to poverty and be content with poverty as their lot in life. In Europe, men will no longer tolerate seeing land going out of cultivation while their children lack food, or factories idle while their families live huddled together in disease-ridden slums. But it is in the underdeveloped countries that the greatest adjustment must and will take place...[17]

But access to enough food did not mean healthy nutrition. Several technical reports indicated that even in the best fed countries, between 20 to 30 percent of the population lacked food for a healthy, balanced dietary standard. Poverty and cooking traditions were to be blamed. In the underdeveloped countries much of the population, even before the war, suffered from food shortages and at times from actual starvation. If sufficient food should have been produced during the post-war years to feed all mankind to healthy standards, a great expansion of agriculture in all countries would have taken place. Even in the United States and in the United Kingdom, the production of the more expensive foods – animal products and fruit and vegetables – was not considered to be enough and an increase from 15 to 75 per cent was calculated.

In the late 1940s Boyd Orr argued that, considering the food problem in its global dimension, the production of the most expensive foods would need to be nearly doubled.[18] Under those circumstances, the role of industrialisation of food production appeared as a nuclear point and probably the only realistic prospect. The necessary amount of food could not be produced without an enormous quantity of industrial production, not only of agricultural implements and fertilisers but also,

---

17 Orr, John Boyd, "Can mankind make good? The answer depends on our supplying the world's paramount food need, says the Director General of the UN's FAO..." Survey Graphic, March, 1948, p. 97.

18 *Ibidem.*

for example, of capital equipment for irrigation and flood control and for the improvement of the means of transporting, storage and food preservation. The increase in the social level of the peasantry was essential, since food would not be produced "unless the man on the land has a standard of living comparable to that of workers engaged in other industries".[19]

The political economy of hunger and food was born at the end of World War II within the context of a dramatic landscape, one in which state governments and international organisations were called upon to save mankind from the huge risks lying ahead: science, technological power and moral and intellectual degradation.

> The Food and Agriculture Organization of the United Nations was established to enable nations to work together in carrying out a world food plan... The Two World Wars marked the convulsive end of an era. The atomic bomb, which fell in Hiroshima was both the death kernel of a passing age and the herald of the birth of a new age. This crisis in our civilization is due to modern science, which has advanced more in the last forty years than in the previous two thousand years. The great forces which science has let loose are pushing man into the new age for which he is ill prepared, morally and intellectually.
>
> The issue which he must now face is whether he will use science to destroy human society, or realize that the only hope of survival is the acceptance of the futility of war, and effective cooperation among nations to build a new civilization in which man can attain a level of physical and spiritual well-being beyond the dreams of the Utopians.[20]

The First Session of the Conference of the FAO, held in Quebec (October-November, 1945) established a primary objective for the organisation: to improve the levels of nutrition throughout the world, in order to ensure not only that all the population was out of any danger of starvation and famine, but also that they obtained the kind of diet essential for maintaining health.[21] To fulfill this target, a Nutrition Division was created in 1946 and a Standing Advisory Committee on Nutrition was convened to advise the Director-General of the FAO on the organisation's nutritional activities. At its first meeting, the broad lines of the FAO's nutrition programme were laid down.[22] The Standing

---

19 *Ibidem*, p. 98.

20 *Ibidem*

21 FAO, *Report of the first session of the conference,* Washington, 1946.

22 FAO Standing Advisory Committee on Nutrition, *First Report to the Director-General*, Rome, FAO Archives, Con 2/Un 1.

Advisory Committee on Nutrition also met in 1947 and 1948 to review the progress made and to recommend further projects and activities.

CHAPTER 8

World Food Surveys (1946-1960): Economy, Science, and Politics

At the end of World War II millions of people suffered from starvation and malnutrition was widespread in many regions in the world. Many of those who were undernourished were simply not getting enough food, yet a significant number of them were not really suffering from hunger at all; they were just not receiving the diet they needed for optimum health. FAO experts recognised in their first World Food Survey that vague knowledge confirming the existence of such a situation was not enough: "Facts and figures are needed if the nations are to attempt to do away with famine and malnutrition".[1] The issues that required more definite information in order to take practical action that would eradicate hunger, famine, nutritional diseases and malnutrition were: food consumption, food needs, shortages (ways to address these and other problems within a reasonable time) and adequate food production to satisfy global needs.

One of the FAO's early pieces of analytical work, which resulted in one of its first publications, was the first *World Food Survey*, published in 1946, just a few months after the end of the war.

> Given the complete breakdown of statistics during the war, the approach used was to estimate a baseline of pre-war calorie availability and compare them with postulated minimum nutritional standards. The baseline conclusion was that over half of the world's population had access to less than 2,250 calories per day; one-third had access to over 2,750 calories per day. And the remainder was in between. Thus, between half and two-thirds of the world population were undernourished before the war. The analysis concluded that things were worse after the war.[2]

As has already been discussed in previous chapters of this book, the world trading system prior to the big crisis of the 1930s – based on the gold standard and relatively free trade, which forced nations to adjust to

---

1 *World Food Survey.* Washington, Food and Agriculture Organization of the United Nations, 1946, p. 5.

2 McCalla, A.F., Revoredo, C.L., *Prospects for Global Food Security: A Critical Appraisal of Past Projections and Predictions*, Washington, DC, IFPRI, 2001, p. 26.

an international gold standard – finally collapsed in the 1930s, with competitive currency devaluations and increases in trade barriers. The failure of classical economic paradigms opened the door for the Keynesian turn, which focused economies on national variables of fiscal and monetary policy. International policy therefore had to adjust to domestic concerns. Thus, even under the exceptional circumstances of the post-war period, market economy development paradigms had to accept the role of the state as a dominant agent in managing the economy, with a focus on domestic planning. During those critical years, emphasis was placed on import-substitution and industrialisation programmes.

The implementation of this dominant economic development paradigm focused on the recovery of physical infrastructure because that was what the war had destroyed to a great extent. It also assisted national governments in pursuing appropriate policies and getting access to capital and technology for domestic industrial development. The beginnings of foreign assistance came with the implementation of the Marshall Plan, and later other bilateral assistance programmes followed, all of which stressed engineering and physical capital and advised a limited role for economic policy and particularly for social investment.

The idea that the expansion of the trade market was a path to development had not been discussed, and in many cases trade was seen as a source of inequality and exploitation. Therefore, protectionist policies were considered a legitimate part of national policy instruments. Agricultural development was predominantly seen as mainly a technical issue with a focus on machinery, dams, irrigation systems, roads, fertilisers and other facilities. Farmers and peasantry still represented a backward sector of the society, needing to be educated to use better and more advanced technology, which would lead to increased production and improve their incomes and standard of living. This opinion was a combination of a series of accepted ideas: that increases in the production of food were critical; that agriculture was technically backward; that the principle focus of economic policy should be inward looking; and that the nation state was responsible for feeding its people, leading inevitably in most people's mind to a food security paradigm of self-sufficiency.[3] But trading exclusively for one's food supply was a dangerous policy, as clearly many countries should have learned after two World Wars.

Once the idea of global governance was abandoned, and the project for a World Food Board set aside, how were the critical issues to be

---

3 *World Food Survey*, 1946.

addressed given the prevailing economic and political paradigms? The predominant economic ideology required the creation of an international network that preserved national sovereignty but encouraged and helped nations adjust to a more open and freely functioning set of international markets for goods, services and capital. While an individual nation might fear the liberalisation of trade if it thought that no one else would do likewise, and if there were a mechanism where all nations could agree and do it together, every one would be better off. If a country realised that its currency was over valued, it needed a structured mechanism to do the needful. The genius of the Bretton Woods Institutions and later GATT was to create organisations that could help to stabilise international markets while leaving in place the idea of national sovereignty over economic policy.

By offering monetary assistance, opportunities for growth and technical advice, the IMF, GATT and the World Bank supported national policy makers to become more outward looking. If nations could meet and debate their differences and approximate positions, and even though agreements were not attained, the chances of conflict would be lessened. If the better off could help the ravaged and the less well off grow more rapidly, peace would be more likely. Thus the United Nations itself and its specialised agencies such as the World Bank, the FAO and the WHO could provide technical assistance, policy advice and long-term capital for reconstruction and development, without interfering with the internal policies of the states.

In agriculture, if the global community wanted to help, the best way was with technical, biological and mechanical assistance and funds for domestic investments. After the failure of Boyd Orr, and a more ambitious programme of global governance of food markets, the FAO focused on creating the best conditions for technical relief. External relief was a major necessity in many regions in the world. A noteworthy fact is that it would take at least 15 years for the World Bank to start to show much interest in agriculture. The United Nations and its then emerging specialised agencies, such as the FAO, dominated the landscape. The developed countries that were not deeply damaged by the war played a part. By far the most dominant was the United States, which provided capital, technical assistance and policy promotion in many ways, including the Marshall Plan, which swamped efforts to move capital by the newly created World Bank. Other countries such as Canada, Australia and South Africa provided funds and technical assistance. The European pre-war colonial powers such as the United Kingdom, France and the Netherlands had tropical agricultural research organisations, which potentially could help developing countries and

Latin America, and the Rockefeller Foundation developed agricultural programmes in Mexico and other countries.

The First World Food Survey (1946): the Pre-war Food Picture and Strategies for the Short Term

The First World Food Survey published in 1946 was prepared by two working groups, one in charge of nutrition targets and the second devoted to reporting on the food consumption before the war. Two working groups were appointed, with the following experts:

1. Nutrition targets:

- Boudreau, Frank, G. Executive Director of the Milbank Memorial Fund, New York

- Cassels, John M., Office of International Trade Operations, Department of Commerce, Washington

- Maynard, John M., School of Nutrition, Cornell University, Ithaca, New York

- Miranda, Francisco, Director of National Institute of Nutrition, Department Public Health, Mexico DF

- Phipard, Esther F., Bureau of Human Nutrition and Home Economics, Department of Agriculture, Washington

- Roberts, Lydia J., Director Home Economics, University Puerto Rico, Río Piedras

- Stiebeling, Hazel K., Chief Bureau of Human Nutrition and Home Economics, Department Agriculture, Washington.

2. Pre-war Food Consumption:

- Becker, Joseph A., International Commodities, Office Foreign Agricultural Relations, Department of Agriculture, Washington

- Gibbons, Charles A., Bureau of Agricultural Economics, Department of Agriculture, Washington

- Klatt, Werner, Senior Statistician, Ministry of Food, London, England

- Knight, H.V., Senior Statistician, Ministry of Food, London, England

- Malenbaum, Wilfred, Special Assistant to the Director, Office of Intelligence, Coordination and Liaison, Department of State, Washington

- Peter, Hollis W., Head of Food and Agriculture Section, International, Functional, and Intelligence Division, Department of State, Washington

- Wells, O.V., Chief, Bureau of Agricultural Economics, Department of Agriculture, Washington.

The expert committees examined the information available for 70 countries in the pre-war period and they observed great variations both in the calorie intake and in the dietary patterns among the population in these countries. The reports indicated that the food supply of over half of the world's population furnished an average of less than 2,250 calories per caput per day. At the other extreme, less than a third of the world's population had an intake of more than 2,750, and the rest, affecting about one sixth of the world's population, were between these two levels. The high calorie intake areas included most of the Western countries, Oceania and the USSR, but only three countries in South America.[4] The medium-calorie regions included most of the Southern European countries, three countries in Asia, a part of the Middle East, a part of Africa and a part of South America, whilst the low-calorie regions included most of Asia, a part of the Middle East and all of Central America. Some parts of South America and Africa were not included in the survey due to the absence of reliable records. With this data it was easy to come to the conclusion that the world food situation was in dire straits. The experts stressed the fact that the average calorie intake of a country served as a general guide only and that it was important to understand that some people obtained considerably more than the average, while a large number had less; even in the countries with the highest rates of calorie intake a considerable part of the population was not well nourished in accordance with health standards.

The areas of greater deficiency were Central America, most of Asia and probably many parts of South America and Africa not covered by the survey.

> Many of the low-calorie countries are located in the tropics and subtropics. In these countries, food energy requirements may be lower than in colder countries. The average body size of the people is usually smaller. Demographically, the proportion of children in the population is usually greater as well, due to high birth and death rates. These factors, however, cannot account for the great difference in the per caput daily calorie intake between the lowest and the highest-intake countries. A population with a high percentage of children, for example, would require 100-150 fewer calories per person per day (but relatively more minerals and vitamins) than a population with an aging demographic profile now typical of Western civilization. As noted earlier, the actual difference is around 1,000 calories

4 *Ibidem*, p. 6-7.

per person per day. Calorie intake in the low-calorie countries is only two-thirds of that seen in high-calorie countries.[5]

It was evident in the first WFS that before the war about half of the world's population was subsisting at a level of food consumption that was not high enough to maintain health standards, allow for normal growth of children, or furnish enough energy for normal work. Poor nutrition was associated with high death rates and a low life expectancy, high infant and child mortality, increased susceptibility to many diseases such as tuberculosis and impaired working capacity.[6]

In addition to calorie intake, the composition of diets showed great variation that depended on food habits and the availability of food supplies. Obviously, when the average calorie levels were around 3,000 or more, diets were generally balanced. The United Kingdom, Scandinavia, the Netherlands, Switzerland and Germany were in this group. In all these countries the consumption of cereals in relation to that of other foods represented about 1,000 calories, while milk and meat consumption were comparatively high, with animal protein accounting for about 50 grammes.

This dietary pattern contrasted sharply with that of countries where the average total calorie supplies were around 2,000 calories or less. This group included Far East countries such as India, Indonesia, the Philippines and Korea, as well as some Middle East countries (Iran, Iraq, and Transjordan), Central America (Mexico, El Salvador, Costa Rica) and South America countries (Colombia). In this group of countries a high proportion of calories was obtained from cheaper foods rich in carbohydrates, especially cereals. The evidence put forward by the first WFS was clear: that poverty was the chief cause of malnutrition. The survey compared pre-war calorie consumption with national incomes per capita, and all the countries in which the supply of calories was less than 2,250 per person per day were countries in which the average income was less than $100 per caput per year.

Once the world food consumption had been examined by groups of countries and world regions, the next step forward was to set up nutritional targets that showed the changes in food supplies, which were considered necessary to provide the population with a better and healthier diet. The spread of dietary standards for international application became one of the fundamental concerns of the FAO and the WHO during the post-war years. In the USA, the recommended daily

5 *Ibidem*, p. 8.

6 *Ibidem*.

allowances of the National Research Council were widely accepted and applied by official agencies. However, the experts considered these standards provisional as they represented the consensus of experts at a given time and were subject to modification, as was scientific knowledge itself.[7]

In practical terms, in those countries, regions or social groups where food consumption was considered to be quantitatively adequate, the so-called *optimum standards* could be applied as a target, to determine the changes in food supply that were needed to improve the quality of national diets. In many of the countries with a medium calorie intake, and especially in all those with low intake rates, consumption goals had to be set considerably below the optimum levels, if they were to be achieved in a reasonable amount of time and at the required proportion. Those intermediate steps were considered to be milestones or intermediate goals that generally improved world nutrition.

A small group of nutritional experts convened by the FAO in 1946 to discuss the question of targets took as a point of reference the pre-war standards, agreeing that weight should be given to the 1946 position regarding the production and supplies of various foods. Targets called for the modification of existing dietary patterns rather than for revolutionary changes. They suggested the following principles:

a) A calorie intake between 2,550 and 2,650 was to be considered a minimum level to which intake should be raised and the quantities of additional foods required should be estimated on this basis.

b) If calories from cereals fell between 1,200 and 1,800, no change was recommended, but if they fell below 1,200 and the total calorie intake was below 2,600, some increase in cereal intake was recommended, unless the total calories from cereals, starchy roots, tubers, starchy fruits, sugar, fats, and pulses exceeded 2,000 to 2,100. If calories from cereals exceeded 1,800 and total calories were high, decreasing the former was considered the best solution.

c) An intake of 100 to 200 calories from starchy roots, tubers and starchy fruits (such as bananas) was set as a desirable objective, although a larger amount was advocated if intake of cereals was low and adequate amounts of protein could be obtained from pulses, milk, meat and fish.

d) Intake of sugar should not exceed 10 to 15 per cent of total calories.

e) Total daily calories from fats should be at least 100 and preferably 150 to 200.

---

[7] *Ibidem*, p. 11.

f) In countries where pulses constituted an important part of the diet, calories from this source could reach 250 to 300 daily. Meat supplies in these countries were under 150 calories and animal proteins limited. Even when meat calories amount to 200-250, calories from pulses might be pushed to 200-250. Pulse intake should be considered in relation to the intake of cereals, starchy roots, tubers, starchy fruits, milk and meat.

g) Calories from fruit and vegetables should total at least 100 per caput daily. Leafy green, yellow vegetables and fruit rich in vitamin C were the best option, with the recommended quantities calculated in relation to their nutritional value: their vitamin and caloric content.

h) Meat, fish and eggs should amount to no less than 100 calories per caput daily and preferably 150 to 200. If the intake of milk and pulses was high, the contribution of fish and meat calories could be proportionally reduced to balance each other.

i) The minimum desirable level of consumption of milk and milk products was calculated between 300 and 400 calories per caput daily. Milk consumption as well as intake levels could be compensated by a combination of pulses, leafy green and yellow vegetables, providing important nutrients of milk.

On the basis of the criteria proposed by the FAO Nutrition Committee, and according to the principles of the experimental science of nutrition, specific targets were drawn up for 18 areas. This covered 70 countries, in terms of total calorie intake and calories from various food groups, taking into consideration pre-war standards of consumption in each of those countries and areas, for purposes of comparison.

> Because of the great variation in existing consumption and in the nutritive value of national diets, it was considered impracticable to put forward targets calling for a uniform degree of nutritional adequacy. In countries in which food supplies were insufficient in quantity as well as unsatisfactory in quality, the first step was to consider the increases in food supplies necessary to raise calorie intake to a reasonable level of sufficiency. Targets for countries in which pre-war food supplies yielded less than 2,600 calories per caput daily have been adjusted to bring the calorie level to 2,600 (plus or minus 50). For countries with calorie supplies above this level, adjustments were made to improve the quality of the diet while the same energy value as in the pre-war period was maintained.[8]

In the WFS, the experts stressed that improving nutritional quality was more necessary than increasing total food supplies; a satisfactory distribution of food and a change in food habits was considered a

8 *Ibidem*, p. 14.

priority as well. Countries with inadequate food supplies were called on to obtain the additional food needed to raise nutritional levels by importing from other countries, increasing their own production or a combination of both. Great Britain represented the first case in the post-war period, since the supplies produced by its own agricultural activities could not meet the requirements of the population. It was able to satisfy its needs by exchanging goods and services for food from other countries. A meaningful expression of this policy is that during the war the United Kingdom increased its food production by about 70 per cent in terms of calories due to an adequate policy of rationing and food management.

Although many thought that international trade would become increasingly important after 1946, much of the additional supplies required by the low-calorie intake countries to reach the consumption goals would have to be obtained by expanding their own food production. In most of the less developed countries people lived mainly on a vegetarian diet, which often lacked sufficient quantities of proteins, important vegetables and fruit, and therefore the targets required diets containing more foods of animal origin. Yet this issue was not free of controversy. Nutritional experts introduced the term *original calories*, to mention calories yielded by crops. When crops were used to feed animals instead of being eaten directly by humans, about seven of these *original calories* were required to produce one calorie from animal products.[9]

As the experts believed that by 1960 original calories would have to be increased by 90 per cent in comparison with the pre-war value, with 55 per cent of this increase accounted for by improvements in the diet and 35 per cent by population growth, improvements in farming efficiency were seen as being essential to meeting their goals. The instruments needed to face the challenge included more efficient fertilisers, better varieties of crop plants and seeds, plague and parasitic control, efficient tools and new machinery. This was summarised as a need for better land use all over the world.

The political dimension of the programme was evident and a worldwide agricultural reform was deemed to be the only solution: land ownership, funds, technical improvement and price regulation were some of the issues discussed by the international experts as being central to the economic reforms required to solve the international crisis after the war:

9 *Ibidem*, p. 19.

> Since food production is the most important aspect of the whole economy and way of living of most peoples, a wide range of economic and social changes will be involved in making extensive improvements. For example, unjust and oppressive systems of land tenure which give the cultivator neither opportunity nor incentive to improve his lot will need to be swept away. Since most methods of increasing food production necessitate an outlay of capital, satisfactory systems for supplying credit to farmers are essential; in most countries they do not exist. The capacity of the farmer to develop his land depends to a large extent on the price of primary agricultural products; he must therefore obtain a fair return for the food he produces, and consumers must have the purchasing power to give him a fair return.[10]

Increasing individual productivity was identified as being at the heart of the problem. Some European countries had a large population in relation to land area and enjoyed relatively high standards of living because their production of wealth in the form of goods and services was relatively high. In some European countries a fifth of the population was devoted to agriculture, producing foodstuffs that were capable of supplying around 8,000 calories per caput daily: one farm family could feed itself and four other families at a comparatively high nutritional level. If new technologies were applied this proportion would improve. By contrast, in many poor countries, two thirds or more of the population produced an inferior diet of 2,800 to 3,000 original calories for the country as a whole, and one farm family managed to produce only enough to feed itself and half of another family.[11]

Land resources for agricultural production were limited, and when population growth was high, rural underemployment and inefficiency were inevitable. This critical situation prompted experts to call for rapid, large-scale development of industry and trade, as well as the implementation of instructive programmes oriented to peasants and farmers and the modernisation of all services involved. To do this, a large investment of both capital and technical skills was needed. "All nations will gain by world advances in human health and wellbeing and in production and trade, and all must participate in bringing them to pass".[12]

The experts mentioned the enormous achievements of a significant number of Western nations during the war as proof that improvements in technical tools and skills, as well as great economic expansion, were

[10] *Ibidem*, p. 22.

[11] *Ibidem*, p. 24.

[12] *Ibidem*, pp. 24-25.

realistic. However, during the post-war years, the need for adequate international action was considered to be not only convenient but also necessary to avoid a regression to the trends of the 1930 crisis. Altogether, between 1929 and 1939, the world failed to deal with the situation created by the application of science to agriculture and was unable to absorb the increased food supplies thereby made available. The WFS partly attributed this to disorganisation in food production, instability and fluctuations in the whole economic system. Solutions could not come from separate initiatives of individual nations acting alone and from attempts to deal with commodities separately, without global coordination. Food experts were convinced that unilateral action would inevitably worsen the general situation, creating barriers, new problems and competition instead of complementation.[13]

The political economy of scientific knowledge required global governance and new directions: "After the failure of the World Economic Conference in 1933, a new approach was developed in the international sphere. The science of nutrition had advanced far enough to make it possible to define with some accuracy the kinds of diets needed for health, and it had become clear that the greater part of the world's population was getting far less than good nutrition required".[14]

As has been discussed in a previous chapter, in 1935 the Assembly of the League of Nations authorised the League to report on the effect of improved nutrition upon health and the relation of nutrition to agricultural and economic problems. In the years that followed the Mixed Committee on Nutrition of the League of Nations reviewed these problems and urged governments to develop food policies that would improve nutrition, especially in the lower income groups, and simultaneously reduce agricultural surpluses. As a result, a number of nations established national nutrition organisations to advise governments on policies for nutritional improvement. However, the war interrupted the initiative before much progress was made.

At the end of the war it was clear that a food crisis had swept the world. The food situation rapidly deteriorated and the experts foresaw that the shortages of fats, meat, dairy products and sugar would remain acute for a considerable amount of time; the supply of grain was seriously insufficient at the end of 1945. Among the main causes that led to this shortage were obviously the devastation produced by the war, but also the serious dislocation of the world agricultural economy and trade and the war's dismantling of the world's transport system. The

13 *Ibidem*, p. 27.

14 *Ibidem*, p. 28.

series of droughts from 1945-46 added to the negative context, becoming culminating factors.[15] Moreover, the post-war food crisis was expected to last. To address the situation and minimise the effects, an International Emergency Food Council was set up to replace the Combined Food Board, the result of a Special Meeting on Urgent Food Problems called by the FAO in May 1946. Although local governments and nations were forced to take immediate decisions to solve short-term problems, it was evident that global food policies required international action. The First World Food Survey (1946) supported the idea that the world's needs required planning and organisation in the field of production, trade, marketing and finance, which neither producers nor nations acting by themselves could carry out. The experts supported the arguments contained in the *Proposals for a World Food Board*, the first big disappointment in the implementation of a globally managed political economy of food and hunger after World War II.

Surveys on the State of Food and Agriculture in Europe (1948-1949)

Three years after the termination of hostilities and the founding of the FAO, a survey of world conditions and prospects concerning the state of food and agriculture was published.[16] In 1948 experts and politicians became aware that the short-term crisis announced for 1945-47 had been underestimated. Full employment was found almost everywhere in the recovering countries of Europe and the Far East, in the developing countries of Latin America and in countries undergoing expansion, such as the United States and Canada. Although large amounts of money were generated, the output of consumption was inadequate to match the level of consumer purchasing power.

> The experiences of the war have brought food to occupy a central position in government policy in many countries and it may ultimately take such a position in all countries. Furthermore, the persistent scarcity of supplies and the emergency of special problems, which will presently be discussed, impelled governments at the last session of the FAO Conference to recognize the need for periodic discussion of the state of food and agriculture.[17]

---

15 *Ibidem*, p. 29.

16 *The State of Food and Agriculture-1948. A Survey of World Conditions and Prospects*, Washington, Food and Agriculture Organization of the United Nations, [September] 1948.

17 *Ibidem*, p. 2.

In the report on the state of food and agriculture published in 1948, a chapter was devoted to Europe as one of the higher-income, densely populated regions, emerging from World War II with important losses that, according to the experts, had been underestimated:

> Because industrial production, apart from Germany, is back to the pre-war level, because bridges have been rebuilt and the railways are operating again, there is a misleading impression that Europe is already far along the road to recovery. On closer examination the situation is more serious. Some of the capital losses can never be replaced: for example, most of the overseas investments, which were liquidated. Some of the industry cannot be rebuilt, but must be replaced by new industries, which have a better chance of finding new export markets. And behind this lies the immense backlog of investment needs in houses, schools, hospitals, and other public services.[18]

Europe faced two main agricultural problems associated with production on the one hand and distribution of the products on the other. European countries aimed to recover and exceed pre-war levels, especially in the production of milk, cereals and potatoes. Eastern European countries planned for a substantial expansion in food production. Most European countries achieved a comparatively high standard of living through intense specialisation and the exchange of large amounts of manufactured products for raw materials and food. But food was still scarce and expensive because of an increased retention for consumption in food-exporting countries. This situation gave rise to the problem of international trade. Indeed, the European reality was plural and variable, with contrasts between highly industrialised countries mainly in the Northwest and predominantly agricultural countries in the South. For example, the population density ranged from 291 inhabitants per square kilometre in the Netherlands to as low as 42 inhabitants per square kilometre in Albania, and income levels varied greatly from over $500 per caput in the United Kingdom to just over $50 in Greece and Yugoslavia.

Prices of farm products had risen sharply in almost all European countries during and since the war and governments intervened to fix them. In those countries where price controls were maintained, the differences largely reflected the increased costs of livestock production arising from the scarcity of protein feed. At this juncture, production prospects for 1948-49 were favourable throughout Europe:

> From preliminary returns now available, it would appear that the production of bread grains in Europe this year will exceed 1947 production by about 15

18 *Ibidem*, p. 98.

> million tons. About 75 per cent of this increase affects importing countries. Noteworthy examples of better prospects are France and Italy. The new crop in France is estimated to be over twice as large as in 1947. These results are due to exceptional weather, however, and somewhat exaggerate the degree of recovery really attained by this date.[19]

Notwithstanding the social crisis derived from the war, in Western Europe in 1948 there were some 11 million more people than before the war on the reduced land area resulting from the change in the frontiers with Germany. In Eastern Europe, the production of foodstuffs was extremely slow and many countries in the area were anxious to import goods from outside Europe in order to maintain food consumption at least at a minimum level. Average levels of imports from 1946 to 1948 compared with pre-war levels were as follows:[20]

- Imports over 100 per cent of pre-war levels were registered in Germany, Italy, Spain, Portugal, Poland, Czechoslovakia and Romania.

- Imports between 80 to 100 per cent of pre-war levels for Finland, France, Yugoslavia and Greece.

- Imports between 60 to 80 per cent of pre-war levels in Norway, Sweden, United Kingdom, Belgium, Luxembourg and Switzerland.

- Imports under 50 per cent of pre-war levels in Denmark, Netherlands, Ireland, Austria, Hungary and Bulgaria.

In Western Europe, during the period 1946 to 1948, the imports of grain, sugar and fats were lower than pre-war imports and those of meat, eggs, and dairy products were higher. One must take into consideration that imports of grain, sugar, and fats were constricted by physical limitations and were subject to the allocation procedures of the International Emergency Food Committee. Conversely, the increased imports of animal products represented a partial compensation for the great fall in exports within Western Europe. Only a few countries had surpluses, such as Denmark and Ireland, with the levels not much more than half of what they were before the war. The level in the Netherlands was much lower. During the post-war years a substantial shift occurred in Western Europe's sources of food; before the war a quarter of food imports came from other European countries, while in 1948 this European trade had almost disappeared.

As regards consumption, in 1948 the consumption of bread, potatoes and milk in Western Europe had declined significantly, showing great differences between several regions and countries. In most countries the

19 *Ibidem*, p. 100.

20 *Ibidem.*

percentage of calories obtained from cereals and potatoes remained very high, with an intake of animal protein that was abnormally low compared with the pre-war period, particularly in Austria, Hungary, Finland, Yugoslavia, Spain and Germany.[21]

There was, however, a steady improvement in the state of health of the European population since 1947. In most countries, the average heights and weights of children were found to surpass the levels of the previous post-war years, although many could not attain pre-war levels. School-age children were usually found to have improved more than adolescents. While in the Netherlands the average heights and weights of school children were back to pre-war levels, the evidence showed that in the United Kingdom adolescents were on average lighter in 1947 than they were in 1945. In Finland, Greece and Germany, adolescents appeared to be the most underweight and under height.[22] A positive indicator was the declining tendency of infant mortality rates, as the following table shows:

Infant Mortality Rates in Selected European Countries (per 1000 births)

Country	1937	1946	1947
Austria	92	81	76
Belgium	83	75	75
Bulgaria	150	124	
Czechoslovakia	117	109	
Denmark	66	46	
Finland	69	56	59
France	65	73	66
Hungary	134	114	111
Italy	109	84	82
Netherlands	38	39	34
United Kingdom	61	43	

Source: The State of Food and Agriculture - 1948

21 *Ibidem*, p. 108.

22 *Ibidem*.

Tuberculosis was mentioned as a major problem in some countries, and deficiency diseases such as pellagra affected Romania, although the rate of undernourishment was considered to be lower than in previous years. In 1948 rationing of basic foods was still in force in most European countries:

> Some countries make allocations according to physiological needs, as in the United Kingdom; others use rationing as a form of wage supplements, as in Poland, or to provide incentive for work of certain types, as in Germany. Most countries, however, make provision to some extent for the vulnerable groups in the population, and some have steeply differentiated allowances, especially of milk, as in Germany and Finland. While some countries, like Italy, are completely or partially de-rationing certain foods, others are finding it necessary to impose more stringent controls. Greece plans to include a greater number of foods in its ration scheme and Czechoslovakia has had to ratio potatoes, vegetables and cheese and to cut rations of other foods drastically.[23]

Community feeding was expanding in Europe. Many countries had previous experience from the economic crisis of the 1930s and older schemes based on public canteens chiefly devoted to children, pregnant and nursing women and workers were again implemented. The programme *International Children's Emergency Fund* was established by the United Nations and operated in 12 European countries, mostly in Eastern, Central and Southern Europe. The neediest children received a meal consisting of protective foods provided by UNICEF, notably dried skimmed milk, matched by local foods of equal caloric value provided by the government of the country. In 1948 the scheme helped four million children, who received basic meals such as breakfast. This was successfully implemented in Greece and consisted of a milk drink and a slice of milk raisin bread.

The number of school children receiving school meals in the United Kingdom had grown spectacularly, from four per cent of the total in pre-war time to 52 per cent in 1948. In addition, 88 per cent of school-age children received free school milk as well. After the war, Finland introduced a decree making it compulsory for schools to supply meals. In Norway, the so-called *Oslo breakfast* was served to 91 per cent of school children for free and consisted of a simple nutritious meal. At the end of the 1940s half the children in Germany enjoyed a ration-free school meal as well. All these different school feeding programmes were widespread among all European countries. The initiative was

---

[23] *Ibidem*, pp. 108-109.

shown to have a beneficial effect on the health and growth of children in European countries, mitigating the critical post-war food situation.

Food for workers, on the other hand, was implemented in many cases as an emergency measure during the war, and in the years that followed, the scheme was maintained to minimise the negative effects of acute shortages on the health of the population and worker strength and productivity. The initiatives spread throughout Europe, becoming a permanent institution in many countries. Much experience had been accumulated since the first initiatives that were put in place during the crisis that affected the 1930s.

Due to the critical situation of the post-war years, there was widespread interest in nutrition education in Europe, an approach requiring staff, funds and a cooperative attitude among all the groups involved. A number of countries, including the Netherlands and the United Kingdom, established permanent organisations for nutrition education; others, like Greece, started work in the same direction. Most of the National Schools of Public Health, as in the case of Spain, developed specific programmes to spread nutritional information, preparing propaganda and popularisation programmes in the rural districts and specific programmes for mothers on dietary needs, cooking and the feeding of children. Some experts working in national institutes became specialised in nutritional popularisation, writing books for the public-at-large, with lectures, films, leaflets and audiovisual materials.[24] If Carrasco Cadenas is a typical example in Spain of this new figure of doctor-nutritionist devoting intense activity in educating the population, many academics and rural doctors developed similar initiatives. This was the case of Isadore Julius Wolf, a family doctor and professor at the Kansas School of Medicine, and author of a well-known book that popularised dietetics.[25] Teaching nutrition to medical students and public health specialists was another initiative, as well as the creation of university degrees in this field. We shall take a more in-depth look at these programmes in the years that followed in a later chapter.

All European countries designed policies and programmes during the post-war years, not only to restore the pre-war level of food production, but also to increase agricultural efficiency. In Eastern and Mediterranean

24 Carrasco Cadenas, E., *Ni gordos, ni flacos. Lo que se debe comer*, Madrid, Diana, 1935; Carrasco Cadenas, E., "Escuela Nacional de Sanidad. Sección de Higiene de la Alimentación y de la Nutrición y Técnica Bromatológica. Su orientación y programa de trabajo al año y medio de su organización", *Revista de Sanidad e Higiene Pública*, 1933, Vol. 8, pp. 258-260.

25 Wolff, I.J, *The Human Fuel*, Boston, Chapman & Grimes, 1936. I want to thank Kathy Fabiani-Wolf for information about the man, his activities and publications.

Europe, emphasis was placed upon increasing crop yields, diversification of production and improvement in the quality of livestock, notably dairy cattle, whose milk yields were less than half of that in the West. In Western Europe the emphasis was placed mostly on better use of grassland, better livestock and increased cultivation of fruit, vegetables and other specialty crops.[26] Western European farming depended heavily upon the use of large supplies of raw materials, such as fertilisers and feed, most of which were normally imported from abroad. Future programmes envisaged a substantial increase in production and in the use of tractors and other forms of mechanised agriculture. Indeed, the outstanding tendency in Eastern European programmes at the end of the 1940s was to increase industrialisation and efficiently organise the absorption of agricultural populations into other occupations. This trend indirectly aided agriculture by leaving remaining farm families with more farmland; hitherto, their holdings had been, on average, notably smaller and less economically efficient than those of Western Europe.

Agricultural production faced a great challenge: it needed to be intensified, adapted to the requirements of growing urban populations and to the export markets. However, the extension and output of cereals in 1950-51 was expected to be still below pre-war figures. The aim was to increase potato yields, with the exception of Poland and Czechoslovakia, where the pre-war production was considered to be excessive. The programme aimed for more sugar beets, oilseeds and industrial crops such as flax, hemp, cotton and tobacco. While the intention was to increase yields far beyond pre-war averages, this was not expected to happen before 1951.[27] The number of horses and other draft animals had not recovered in Eastern Europe, even though programmes that favoured the introduction of tractors had not been fully implemented. The number of cows had not fully recovered either, although the number of pigs and poultry was expected to be well above pre-war figures. Meat production had largely recovered, especially pork. More fish was also available, but milk and dairy products were significantly below pre-war standards. In the whole of Europe the grain-producing area and the output in 1950-51 was expected to be slightly lower than pre-war figures. In contrast, more potatoes, sugar, fruit and vegetables were expected. In France and the United Kingdom, yields were expected to be higher than pre-war levels, and in other countries

---

26 *The State of Food and Agriculture-1948.*

27 *Ibidem*, p. 111.

more ambitious plans for agricultural growth and efficiency in production were established.

Considered as a whole, these production programmes aimed for an extremely rapid recovery from the condition in which agriculture was left at the end of the war, but it was not expected that livestock production goals could be reached before 1953. In 1948 European governments were collaborating under the auspices of the FAO to solve a number of technical issues in the agricultural and food production programmes. For instance, conferences on soil conservation and infestation control were held in Italy, and others took place at the end of November 1948 in Poland on animal diseases and in the Danube countries on the dissemination of hybrid corn.

In addition to the issues involved in improving food production, others existed concerning international trade, an essential aspect of the problem. Yet this depended to a greater extent on factors outside the control of the national governments, and therefore plans calling for coordination of nations formulated by international organisations could not be precise or possess executive power. It was expected that Eastern European countries would again become part of a food-exporting area, although in 1951 net exports of grain were not expected to exceed one million tons, compared with three million in the pre-war period. Yet the exports of meat, eggs and sugar were expected to be substantially above pre-war levels, particularly in Poland, Hungary and Yugoslavia. This was a consequence of the intensification of agriculture, with the challenge for these countries being to process primary agricultural products, such as cereals, and redirect them into exports instead of livestock products. In Eastern Europe, the pressure of increasing internal demand as a result of a certain degree of industrial development might have reduced the export surpluses, and trade tended to be mostly focused on the Soviet Union rather than other parts of Europe. The industrialisation programmes implemented in Eastern European countries required high imports of machinery and other production equipment, which could be obtained from Western Europe, this becoming a source of intra-European trade.[28] On the other hand, in Western Europe food imports were expected to be greater than in pre-war years, particularly for grains, sugar, meat, cheese and processed milk. But the imports of rice and fats remained below pre-war levels.[29]

Food production and international trade was a key issue for economic recovery after the war. However, the main point from a health

[28] *Ibidem*, p. 113.

[29] *Ibidem*, pp. 113-114.

perspective was the recovery of the poor levels of consumption. In both Eastern and Western Europe, the general trends showed that the average caloric supply of the population was expected to return to pre-war levels in 1951, being already somewhat above that level in Poland and Czechoslovakia, and significantly lower in Finland, Germany, Austria, Hungary and Yugoslavia.

> The diet in most countries should be better balanced than at present, particularly in certain countries with previously unsatisfactory nutritional standards. In Eastern Europe, a significant increase is anticipated in consumption of sugar and fats, which formerly was very low, and consumption of vegetables, fruits, and eggs will probably increased. In most western Europe the wartime increase in potato consumption is likely to disappear and consumption of milk, vegetables, and fruits to rise. However, most governments have milk consumption targets, which cannot be fully realized as early as 1950/51.[30]

Countries envisaged nutritional surveys on the diet and nutritional status of the population and educational campaigns as the basis for national food-distribution programmes. Similarly, nutritional education was considered to become an essential tool in improving health and living conditions. "Some countries such as Poland, Czechoslovakia and Italy are making a start in collecting data. During the past year Greece and Belgium have set up national nutrition organizations. There is an urgent need for standardization of field methods and agreement on criteria of nutritional status as the present results often convey no clear meaning".[31]

Indeed, the future level of food consumption in Europe depended in large measure upon the extent to which these countries could expand their national production of industrial and other goods, as well as on the success in obtaining export markets for a part of their output. "Europe's pre-war standard of living, although unsatisfactory in many countries, was as high as it was only on the basis of considerable specialization of labour".[32] Even if the development of industries in other continents made it increasingly hard for Europe to find new fields of profitable specialisation, the rapid recovery of industrial production in 1948, coupled with a significant recovery in exports, led experts to believe that Europe might find ways of recapturing and even improving on its former standard of living, in the different conditions of the post-war

---

30 *Ibidem*, p. 115.

31 *Ibidem*.

32 *Ibidem*.

period. Technical analysis of the political economy of food and health was abundant during post-war years.

A second survey was published by the FAO expert committee in 1949, devoted to the state of food and agriculture.[33] A specific section discussed the situation in Europe. It seemed evident to the experts that there had been a notable improvement in those European countries in which diet and the nutritional state of the population were already satisfactory before the war. In contrast, for those nations in which food intake had been traditionally low, the situation was notably deficient. From a global perspective, these regions contained most of the world population. Total food supplies were still highly inadequate and inequalities in the distribution had increased. It was therefore extremely important to pay attention not only to the resources available to stimulate agriculture, improve efficiency and establish better channels for food trade, but also to providences that could bring about an improvement of available foodstuffs, considering their nutritional value. The international experts suggested a series of strategies that would globally address improvement in food policies:

a) The implementation of food rationing schemes. In certain countries, especially in the United Kingdom, food rationing had allowed for a better use of food provisions in periods of scarcity. However, it should be noted that effective rationing programmes could be hardly implemented within those countries, which mainly depended upon foodstuffs produced locally and also when there existed great differences among social groups. In any case food-rationing schemes provided the national authorities with an instrument that safeguarded official distribution paths and ensured minimum access to food to avoid exclusion.

b) Beneficial methods to improve diet. A diet mainly based on extensive production of cereals could lead to deficient nutritional levels. However, foodstuffs enhanced with vitamins and minerals may be rejected by the public. As these beneficial actions were the result of industrial procedures under sanitary control, any resistance to these products on the part of the public could be minimized with the implementation of well designed information and education campaigns.

c) A specific instance of the previous point was food enriched with vitamins and minerals, which was thought to provide unquestionable benefits to a healthy diet.

---

33 *El Estado Mundial de la Agricultura y la Alimentación. Las condiciones actuales y sus perspectivas*, Washington, Organización de las Naciones Unidas para la Agricultura y la Alimentación, [octubre] 1949.

d) Education programmes for better nutrition for the entire population and other programmes oriented to specific groups such as farmers, peasants, housewives, mothers, teachers and doctors. Any change in dietary habits and cooking practices was usually the result of a slow and difficult process, which was, on the other hand, highly recommended. Nutritional education tended to stimulate the demand for different dietary products of higher nutritional value, although it could also increase profit from existing provisions.

e) Supplementary feeding. Nutritional deficiencies were not a result of foods with relatively poor nutritional value alone, they might also arise from a physiological need for more nutrients under special conditions, such as quick growth, pregnancy or heavy work. Therefore, supplementary feeding programmes became more important for children and adolescents, pregnant and nursing women, as well as for industrial workers.

Nutrition programmes were to be based on solid knowledge about the nutritional state of the population in a country, region or rural area, according to the information contained in food surveys and the knowledge derived from research on the nutritional value of available foodstuffs. It is remarkable that in 1950 the implementation of nutritional programmes was absolutely necessary, not only in those countries in which the population was poor and undernourished but even in other countries with apparently sufficient food provisions; these countries might have been suffering from poor distribution, which may have led to poor nutrition among a significant proportion of the population. It was only through programmes of this type that people in either of these situations were able to prevent nutritional deficiencies and increase health standards.

The Second World Food Survey (1952)

After the two surveys on the state of food and agriculture published in 1948 and 1949, a second *World Food Survey* was published by the FAO in 1952, showing, once more, a critical picture of the world food situation. The survey touched on three aspects in particular: food production, trade and consumption. Thus, the 1952 World Food Survey showed the overwhelming interest of FAO experts in the importance of increasing food production in areas previously ravaged by the war and in the growing numbers of newly independent countries – India, Pakistan and Indonesia being some of the early states to gain independence in the late 1940s.

But by 1950 concern over growing grain surpluses in richer countries increased, in part due to rapid agricultural recovery in Europe and Japan. Therefore an early divide between the rich and the poor regions in the world emerged. This converse situation and its substantially different challenges made these countries – the FAO's main source of funding – question the organisation's emphasis on increasing production in the face of surpluses.

To start with, Norris E. Dodd, the FAO Director-General, qualified the First World Food Survey of 1946 as the first major accomplishment of the FAO since its creation. Several years later FAO authorities thought it necessary to gauge the progress made towards the previously defined objectives and discuss the prospects for the future. The Second World Food Survey was essentially concerned with the same basic questions, now examined in the light of changes that had occurred in the post-war years and available knowledge. Nevertheless, the general assessment advanced by Norris E. Dodd was far from being optimistic:

> The new information gives no ground for complacency. The average food supply per person over large areas of the world, five years after war was over, was still lower than before the war. The proportion of the world's population with inadequate food supplies has grown appreciably larger. World food production has indeed expanded since the end of the war, when it fell to a low point, but much of this achievement represents merely a recovery from wartime devastation and dislocation. Clear signs of any far-reaching changes in the entire scale of food production, essential for the improvement of nutrition on a wide scale, are lacking. Annual increases in food production are barely keeping pace with the increasing population. The intensification of health measures in under-developed countries, in particular the use of new methods for controlling mass diseases such as malaria, is likely to lead to a still more rapid growth in numbers. Further, since the Second World War birth rates have been relatively high in most of the well-developed countries, including those which at present produce surplus food. The whole demographical picture, though still imperfectly understood and interpreted, adds a note of urgency to the task of expanding world food production.[34]

All these facts, taken together, were interpreted by FAO authorities as scarcely presenting an encouraging picture of the world situation in 1952. The low level of food production in the less developed regions of the world, and the wide disparities between food consumption in these areas and in the more advanced countries, had long been recognised as outstandingly grave aspects of the world's food and agricultural situation. The effect of World War II was to aggravate these problems acutely. Destruction of livestock, farm machinery and buildings, and storage and processing facilities had occurred on an immense scale,

---

[34] *Second World Food Survey*. Rome, Food and Agriculture Organization of the United Nations, 1952.

whilst soil reserves and in certain cases agricultural manpower were seriously reduced. Most fishing grounds were closed and the best craft were converted for war purposes. Important sources of supply and trade distribution were cut off. The immense burden of supplying the Allied Powers with food and other requisites for the war effort fell upon the few areas in which supplies were accessible, especially those in which the output could be increased rapidly. Under these parameters, post-war dependence on the surpluses from North America and Oceania emerged and the world food situation during the post-war years was essentially that of an exhausting struggle to increase agricultural production all over the world, and to restore some balance in the patterns of production and international trade. From a purely technical perspective, success was possible, but it had been obstructed by political interference, crisis in foreign exchange mechanisms, the negative influence of recurrent shortages of raw materials and other means of production.[35]

The figures for 1946-1947 showed a heavy decline in grain, potatoes and sugar production in Europe, a fall in rice production in the Far East and an increase in grain and sugar output in North America. Taken as a whole, the change in global yield per hectare was the major factor. In Europe, the cumulative wartime shortages of fertilisers depleted soil reserves to the point of exhaustion, sharply reducing yields. The pattern of livestock production emerging from the war was broadly similar to that for crops, with heavy losses in cattle, pigs, and sheep, especially in Europe, but also in many parts of Asia. The supply of livestock products in food deficit areas was affected more deeply than that of vegetables, and the overall food shortage was so severe in certain areas that little grain could be spared for feeding livestock. The majority of the increased feed grain and livestock output in the surplus areas had to be retained to supply an increasing population, whose demand for meat and other livestock products was steadily expanding. The early post-war shortage of livestock products, especially meat and eggs, was particularly severe in Europe.[36] The shortage was responsible for large and widening margins between prices paid to farmers for grain and those prevailing for meat and eggs on the free and black markets.

The following table shows the evolution in food production per caput in the various world regions since the end of World War II, according to the FAO survey:

---

35 *Ibidem*, p. 3.

36 *Ibidem*, 1952, p. 4.

Indices of Total and per Caput Production of Food Crops[37]

Region	Average 1946-1947		Average 1949-1951	
	Total	**Per caput**	**Total**	**Per caput**
Europe	71	68	96	90
North & Central America	143	124	150	124
South America	106	87	93	72
Far East	93	85	99	87
Near East	103	91	115	95
Africa	110	96	125	105
Oceania	104	94	116	103
World (excl. USSR)	100	91	111	97

Source: *Second World Food Survey*, Rome, Food and Agriculture Organization of the United Nations, 1952

The table shows that in many parts of the world the per caput food production in 1951 remained below pre-war levels. A few countries, such as the United Kingdom and Japan, largely dependent on food imports, had managed through strenuous efforts to increase domestic food production. Recovery was generally greatest in the regions that had suffered the steepest declines during the war. Aided by more abundant fertilisers, increased supplies in farm machinery and other agricultural innovations given aid under the Marshall Plan, Europe was able to make the most impressive recovery. By 1950-51 the agricultural production in OEEC countries, considered as a whole, was more than 10 per cent above pre-war levels. Fish production recovered fast, and by 1950 the capacity to produce fish was larger than ever, although in Austria and Germany, the division into different zones of occupation, territorial changes as a consequence of the war and other political and economic factors delayed recovery. Food production in Eastern Europe immediately after the war was much lower than in Western Europe, and so was the recovery in most of the countries in Eastern Europe. Conditions of chronic food shortages in countries of Southern and Eastern Europe were frequent.

Competition between the demands for agricultural resources for direct human food and for feeding livestock characterised much of the struggle for recovery in post-war years. According to the international

37 The eight main crops are: wheat, rye, barley, oats, maize, rice, sugar and potatoes.

surveys, this competition was particularly severe in Europe, where programmes for expanding the area had to be repeatedly abandoned or postponed to prevent recurrent food shortages, sometimes reaching dangerous proportions. Countries were compelled to seek economies by finding alternative and less expensive foodstuffs, improved silage and more efficient methods of feeding and handling grassland. These strategies led to higher milk production per animal in the early 1950s.

Consumption, Nutrition and Health

Technical reports handled by FAO experts, to discuss the world's situation and draw up new programmes, were essentially based on a *Food Balance Sheet Method.* This was an instrument that contained national average food supplies available for human consumption, which allowed for estimation of the caloric and protein contents of a given diet. The pre-war estimates used in the Second World Food Survey mostly referred to the period 1934-38. They were similar to those used in the first WFS and included several improvements in the accuracy of the statistics. The broad picture presented by the earlier statistics remained unchanged and estimates for the post-war period included 52 countries. Taken as a whole, average food supplies, measured in calories, were six per cent lower in 1950 than in pre-war years. Shortages led many countries to take exceptional measures to maintain food supplies. Milling extraction rates were high, the admixture of coarse grains such as barley, oats and maize in bread was appreciably increased and products normally limited to industrial uses, such as oilseeds, were now used for human consumption. By far the largest economy was achieved by the diversion to human consumption of crops normally reserved for feeding stock.

Since caloric intake was considered a quantitative measure of a diet, the 1951 survey considered the adequacy of national average food supplies in relation to estimated physiological requirements. The method used to assess energy requirements included environmental temperature, body weights, and the age and sex of the population. It was thought to provide a better average of calorie requirements of different population groups than any uniform standard applied to the whole world. The results for some European countries offered by the survey are the following:

Calorie Supplies Measured Against Requirements

European Countries	Recent level	Estimated Requirement	Difference
Belgium-Luxembourg	2770	2620	+5.7
Denmark	3160	2750	+14.9
France	2770	2550	+8.6
Greece	2510	2390	+5.0
Italy	2340	2440	-4.1
Netherlands	2960	2630	+12.5
Norway	3140	2850	+10.2
Sweden	3120	2840	+9.8
Switzerland	3150	2720	+15.8
United Kingdom	3100		+16.9
USSR	3020	2710	+114.

Source: *Second World Food Survey*, 1952, Rome, Food and Agriculture Organization of the United Nations, 1952

However, the situation in Europe represented an exception to the global picture, since shortages were significant in many parts of Latin America, the Near East, the Far East and Africa. Nevertheless, no relatively simple unit like the calorie could be used for measuring diet quality, which was principally determined by the presence of nutrients, vitamins and minerals in satisfactory amounts. The amount of proteins consumed per caput tended to be considered the best available indicator: "Where the food supply is sufficient in calories, it has usually a high protein content, a good proportion of which is derived from animal products. On the other hand, when calorie supplies are inadequate, the total amount of protein in the diet is usually small and supplies of protein from animal products frequently do not reach 10 grams per caput a day".[38]

The tendency to consume less cereals and starchy roots and more nutritionally rich protective foods such as meat, milk, eggs, fruit and vegetables was apparent in countries that were enjoying an increase in real national income. It has been discussed previously in this book how special efforts had been made in many countries to increase the consumption of milk in order to safeguard the health of nutritionally

[38] *Second World Food Survey*, 1952, p. 14.

vulnerable groups such as infants, children and nursing and pregnant women.[39] During the post-war years the volume of international trade in dried and condensed milk had more than doubled, with these products playing a role in the international food trade as well as in a more balanced diet, according to medical experts.

Governments had become increasingly aware of their responsibility in safeguarding the health and nutrition of the more vulnerable members of the population. This protection was ensured through food rationing and price control during the war and much of the post-war period; the results were considered to be satisfactory when efficiently organised. Rationed items included not only bread and cereals, but also protective foods like meat, milk, cheese and eggs. In addition, European governments assumed the burden of food subsidies to ensure that essential supplies arrived to the most needy sectors of the population. As the food situation gradually improved, rationing in most countries was abolished or at least substantially reduced. In some cases, political and social perceptions led to the premature abolishment of rationing, which was quickly reintroduced when new acute shortages reappeared. Again, the provisions of supplements and special foods to infants, school children, expectant and nursing mothers and heavy manual workers showed excellent results and was widely applied in many countries.

Food Consumption Targets for 1960

Among the basic ideas that led to the creation of the FAO, food production targets related to nutritional requirements and the health of a population were of special significance. The Hot Springs Conference (1943) distinguished two kinds of targets: first, governments were urged to adopt as their ultimate nutritional goals "dietary standards or allowances based upon scientific assessment of the amount and quality of food, in terms of nutrients, which promote health". Secondly, it drew the attention of governments to the need for more immediate consumption goals, "which necessarily must be based upon the practical possibilities of improving the food supplies of their populations".[40]

---

[39] Research on the case of Spain: Castejón-Bolea, R., Perdiguero-Gil, E., "The closest thing to a mother's milk": the introduction of 'formula milk' and bottle feeding and their medical regulation in Spain (1926-1936)", *Food & History*, No. 6, 2008, pp. 247-276; Castejón Bolea, R., Perdiguero Gil, E., "Médicos, regulación estatal y empresas alimentarias en la introducción y consumo de las fórmulas infantiles en España (1900-1936)", in Bernabeu-Mestre, J., Barona, J.L. (eds.), *Nutrición, salud y Sociedad. España y Europa en los siglos XIX-XX*, Valencia, SEC/PUV, 2011, pp. 323-369.

[40] *Second World Food Survey*, 1952, p. 17.

According to the commitments expressed in its constitution, the FAO was established with the general goal of raising nutritional levels throughout the world. As we have just discussed, the 1951 WFS established a series of very detailed targets related to food production, trade and consumption of all types of food. Those targets were considered to be a compromise between what might be desirable from the standpoint of nutrition and what might be feasible in practice. The targets were a consequence of this central point and feasibility was a permanent condition. They tried to represent quantities and patterns of food supplies, which, if made available, would improve the levels of nutrition of the people consuming them. It was therefore essential to adopt certain nutritional principles, considering practicability and feasibility, so that in general the targets represented a compromise between the nutritionally desirable and the analysis and recognition of hard existing facts and problems. The specific targets referred to particular aspects of human nutrition such as caloric intake, animal and vegetable protein and other nutrients, as well as food groups: animal origin, pulses, vegetables, fruit, cereals, starchy roots, fats and oils and sugar.

The 1951 WFS targets tried to establish a meeting point between the science of nutrition and the organisation of food production. It tried to discuss not the ideal nutritional goals for 1960 but rather the general direction that improvement should take.

> Some targets demand so large an increase in production that their achievement calls for the most determined efforts. Further, these efforts must cover a wide field, including within their scope such measures as the reform of systems of land tenure, provision for agricultural credit, appropriate adjustments in land taxation, the fostering of cooperatives and the development of extension services. In many instances possibilities of attainment will be influenced by price levels, purchasing power and the readiness of people to change consumption habits. It is clearly impossible to consider each article of food in each individual country, and decide on the chance of its production being increased and its distribution improved in the light of all relevant circumstances, many of which are unpredictable and imponderable.[41]

The FAO experts recognised that national governments were in a better position to assess the influence of the relevant conditioning factors than the experts of any international organisation. The establishment and achievement of satisfactory targets indeed represented

41 *Ibidem*, p. 21.

a challenge both to national governments and also to FAO technicians, calling for a collaboration that required exchange of information and common work. An Expanded Technical Assistance Programme was settled to formulate plans for further implementation.

In the field of food production, the FAO experts established a series of goals open to criticism, which proposed changes and adjustments in national and world food supplies. Considering 1960 as a deadline, the targets were likely to succeed only if the following assumptions were made:

a) There would be no major world war or similar disasters.
b) Average climatic conditions would continue to prevail.
c) The volume of international trade will at least not decrease and such trade would continue to have roughly the same relationship to production as at the present.
d) National plans and programmes to develop food production would be pushed forward vigorously.
e) Technical advances in methods of food production and their application in practical terms would be accompanied by simultaneous advances in other fields, such as social, educational, economic and administrative improvements.
f) International assistance to under-developed countries, both technical and financial, would continue to increase.

Those were the 1960 targets for Europe regarding the calorie intake:

Targets for calorie supplies measured against requirements for 1960

European countries	1960 targets	Estimated requirements	Difference
Belgique-Luxembourg	2880	2620	+9.9
Bulgaria	2800	2630	+6.5
Czechoslovakia	2810	2640	+6.4
Denmark	3120	2750	+13.5
Finland	3130	2830	+12.4
France	2890	2550	+13.3
Greece	2634	2390	+10.2
Hungary	2730	2650	+3.0
Iceland	3240	2800	+15.7
Italy	2680	2440	+9.8
Netherlands	3030	2630	+15.2
Norway	3190	2850	+11.9

Poland	2780	2660	+4.5
Portugal	2730	2450	+11.4
Romania	2680	2650	+1.1
Spain	2700	2460	+9.7
Sweden	3120	2840	+9.8
Switzerland	3120	2720	+14.7
United Kingdom	3120	2650	+17.7
Yugoslavia	2440	2630	-7.2

Achieving the targets meant an adaptation of food production, trade distribution and food consumption to the estimated population for 1960. To these estimates, the FAO expert committees added allowances for processing and wastage from the stage of production to the retail stage, and for the quantities that would be used for animal feed, seed, manufacturing and other non-food purposes. Many of those allowances were admittedly speculative, since the pattern of crop utilisation for feed and non-food purposes in 1960 could not be accurately predicted. In making those predictions, account was taken both of the present and pre-war patterns of utilisation and the additional supplies needed to meet the targets for livestock products. The estimates considered national food production – more imports, less exports – because if imports and exports were balanced for the world as a whole, global food supplies should bear some relation to world food production.

Globally speaking, the estimated increase in gross supplies that were needed to attain the targets was far in excess of the estimated increase of the population, particularly for pulses and livestock products. However, "to achieve the targets, it is vital that the largest increase in production should occur in the areas where the need is the greatest".[42] At best, the surplus areas could provide only a small fraction of the needs of the major deficit regions. These needs could only be met almost entirely from their own production and therefore a great expansion of the food supply was required, especially in the Far East, Near East and Africa. In these regions, the increase in the supply of cereals had to be twice as large as the expected increase in the population, while for pulses, milk, meat, eggs and fish the increase had to be proportionally even greater. In

42 *Ibidem*, p. 26.

Latin America and Europe, except for pulses, the increases called for were smaller, but the estimates for livestock products called for a level of expansion that was substantially greater than the estimated population increase. Obviously, the targets did not represent the full satisfaction of nutritional requirements. If they did, the increases called for in the supply of many foods, especially livestock products, would be much larger and far in excess of what could be achieved by 1960 under the most favourable conditions.

In most of Europe, chiefly in Western Europe, post-war recovery had greatly outpaced the increase in the population, especially with regards to the production of sugar, cereals and potatoes, but also in the turn towards livestock products in the 1950s. A large part of Europe's food requirements, however, had to be met by food imports. Unless such imports were heavily expanded, Europe's own food production had to continue to climb at a rate far exceeding the growth in population. This particularly applied to livestock products, the consumption of which had still not attained pre-war levels.

A few questions were discussed by the FAO experts but no clear solutions were proposed: could fish culture be expanded and to what extent? Have the efforts made so far – to increase yields per hectare and per animal through the use of more and better fertilisers; new irrigation systems; improved methods in animal husbandry and fishing; and land reforms and the like – achieved much higher yields than those duing the pre-war period? These were considered crucial for a substantial increase in food production. Regarding the expansion of food crops, in Europe the extension was lower in 1951 than it was in the pre-war years. On the other hand, if a substantial increase in farmed area had been required in under-developed and food-deficient areas of the world, an immense amount of capital investment was also be required, especially for irrigation and drainage.

Conversely, increasing crop yields appeared to be more feasible. In the more advanced countries, yields per hectare had increased over pre-war levels through greater mechanisation, more fertilizers and new technologies. In Europe, even among countries where yields were already high due to intensive production, some noteworthy increases had been achieved. Wheat yields were mentioned as being 10 per cent or more above pre-war levels in Belgium, Denmark, Western Germany, the Netherlands and the United Kingdom. To some extent this was due to cultivation being confined to more favourable land. For the most part, however, the rise in food production was the result of using more and better fertilisers and improved agricultural techniques.

From a worldwide perspective, achieving a substantial increase in the output of livestock products remained one of the most important long-term problems, especially in the less developed regions. The 1952 WFS stressed that when crops are fed to animals instead of directly to humans they lost between 80 and 90 per cent of their caloric value before they produce animal calories. But the prospects for 1960 considered that to a large extent animal and crop production should be deemed complementary rather than competitive and a mixed system of farming gave better results for both.

In many areas of the world animals still constituted the main form of draft power without which crop production would seriously suffer. The 1951 survey considered that in many countries the output of livestock products could be at least doubled, without detriment to the production of food crops, by applying better crop rotations, improving grassland unfit for cultivation, using more efficient crop residues for inedible by-products, and by reducing livestock losses from diseases and parasites. Western European countries were presented as a model to follow as they had attained that with much less reliance on imported feeds than before the war. Milk and meat yields per animal had risen steadily by about two per cent per annum during the last years before 1950 and in a number of European countries they appreciably exceeded pre-war levels.

As a realistic assessment, FAO experts considered that despite the immensity of the problem, progress was possible if all potentially productive resources – land, farm machinery, fertilisers – were fully mobilised. They appreciated the increasing attention given by national governments to the implementation of agriculture development programmes, research and extension work focused on the farmers as an encouraging sign. But they considered that the scale of the effort still remained inadequate, much below that needed if the 1960 targets were to be attained.

> It has indeed become increasingly clear that development programs, land reforms, the setting up of research stations and training schools, agricultural co-operatives and the like, are only the framework within which expansion in production may be possible. They cannot by themselves assure the accomplishment of the task, unless the individual farmers, who are ultimately responsible for food production, are convinced by demonstrations and results of the value of the best techniques appropriate to their circumstances. A tremendous expansion in extension and demonstration work is needed if existing knowledge is to overcome the deep-rooted traditions, prejudices and distrust of farmers whose primitive methods have often remained unchanged for many hundreds of years. For this reason, the Sixth Season of the FAO Conference called on all Member Governments a) to establish adequate extension and demonstration services which are brought down to the level of the man on the land linked with local administration and education in their own countries; b) to ensure that the

> necessary supplies and equipment are available for effective demonstration work; c) to promote where necessary the development of pilot schemes and subsequently demonstration areas in the organizational development of small farmers on a group basis; and d) to provide adequate services to ensure the improvement of home economics in rural areas.[43]

The expansion of trade and the shaping of an efficient and steady world trade market was without doubt a necessary step, but for the FAO experts the primary obstacle to the improvement of the diet of the many millions who still suffered from under-nutrition and malnutrition was their low economic status and the lack of purchasing power. For any population living at bare subsistence levels, food choice was severely limited and even non-existent. Their foremost need was just to satisfy hunger and obtain enough calories in the form of energy-yielding foods. Under those circumstances, real dietary improvements could scarcely take place without economic development. It was only when minimum calorie requirements were satisfied that serious attention could be given to other aspects of dietary improvement: "Where the simple need is for enough food to keep alive, *nutritional balance* is often largely of academic interest".[44]

Conversely, the FAO experts considered that much could be done to improve the diets of populations living at intermediate economic levels, not oppressed by extreme poverty. Being poor is the essential factor of hunger, but faulty food habits arising from deep-rooted traditions, prejudice and ignorance were considered to be responsible for much malnutrition as well.

> A serious deficiency disease called beriberi is found in Asia and elsewhere among people whose staple food is highly milled rice, which has been deprived of the essential vitamins because of the mechanical milling of the grain to a high degree. Although the solution of the problem obviously lies in avoiding the use of such rice, there are several obstacles, mainly of a social and psychological character. People accustomed to highly milled white rice do not take kindly to other kinds of rice, such as under-milled and parboiled rice, which are more nutritious but less attractive to the eye and the palate. Many other examples of social or cultural obstacles could be quoted. These may be religious taboos, such as those which prohibit eating meat from the cow or the pig, or they may be individual and collective prejudices, e.g. against the consumption of milk, fish, eggs and so on. Sometimes the taboo or prejudice is not related to the consumption of particular foods but to their production or distribution. For example, raising vegetables is considered as an inferior occupation in some areas and is

43 *Ibidem*, p. 31.

44 *Ibidem*, p. 33.

therefore undertaken only by immigrants. Another important obstacle to improving diets is the difficulty of popularizing new and unfamiliar foods. General experience indicates that such popularization, while by no means impossible, inevitably takes time. The speed and nature of proposes dietary changes, however desirable these changes might be from the nutritional standpoint, must necessarily be adjusted to prevailing food habits.[45]

The need for an integrated approach – national, regional and international – was pointed out in the 1952 WFS. In the less developed areas, the vicious circle of poverty, hunger, malnutrition, disease and physical inefficiency was not broken in the 1950s. The international experts stressed that people were less tolerant with hunger and famine, and danger of social upheaval was real.

Land reforms must be planned not only to remove injustices that have made progress impossible, but also to ensure that farming efficiency is preserved and increased, and that the transition to new systems of land tenure is made without a disruption of the country's economy. Agricultural programs must be closely linked with nutritional policy to ensure that the right kinds of food as well as enough food are produced. They must be closely co-ordinated with plans for industrial development to attain a balanced expansion in the country's economy, including a growing interchange of products between farm and city. Finally, steady advance in these fields cannot be assured without a parallel advance in many others, including education, health and hygiene, housing, transport and the like.[46]

The diagnosis for the 1950-60 decade was based on planning, modernisation and public control. In a world with a growing population, and a growing multiplicity and complexity of wants and needs, where land and natural resources were still ample in relation to population, modern techniques could be applied. In Europe, the experts considered that national units had become too small for full advantage to be taken of modern forms of industrial organisation and techniques. National protectionism and trade barriers had brought about diminishing results to a point at which economic standards could scarcely be maintained. In this context, greater pooling of resources, technical innovation, scientific knowledge and experience had to take place within the whole region. National plans and programmes had to be coordinated within a regional framework to ensure that output was expanded; trade and other restrictions within European regions had to be reduced to a minimum to obtain a ready market for increased production.

45 *Ibidem*.

46 *Ibidem*, pp. 33-34.

This integrated approach claimed for the European population was similarly essential at the international level. Available expert knowledge could not benefit the less advanced regions unless the natural resources of these poor countries were more efficiently mobilised. However, development programmes required capital investment on a scale far beyond the resources of individual countries, and especially for those living under the poorest conditions. Since private organisations could not lend funds and assume risks, international collaboration was needed to ensure the orderly marketing of foodstuffs at reasonably stable prices. Steps had to be taken to avoid the dangers of recurrent world food shortages and, in the same direction, special efforts were necessary to mobilise great food surplus regions to meet the urgent needs of the deficit areas. International machinery and immediate relief when famines arise were considered necessary.

In the industrially developed countries, the trend of declining birth rates came to a halt in the early 1930s, and was sharply reversed during the years following the world economic depression and in the post-war years.[47] This change was responsible for an exceptional upsurge in the population of developed countries, which was considered to persist until 1960. In densely populated and less developed areas, the potential effect of modern medical technologies (preventive methods, vaccination, antibiotics, etc) on the population was expected to be enormous and to have a direct effect on demographic growth:

> The accumulated knowledge available to medical science and the technical facilities at its disposal has, however, made it possible to reduce mortality rates far more rapidly than was possible in the past. Because "mass diseases" like malaria, tuberculosis, etc… affect such a high proportion of these populations, the control of these diseases alone, now possible at relatively little cost, can bring about a striking reduction in mortality. For example, in Ceylon the death rate, recently reduced mainly by successful measures against malaria to nearly one-half of its previous level, now approaches the death rate prevailing in industrialized countries. Similar results are being achieved elsewhere. Since, however, birth rates are still in the main determined by longer-term factors relating mostly to economic and social attitudes, they are not susceptible to equally rapid change.[48]

The FAO expert report alerted to the possibility of a rapid increase in the world population. They considered the problem could be eased by improved efficiency of successful health measures. In some cases, an increase in food production was achieved entirely through improved

47 *Ibidem*, p. 35.

48 *Ibidem*, p. 36.

efficiency following successful attacks upon disease. A global mentality would emerge that included the belief that better-off countries must assist the comparatively poorer nations, not merely for humanitarian reasons, but also to safeguard their own living standards. This also required a greater understanding, to some extent translated into action, of the need for integrated planning at all levels to achieve higher living standards for people all over the world.

CHAPTER 9

Joint FAO/WHO Nutrition Committee

As an inter-governmental health agency, the World Health Organization (WHO) was the culmination of a long tradition in international health that started in the mid 19th century and was institutionalised for the first time decades earlier with the founding of the *Office Internationale d'Hygiène Publique* (1907), the Health Organization of the League of Nations (1920) and the Health Division of the UNRRA.[1] The WHO originated in the United Nations Conference held in San Francisco in 1945 and was a logical consequence of the shaping of an international sphere after World War II. One year later representatives of 61 governments met at the International Health Conference in New York to draft and sign the WHO Constitution, establishing an Interim Commission to serve until the constitution could be ratified by the 26 member states of the United Nations. The Constitution came into force on April 7, 1948, and the first World Health Assembly took place in Geneva in June 1948, with the permanent organisation being officially established in September 1948.

From the outset, the work of the World Health Organization was carried out by three bodies: the World Health Assembly, the supreme authority, to which all Member States sent delegates; the Executive Board, the executive organ of the Health Assembly; and the Secretariat under the Director-General.

> The scope of the WHO's interests and activities exceeds that of any previous international health organization and includes, in addition to major projects relating to malaria, tuberculosis, venereal diseases, maternal and child health, nutrition, and environmental sanitation, special programmes on public health administration, epidemic diseases, mental health, professional and technical training, and other public-health subjects. It is also continuing work begun by earlier organizations on biological standardization, unification of pharmacopoeias, addiction-producing drugs, health statistics,

[1] A general approach to the shaping of the international sanitary movement in Barona, J., Bernabeu, J., 2008, pp. 27-56. A special mention to the *Office International d'Higiène Publique* in the same book, pp. 83-88.

> international sanitary regulations, and the collection and dissemination of technical information, including epidemiological statistics.[2]

During its first decade of existence the WHO carried out specific technical work in a number of fields related to nutritional health. *Kwashiorkor*, a deficiency disease described in 1935 in Jamaica, was one of the first problems addressed by the organisation. It is an acute form of childhood protein malnutrition, characterised by oedema, irritability, anorexia, ulcerating dermatoses and an enlarged liver with fatty infiltrates. Moreover, attention was paid to endemic goitre and iodine deficiency, pellagra, beriberi, ophthalmic diseases linked to malnutrition, heart diseases and others. The WHO and the FAO started working together to address nutritional deficiencies and malnutrition as direct and indirect causes of a wide range of diseases that mainly affected the population of poor countries. The WHO focused mainly on nutrition as affecting health, and the FAO tried to increase levels of nutrition, improve living standards, and attain improved efficiency in production, trade and distribution of foodstuffs and agricultural products. Both shared a common target, used a similar rhetoric, notwithstanding the fact that they focused on the problem of hunger from different and complementary perspectives.

First Steps towards a Joint FAO/WHO Nutrition Committee

Soon a Joint FAO/WHO Expert Committee on Nutrition was created and met for the first time in Geneva in October 1948. The session was opened by Brock Chisholm, Director-General of the WHO and chaired by Lord Horder. The members of the Committee were:

FAO Representatives:

- Professor M.J.L. Dols, State Adviser on Nutrition; Professor of Nutritional Science, University of Amsterdam, Netherlands

- Lord Holder, Adviser to the Ministry of Food of the United Kingdom, London, UK

- Dr. V.N. Patwardhan, Director, Nutrition Research Laboratories, Coonoor, India

2 *Joint FAO/WHO Expert Committee on Nutrition. Report on the First Session*, Geneva, World Health Organization Technical Report Series No. 16, 1950, p. 1. A first version of the report on the first session in document WHO/NUT/2, 1 November 1949, WHO Archives.

- Dr. Hazel K. Stiebeling, Chief Bureau of Human Nutrition and Home Economics, US Department of Agriculture, Washington DC, USA

- Prof. E.F. Terroine, *Directeur du Centre National de Coordination des Études et Recherches sur la Nutrition et l'Alimentation*, CNRS, Paris, France

WHO Representatives:

- Professor G. Bergami, Professor of Biochemistry and Physiology, Director, *Istituto della Nutrizione del Consiglio Nazionale delle Ricerche*, Rome, Italy

- Dr. J.F. Brock, Professor of Medicine, University of Cape Town, Union of South Africa

- Professor J. De Castro, Director, Institute of Nutrition, University of Brazil, Rio de Janeiro, Brazil

- Dr. W.H. Sebrell, Medical Director, US Public Health Service; Director, Institute of Experimental Biology and Medicine, Bethesda, Md., USA

Observers:

- Dr. Lu Gwei-Djen, Department of Natural Sciences, UNESCO

- Dr. M. De Viado, Social Security Section, ILO

Secretaries:

- Dr. W.R. Aykroyd, Director, Nutrition Division, FAO

- Dr. F.W. Clements, Chief, Nutrition Section, WHO

As terms of reference the Expert Committee had two previous agreements adopted by the First World Health Assembly and by the Second Session of the Conference of the FAO, claiming to act as an advisory body to both organisations, working in close collaboration in "those fields of nutrition with which they are mutually concerned..."[3] The FAO had also started collaborative action with the United Nations International Children's Emergency Fund (UNICEF), integrating feeding programmes with nutritional education involving administrators, public-health officers, medical practitioners, nurses and schoolteachers. The WHO-FAO Expert Committee on Nutrition considered programmes designed to raise the level of nutritional education to be one of the most important targets for better nutritional standards. Initially, two main

[3] FAO, *Report of the second session of the Conference*, Washington, 1946.

types of training courses were conducted in member countries and others.[4]

Fellowships were seen as an important part of the general educational work. Three different categories were implemented. First were those granted for extended study, up to a year or more, in a recognised institution, and available to workers who would later participate in nutritional activities and coordinate campaigns in their own countries. They were geared towards medical and public health officers and nurses, administrators, managers associated with food production and food administration. Local leaders called upon to conduct anthropological actions were also included. Other grants went to policy makers and supervisors studying the implementation of nutrition programmes. Finally, other grants were oriented to senior workers in universities and research institutes. The instruction provided by experts in nutrition was considered to be essential for their participation in the programmes promoted by the FAO and the WHO.

Emphasising that the functions of the Nutrition Section of the WHO included the collection, evaluation and distribution of information on recent advances in the science of nutrition, the expert committee recommended that this service be extended to include information on the incidence of deficiency diseases associated with dietary shortcomings. An additional programme of technical assistance to help economic development including food was proposed for 1950 in the ordinary FAO budget, including a provision for nutrition advisory services on a larger scale, training for nutritional workers, the organisation of courses and support for research and provision of equipment and technical innovation at a suitable scale. The FAO Standing Advisory Committee on Nutrition stressed the need for improved food technology, and therefore a Technical Assistance Programme was proposed for further discussion. The WHO presented a nutrition programme for 1951 that aimed to assess a number of nutritional problems, including the evaluation of the nutritional status of population groups, as well as the calculation of caloric and nutritional requirements. Specific diseases, which were considered to represent central problems, were mentioned as a priority, such as: *kwashiorkor*, nutritional disorders affecting the vision and causing neuropathy and blindness; and loss of resistance to parasitic diseases due to nutritional deficiencies and some types of blood dyscrasia associated with malnutrition.

4 *Joint FAO/WHO Expert Committee on Nutrition. Report of the First Session.* Geneva, World health Organization Technical Report Series, No. 16, 1950.

The WHO had made provision for fellowships and a number of them had been granted in the field of nutrition, while the FAO made provision for fellowships in its Technical Assistance Programme. In order to achieve an integrative policy and avoid duplication of duties, the mixed experts committee recommended coordination and prior consultation, the aim being to arrange for the training of the different types of specialists needed to deal with the problems of nutrition in any given country or region. This was so the recipients of fellowships, upon their return, could find adequate support from other specialists to develop balanced nutrition programmes in their countries. Training and education was geared towards administrators, physicians, nurses, social workers and schoolteachers. The pattern for regional and national training courses proposed by the FAO and the WHO was similar, sponsored and planned by national governments and held in national institutions. Some specific symposia and seminars to meet local needs and educational programmes for the general population were also included.[5]

Properly planned and conducted, surveys by the United Nations provided information on social welfare and the economic background. In addition, the FAO published reports and technical surveys on dietary patterns and food consumption levels; the International Labour Organization had published family living studies and the WHO drafted reports on the status of health and nutrition. The experts stressed that the value of this great amount of information on all these subjects was essential and requested coordinated action to publish all information at the same time to ensure its optimum use.

The joint committee also analysed the importance of specific nutritional deficiency diseases and the search for solutions. Endemic goitre was the first one considered. The joint committee urged governments to promote the use of iodised salt in regions in which supplying iodine was practicable as an easy solution with positive results. In association with governments, the WHO planned a further study of all factors intervening in the aetiology of endemic goitre and requested information on areas where endemic goitre had not been prevented by the administration of small amounts of iodine to the population.

Pellagra was a second case that was discussed upon request of the First Health Assembly. The committee had been informed that in some areas classical pellagra had been brought under control by the administration of niacin, even without general dietary improvement. No

5 *Ibidem*, pp. 6-7.

evidence was available to indicate that classical pellagra was of sufficient importance worldwide to warrant its high priority status in the joint FAO/WHO programmes in the immediate future. However, the formal reporting of cases of pellagra was stimulated and considered accurate.

One of the most widespread nutritional disorders in tropical and subtropical regions was a syndrome known by various names, the most popular one being *kwashiorkor*, but it was also known as malignant malnutrition, polydeficiency disease, *m'buaki*, syndrome, *depigmentation-oedème* and infantile pellagra. It was defined as a disease of its own, unlike classical pellagra. The mixed committee rejected the name *infantile pellagra*, since it was not really a variety of *pellagra*. Epidemiologically speaking, it affected mostly children, with the highest incidence of the disease occurring in some parts of Africa. Considerable evidence suggested that it was associated with cirrhosis of the liver, a disease present in significant numbers in some parts of Africa and Central America, where *kwashiorkor* occurred in infants and children. The possible relationship between cirrhosis and the development of primary carcinoma of the liver was also recognised. The Joint Expert Committee recommended an inquiry be held by the WHO on the various signs and manifestations of the disease, including a clinical investigation, in an attempt to define and study clinical features of the disease and food habits, with particular reference being made to diet during pregnancy, lactation, infancy and early childhood.[6] The inquiry was to be extended to areas in which the disease did not occur but which featured the similar diet patterns, in order to establish a correlation between food habits and the occurrence or incidence of the disease, defining the role played by other factors, such as tropical parasitism, in determining the variations in clinical manifestations.

The FAO Standing Advisory Committee on Nutrition placed special emphasis at its first meeting on the nutrition of pre-school children, because in some countries this group felt malnutrition more acutely than any other age group. In many parts of the world, weaned children were usually fed a diet that mainly consisted of cereal preparations, complemented with little or no milk at all. The wide prevalence of the aforementioned syndromes – although their aetiology was not clear – was associated with serious dietary deficiencies during early childhood and the experts thought that the ill effects of malnutrition during this time could be felt during adulthood. Therefore, the committee alerted the FAO to the great need for increased supplies of foodstuffs, milk in

6 *Ibidem*, p. 15.

particular, which could prevent deficiencies in children's diets. "In regions in which an immediate substantial increase in milk supplies is difficult, the production and use of foods and/or preparations which can act as a partial substitute for milk should be vigorously encouraged".[7]

The attention of the joint committee was drawn to a related topic, stated in the following passage in the report of the subcommittee on fat-soluble vitamins of the Expert Committee on Biological Standardization, convened by the WHO in London in 1949: "The sub-committee considers that the value and usefulness of the international standards for vitamins might be increased if suitable methods of estimating the different vitamins in foodstuffs were to be proposed by WHO and FAO and recommended for general use".[8]

Accurate knowledge of the vitamin content of foods was considered a necessity, essential for helping determine the nutrient content of diets. Such knowledge could be obtained only by analytical methods, which, with the technical assistance of the FAO, could be used in the preparation of international food composition tables containing vitamins and minerals. The analysis of vitamins in bodily fluids was another method employed in the assessment of the state of nutrition. Physical, chemical and biological testing methods were used in the analysis of foodstuffs in order to determine the physiological effects and the nutritional value of foods as sources of vitamins for human beings.

From the very beginning the Joint Experts Committee expressed their wish to prepare an international codex of analytical methods that would assist scientific workers worldwide to ensure uniform and comparable data was generated regarding the vitamin content of foods and diets. In a number of countries, certain methods for the detection and assessment of some vitamins were officially recognised, including methods for determining the vitamin content of foodstuffs. A global agreement was absolutely necessary for this and for the development of the pharmaceutical industry as well.

The US Association of Agricultural Chemists set out methods that were revised annually under the supervision of expert committees, and also gave detailed techniques for the preparation of various classes of foods prior to the actual assay.[9] Some countries in Western Europe were initiating a project that would prepare joint proposals for the classification, description and methods of food analysis. All these

7 *Ibidem*, p. 16.

8 World Health Organization Technical Report Series, 1950, No. 3, p. 9.

9 *Joint FAO/WHO Expert Committee on Nutrition. Report of the First Session, 1950*, p. 17.

initiatives were able to facilitate the drafting of an international codex, an issue that was central to the standardisation of knowledge on biological products. As a result, the Joint Committee recommended that the FAO initiate work on analytical methods for the determination of vitamins in foodstuffs by a general survey of the problem and by exploring possible procedural methods. Correspondence with national organisations working in the field of food analysis was one of the options mentioned. Once a preliminary survey was drafted, a small expert committee would convene to consider the scope and to outline the methods to be followed by the FAO. At a later stage small groups of highly qualified specialists might be appointed to consider in detail methods for application to individual vitamins in various types of food. Collaboration with UNESCO and international non-governmental organisations, such as the International Union of Nutritional Sciences, were suggested as well.

The manufacture of synthetic vitamins in underdeveloped countries was also discussed at the first session of the Joint Committee held in 1950. Although the most satisfactory way to improve nutrition was considered to be via the supply of ordinary foods in the quantities and proportions needed to ensure a well-balanced diet, and sufficient amounts of all the nutrients needed for health, the experts recognised that there were circumstances in which the addition of vitamins to foods could be of value to prevent deficiencies. In many parts of the world the amount of food needed to supplement cereals or starchy root-based diets and make them nutritionally adequate was not available at the start of the 1950s. It was not a matter of availability, but its high cost, making the foods inaccessible to the majority of the population. As many years would have to elapse before nutritional requirements could be satisfied by the supply of such foods, synthetic vitamins were able to fill the gap in the meantime and help to minimise some of the existing dietary deficiencies. The Joint Committee endorsed the view of the FAO Nutrition Committee, expressed in its meeting in the Philippines, 1948, with reference to the enrichment of rice by thiamine and other nutrients.[10] A significant reduction in deaths caused by beriberi was the result. At any rate, the experts stressed that enrichment programmes were not enough and should always be accompanied by other active measures to improve nutrition. On the other hand, the value of synthetic vitamins and vitamin concentrates in the prevention and treatment of food deficiency diseases and deficient states was fully recognised, and therefore the need for vitamins and concentrates for therapeutic

---

10 *Ibidem*, p. 19.

purposes became increasingly important in regions in which typical diets were of low nutritive value and deficiency diseases were common.

The Joint FAO/Expert Committee recommended that the WHO assist member governments in deciding whether to undertake the manufacture of synthetic vitamins and provide all the advice needed to establish the industry. Work on calorie requirements had already been completed by the Nutrition Division of the FAO and a report of the Committee on Calorie Requirements was expected after the meeting in Washington, in September 1949. The FAO had intended to continue and expand this work by undertaking the study of nutrient requirements, making full use of data available throughout the world and of the experience gained in different countries. Regional nutrition committees and other nutrition institutions and workers in various regions would be asked to forward any relevant information at their disposal to the FAO.

Naturally, a country's nutrition policy had to be based upon knowledge of the nutritional situation of the population, together with a consideration of dietary patterns, food supply and the economic context. A selected clinical examination of the population was able to give solid information of the nutritional status of the whole, and laboratory tests had also been devised to provide facts about the biochemical and physical state of organs and tissues. In some cases, laboratory tests were considered complementary to clinical findings.

Some countries had established their own methods of clinical testing and had set out standards to assess the nutritional status of the population, but there were others that were unable to do so due to lack of qualified workers and proper equipment. A series of schedules for use in the assessment of nutritional status prepared by an international group of experts would increase the value of national nutrition surveys, allowing for comparisons between conditions in various countries. Countries that had not already conducted surveys would be encouraged to do so.

The committee realised that there was a need for schedules for at least three types of survey:

1. Rapid surveys for emergency purposes, using observation of gross clinical changes.
2. Routine clinical surveys.
3. Clinical surveys supported by experimental laboratory investigations.

Information on food consumption and dietary patterns had to be collected while the nutritional survey was conducted, and the results of the two types of survey correlated.[11] To help these essential research inquiries, FAO experts prepared a booklet on dietary survey methodology and copies were widely distributed among national authorities and experts.[12] As a consequence, the Joint FAO/WHO Expert Committee on Nutrition recommended the spread of standardised methods of assessment of nutritional status with the assistance of the FAO and the WHO and, since levels of nutrition differed all over the world, they suggested inquiries be performed at national and regional levels. Further investigation into nutritional status could be carried out by selecting one or more governments in an advisory capacity in different regions to help determine the most suitable methods for application in the region. At the same time, an international study group was expected to be convened by the WHO with the technical assistance of the FAO, to examine the reports from the various national groups and prepare a comprehensive report.

The Joint FAO/WHO Expert Committee noted that there existed national nutrition committees in many countries. They were under different names, status, structures and functions, falling roughly into five categories: those that were identical to national FAO committees; others which were subcommittees of these; others set up under one or more government departments, or by national research councils; and finally, nutrition institutes equipped with advisory and research functions in the field of food policies.[13] In some countries the national nutrition organisation was an active body participating in nutrition programmes, whilst in other countries it was less effective or inexistent. According to the FAO-WHO nutrition experts;

> National nutrition organizations are an important means of implementing the nutrition policies of FAO and WHO. The committee realizes that each national government must itself decide how this is to be done. It is essential that the various government departments through which FAO and WHO transmit information and requests relating to nutrition should be represented on national nutrition organizations. These organizations can be more effective instruments for the extension of both FAO and WHO nutrition programmes if problems are referred to them by the appropriate government departments.[14]

---

11 *Ibidem*, p. 20.

12 *Dietary surveys. Their technique and interpretation.* Washington, FAO, 1949.

13 *Joint FAO/WHO Expert Committee on Nutrition. Report of the First Session*, 1950, p. 22.

14 *Ibidem*.

The Joint Experts Committee also discussed the role of non-governmental organisations, concluding that any organisation able to influence public opinion on the importance of food for health should be encouraged and supported. Therefore, the joint committee strongly recommended activities that would keep those organisations informed of plans and programmes, encourage them to pay attention to the work of the FAO and the WHO and assist in spreading this information to other national societies, as well as to maintain close ties with international scientific organisations, funds and foundations for mutual exchange of technical information.[15] Similar policy was stimulated among other international organisations, such as the Organization for European Economic cooperation (OEEC), the Economic Commission for Asia and the Far East (ECAFE) and the Department of Natural Sciences of UNESCO in particular. Food and health became an economic, political and international relations issue.

Another subject discussed by the Joint Experts Committee was that of food regulations. Complex and sometimes even contradictory among the different countries, the situation of food regulations constituted a matter involving social conflict between consumers, authorities, producers, traders and other groups. Legal regulations, as well as norms on food preservation, technical terminology, standards of food quality and composition, all of these elements varied widely from country to country. International standardisation was once more the key to any possible solution. New legislation based on scientific knowledge was being introduced in the food industry and in the market. However, the conflicting nature of food regulations might have been an obstacle to trade in foodstuffs between countries and may have affected the distribution of valuable foods. The first Joint meeting was rich in content and in the definition of controversial issues that straddled the boundary between food and health.

A second Joint FAO/WHO Expert Committee on Nutrition met in Rome in April, 1951. During the biennium 1949-51, the FAO had focused its activities in assisting governments in establishing and carrying out food policies through tools and techniques, as well as raising awareness of the importance of the problems of nutrition and the need for effective measures to solve them. Practical aid to individual governments in the field was also included in some cases. Together with the Economic Division, the FAO revised the situation in many different countries and regions and tried to propose suitable technical plans for overcoming critical situations.

15 *Ibidem*, p. 23.

The FAO *Food Composition Tables for International Use* were published and distributed in 1949. They were used to cover proposals for 35 countries, including all the main foodstuffs classified into 11 groups. Those materials were the starting point of the several WFS published by the FAO in this period and discussed in the previous chapter. They included determination of the calorie requirement levels to be adopted in assessing the adequacy of food supplies and the establishment of the guiding principles for the definition of food consumption targets for 1960, examining these variables country by country, to ensure that all particularities were taken into account. Regional meetings were held in 1949 to give careful consideration to trends in food production, supplies and consumption targets for nations in Latin America, the Near East, Asia and Europe. Tables providing information on the caloric, protein and fat content of foods had also been published in the three official languages at the time in the United Nations: English, French and Spanish, and had been put to practical use in a number of countries. In 1951 this work was extended to include the calculation of the mineral and vitamin content of foods for the *Food Composition Tables*. Food technology and technical assistance programmes required closely coordinated work in this field of agriculture, fisheries and nutritional patterns, within the several divisions inside the FAO.

Due to its important strategic function, an international report on school feeding was in preparation when the second joint meeting took place, its main purpose being to increase interest in supplementary feeding and provide technical guidance to the governments when initiating school feeding programmes. An FAO nutrition officer visited different countries in Europe in 1950 in order to collect information on this subject, to discuss relevant problems with appropriate experts and coordinate information about the organisation of the existing programmes in the countries. FAO nutrition officers, in association with UNICEF, had given direct assistance in the organisation of school feeding programmes in Greece, the Philippines and Central America.

As a practical means of helping governments and nutrition workers design and carry out effective educational programmes, a great deal of material on this subject was collected, analysed and set out in the handbook *Teaching better nutrition. A study of approaches and techniques*.[16] Among the questions considered in the book were: the organisation of national programmes of nutritional education devoted to the general public and special interest groups; the training of nutrition

---

[16] *Teaching better nutrition. A study of approaches and techniques*, Rome, FAO, 1950.

workers; the best teaching methods to make nutritional knowledge available; the preparation and handling of teaching materials; and the evaluation of materials and methods implemented to conform nutritional habits to scientific patterns. Information had been directly supplied on request by a number of countries.

On the other hand, following the standardisation aim, a handbook entitled *Dietary Surveys: their technique and interpretation*[17] was published as well. Special attention was paid in the book to the most appropriate techniques to be applied for underdeveloped countries, where little was known about consumption levels.

A nutrition committee for South and East Asia was convened by the FAO in the Philippines in February, 1948, following a second meeting in Rangoon, Burma, in 1950, and two Conferences dealing with the problem of nutrition in Latin America took place in Montevideo (1948) and Rio de Janeiro (1950). Nutritional deficiencies were analysed, as well as training programmes and economic policies regarding prizes, food production, trade, subsidies and other important aspects concerning people's access to food.

The FAO nutrition representative visited several European countries, including the Scandinavian countries, Finland, Ireland, Austria, Yugoslavia and Portugal, to obtain direct information and discuss national plans with the local authorities. The main purpose of these visits was to discuss food and nutrition problems and appropriate practical measures with government authorities, officers and nutrition workers. An FAO officer acted as attaché to the Ministry of Coordination in Greece for three years, to assist with advice and coordination of nutrition activities and the creation of a government nutrition service in the Ministry of Agriculture. The programme was a comprehensive one, including the planning of food production and import programmes based on the nutritional needs of the population, assisting in the development of specific nutrition measures such as school feeding and education in nutrition programmes, and the training of workers to ensure continuity of such activities. The FAO also conducted a preliminary survey of the food and nutritional situation in Turkey in 1949, after a request from the Turkish government for assistance to establish nutrition services. The same FAO delegate working previously in Greece was assigned to Turkey in October 1950. A similar policy was developed by the FAO in Asian, African and American countries.

17 *Dietary Surveys: their technique and interpretation.* Rome, FAO, 1949.

Severe Malnutrition in Times of Disaster

In November 1951 the Joint FAO/WHO Expert Committee on Nutrition published a technical report, previously presented and approved by the Fourth World Health Assembly, on *Prevention and Treatment of Severe Malnutrition in Times of Disaster.*[18] The expert committee responsible for the technical report was composed of the following experts:

- Professor M.J.L. Dols, State Adviser on Nutrition; Professor of Nutritional Science, University of Amsterdam, Netherlands (Chairman)
- Professor W. Halden, Chairman, Food and Nutrition Division, Austrian Public Health Association, Graz-Kroisbach, Austria
- A. Heilbronner, Maître des Requêtes au Conseil d'État; ancien Directeur au Ministère du Ravitaillement, Paris, France
- Miss D.F. Hollingsworth, Ministry of Food, London, United Kingdom
- G. Mathieu, Secrétaire générale de l'ex-Ministère du Ravitaillement et des Importations, Brussels, Belgium
- A.K. Muggli, formerly Chef de la Section du Rationnement, Ofice fédérale de Guerre pour l'Alimentation, Berne, Switzerland

This group acted as consultants for specific sections devoted to food management and organisational aspects. Advice on physiological, clinical and therapeutic aspects was provided by:

- Professor Ancel B. Keys, Director, Laboratory of Physiological Hygiene, School of Public Health, University of Minnesota, Minneapolis, Minn., USA.

Acting as secretaries of the expert committee were:

- Dr. F.W. Clements, Chief, Nutrition Section, WHO
- Miss T. Norris, Nutrition Division, FAO

The Third World Health Assembly had previously considered the subject of prevention and treatment of severe malnutrition in times of disaster. It requested the Director-General to refer it to the Joint FAO/WHO Expert Committee on Nutrition for further study[19], with special attention to the storage of food by governments and private citizens, in order to diminish the risk of severe malnutrition and

[18] *Prevention and Treatment of Severe Malnutrition in Times of Disaster. Report* approved by the Joint FAO/WHO Expert Committee on Nutrition and presented to the Fourth World Health Assembly, Geneva, World Health Organization, [November] 1951. The report was originally issued in mimeographed form as WHO document A4/4, 20 March 1951.

[19] *Official Records of the World Health Organization*, No. 28, 29.

starvation. The Expert Committee was requested to discuss the overall measures to be taken in planning the conservation and distribution of available stocks of food so as to prevent starvation and severe malnutrition in populations living under conditions of severe food scarcity. It was also asked to discuss: the proper treatment of patients suffering from starvation; the measures to be taken during relief activities to prevent the deterioration of the physical and mental state of persons suffering from varying degrees of undernutrition associated with different types of famine; the organisation of general relief activities in relation to nutrition when famine conditions prevailed; and any other measures that were deemed useful in the prevention of disease and death caused by severe malnutrition and starvation. It was considered, for the purpose of the study, that the whole problem could be divided into three main sections: a) food management; b) the physiological, clinical and therapeutic aspects; c) organisational aspects.

The Director-General of the WHO called together the committee members named above to report on food management and organisational matters and requested Ancel Keys – the American physiologist mentioned in an earlier chapter for his implementation in Minnesota of an experimental research project involving humans that dealt with starvation – to prepare the preliminary statement on the physiological, clinical and therapeutic dimensions of the problem.

Food Management

According to the report, "food shortages may arise from the cutting-off of food imports, disorganization of transport, destruction of crops and farm tools and machinery, scattering of agricultural workers, lack of fertilizers, confiscation of food, and various other causes".[20] In addition, the impact of these negative conditions on the food situation in any country depended on a series of internal factors, mainly on the degree of self-sufficiency in food supplies and the potentialities for increasing food production. The Joint Expert Committee mentioned, as a standpoint, the impossibility to propose a standard pattern for meeting food emergencies, one that could be applicable in all countries and for all contingencies. The only general principle was considered to be the setting up of suitable national administrative machinery with enough power to prepare for and deal with emergencies. Plans were to be flexible and made well in advance, because even when a satisfactory broad plan of action had been formulated and was being followed, new

20 *Prevention and Treatment*, 1951, p. 5.

and *ad hoc* action was continually needed to meet current changes in the situation.

An efficient organisation and administration scheme was the first point discussed in the report, considered to be the first step in any country. An appropriate person or collegiate body was supposed to be given the responsibility for drawing up the necessary plans, be an individual, a coordinating ministry or an interdepartmental committee.

> The administrative machinery adequate for the task of handling an emergency should be organized in the preparatory period. In addition, administrative procedures must be prepared so the plans can be put into effect immediately an emergency arises. The creation of a special Food Ministry or a special Food Department in the Ministry of Agriculture, if it does not already exist, may be a necessary step. It is essential that the responsible official or unit should have sufficient authority to review any situation as it changes and take whatever action may be necessary.[21]

The central organisation bearing this responsibility had to rely on standing scientific committees for advice on the nutritional aspects of the food and agricultural programme and for the assessment of the population's nutritional status and general health. When a major catastrophe occurred involving several countries, international cooperation and organisation was essential for the global planning and managing of food policies.

The basis of an emergency plan is the knowledge of the total amount of food needed to feed the whole population affected, a calculation that could be assessed in terms of calorie requirements. The amount needed to cover requirements fully was to be estimated, even though the actual level aimed at might fall below this. However, the relationship between the actual level and full requirements must be known, so that the effects of feeding at the lower level over a given period of time could be anticipated and assessed. Many countries had their own average per caput per day calorie-requirement, although scales recommended by experts included a system for the determination of requirements according to variation in body size, age, activity and climate.[22] A second suggested reference was the average consumption in the pre-emergency

---

21 *Ibidem*.

22 Committee on Calorie Requirements. *Report of the Committee on the Clorie Requirements*, Washington, FAO Nutritional Studies No. 5, 1950.

period, information that was available for European countries but not in all regions.[23]

During the process of making the plans, a decision had to be made on the principal foods that constituted the diet of the population at risk during the emergency period, depending on the habits of food consumption patterns and the potential supplies provided through local food production, stocks and importation possibilities. In general, the experts considered that foods of vegetable origin, which give a high calorie yield, are of primary importance. In addition to calorie requirements, sufficiency of proteins was considered essential for a well-balanced diet and, under critical situations, the quality of proteins became essential. In these circumstances, pulse and leafy vegetables were considered to be important sources of protein that supplement cereal protein. In times of food shortage in Western Europe, encouragement had to be given to the home production of potatoes, vegetables and fruit, to ensure that the needs for proteins, vitamins and minerals of the adult population was met. Simultaneously, suitable measures to keep the intake of nutrients as high as possible were recommended, introducing actions such as margarine enrichment with vitamins or increasing the extraction-rate of cereals. Arrangements had to be made, however, to provide for the special needs of the vulnerable groups, including infants, children, pregnant and nursing women, old people, industrial workers, the unemployed and, in connection with this, particular attention to milk was recommended.

Food production in times of emergency should, as a general principle, be oriented towards obtaining the greatest amount of food in terms of calories. This strategy involved concentrating on crops of cereals, potatoes and other vegetables, as well as oilseeds for direct human consumption, a reduction of the animal population diverting feed crops to food crops, the ploughing-up of pasture and the slaughter of pigs and poultry, which compete directly with humans for cereals. At the same time, once more, it was recommended that account be taken of the need to maintain milk supplies. Measures of this nature were considered appropriate to prevent food shortages and starvation in times of emergency. Storage of food would enable governments to ensure a supply to the people during scarcity periods needed to implement emergency economy measures. The quantities of food stored "in order to diminish the risk of severe malnutrition and starvation" were

23 Organization for European Economic Cooperation, Food and Agriculture Committee, *Food consumption levels in OEEC countries. Report of the working group on food consumption levels*, Paris, OEEC Document AG(50)35.

dependent on food production resources and the imports likely to be possible during the emergency period. On the other hand, geographical location, transport, military considerations and other factors had to be taken into consideration.

Stored foods had to be those that gave a high calorie return per unit of weight and were easily stored without deterioration over long periods of time, such as sugar, cereals, oilseeds and fats. Foods of specific nutritive value to meet the needs of vulnerable groups, such as processed milk and cod-liver oil, had to be accumulated as well. Stocks of foodstuffs that were usually imported also had to be focused on, since a reduction of importation could be expected in times of crisis. Other goods considered just as *psychologically important* for the population included coffee or tea in many countries, or white bread, olive oil and rice, among others.

In most countries, responsibility for food storage was shared by government authorities and private householders. An emergency programme called for extensive guidance to householders to ensure that they knew how to handle, store and periodically change stocks of foods placed in their hands. The most important factor in the building-up of stocks of food was that of time, a decision that had to be made well ahead of an anticipated emergency. Technical aspects also had to be considered to prevent deterioration, avoiding infestation of insects and rodents, using appropriate chemical agents.

The following essential parts of the programme were considered to be the proper, rational use of foods: the way they have to be processed and adapted to the needs of economies in transport and labour. Whether foods were to be directed towards human consumption or to animal feeding was a decision to be made in every country, to guarantee the best economic and effective option. Their use for producing alcoholic drinks or milk had to be controlled. As a general rule, policy management had to be directed towards obtaining the greatest nutritional advantage from the food available. In the case of cereals, an extraction rate of 80-85 per cent for wheat made it possible to allocate to human consumption the maximum food available from the original grain. The remaining 15-20 per cent represented an excellent feed for livestock. The decision to dilute wheat flour with other cereals and potato flour had to be made after due consideration of dietary patterns, cultural habits and to whether or not a better diet could be achieved by this procedure.

Procurement of foodstuffs was the next challenge, since food had to be distributed through a rational and efficient system that was able to ensure that all groups in the population gained access to a minimum healthy diet. However, the experts considered that no system of distribution could operate unless the foods required for distribution through appropriate channels were available and under the control of the authorities. If transport space was limited, it was important to select those foodstuffs that could supply a higher return of calories and nutrients per unit of weight or volume. In order to put in place an efficient distribution system, technical cooperation between food technologists and manufacturers in the exporting and importing areas was needed to solve problems of processing, packaging and storage. Experts warned about the emergence of black markets, a traditional problem that appeared readily in times of food shortage in countries in which attempts were being made by the government to regulate food procurement and distribution. An important factor in the control of black markets was the establishment of a policy of food distribution, which ensured that the available supplies were distributed equitably.

The most difficult problem was considered to be the collection of what was produced and, although no general rules could be applied to solve this difficulty, asking farmers in advance about their production plans. This was expected to help and facilitate verification by local committees, representatives of the administration and farming communities, in order to determine the agricultural production of each farm. It was important to make them aware that a part of the production might be retained for domestic use on the farm and the other part delivered to the common pool. Delivery of each farm's allotted portion could be organised by compulsory methods, but better results were usually able to be obtained by establishing contacts between the producer and the administration by which the latter would guarantee the supply of fertilisers, feeding stuffs and technical equipment to the farmer in return for food. Finally, the price policy followed by the government would exercise a great influence over the production and delivery of agricultural products.

The next stage after procurement was the distribution of foods through an appropriate system to wholesalers, retailers and consumers. Distribution to consumers through a rationing system usually called for considerable changes in normal distribution procedures, although the experts considered it desirable that such changes were reduced to a minimum level and that previously existing channels were used as far as possible, ensuring equitable distribution with the collaboration of manufacturers, wholesalers, retailers and caterers.[24] In times of shortage it was essential to guarantee an efficient distribution to consumers,

24 *Prevention and Treatment*, 1951, p. 12.

according to nutritional needs. Therefore, several points were to be considered in consumer rationing:

a) The system had to be as simple as possible, while taking into account the physiological requirements of various ages, sex and activity groups in the population. The method of establishing a basic ration for the consumer, making special provisions for specific groups, was considered to be the most satisfactory.

b) When supplies were not sufficient to meet demand, a rationing system was necessary to prevent inequitable consumption and health problems, although staple foods, such as cereals and potatoes, should be left out of the rationing scheme, whenever possible. This would enable consumers to adjust their food intake to habits and requirements, something psychologically positive.

c) The ration for any commodity should be set at such a level that it could be distributed throughout the emergency period. According to the experts, the loss of confidence meant an increase in black markets.

d) For high activity groups an extra ration card for foods according to work categories and the supplying of workers with meals in community kitchens or industrial canteens was also proposed.

e) Also, the handling of rationed foods in catering establishments and institutions was considered a suitable measure.

f) The special requirements of vulnerable groups – pregnant and nursing women, adolescents, infants and schoolchildren – for protective food could be appropriately covered by supplementary feeding programmes, such as school meals, and by prioritising the distribution of milk, eggs, cod-liver oil, citrus fruits and juices.

g) The technical report recommended avoiding rigid solutions, because the experts considered that flexibility leaves an element of choice on the part of people in obtaining daily rations and this helps to arrange meals close to the normal food habits.

Cooperation among the various groups involved – agricultural organisations, food processing and distribution industries, consumers and housewives – was considered to be essential. To do so, some specific service had to operate, helping the population to understand the dimensions of the food problem, instructing on the need for the equitable and controlled distribution of foodstuffs, and publicising the need to prevent wastage by proper methods of storage and handling. Teaching the public how to make the best use of the food available, taking into account the physiological needs and planning home economics, was an urgent necessity. The authorities would also give full information about the methods of obtaining rations, priority foods and additional meals, and inform producers and the food industry as well about the regulations and needs for the regular and complete delivery of agricultural and food products to the competent authorities.[25] The establishment of a service to implement this function was most convenient. It would have at its disposal all the available scientific information required for the fulfilment of these duties.

On the other hand, price control was considered to be especially important in ensuring that the lower social groups of the population were neither at a serious disadvantage in times of shortage, nor unable to obtain their rations because of their low purchasing power, always taking account of the nutritional importance of milk and other special foods.

Malnutrition: Physiological, Clinical and Therapeutic Aspects

The medical aspects of the lack of food were a central part of the technical report on the prevention and treatment of severe malnutrition in times of disaster. Ancel Keys' report stressed that the proper treatment of patients suffering from starvation had to attempt to achieve the following goals, as far as possible:[26]

a) Preservation of life.

b) Prevention of irreversible damage to body and mind.

c) Establishment of nutritional and general metabolic conditions leading to maximal recovery.

d) Restoration of morale and promotion of a physiologically healthy state of mind and emotion.

e) Rebuilding of the wasted tissues of the body to the nearest point to the pre-starvation state.

f) Total rehabilitation, for the patient to secure his/her place in the community.

Obviously, the practical measures offered to the population had to be adjusted to the available supplies, facilities and personnel, and this could mean serious constraints to the capacity of action. As a consequence, differentiation was made between an *ideal* treatment and a *proper* treatment, the latter being understood as "the best which could be provided in a given situation". Experience gained from the extreme exhaustion provoked by World War II in Greece, the Netherlands, Leningrad, in prisons, and concentration and internment camps, could be applied to future extreme situations caused by wars or natural catastrophes. In fact, Keys tried to follow such experiments in post-war

---

25 *Ibidem*, p. 15.

26 *Ibidem*, p. 16.

peace times. The Joint FAO/WHO Experts' Committee looked to give practical advice for the treatment of victims living under starving conditions.

> Suffering and death among starving patients and in the general population during famine are not solely the direct result of food shortages and calorie inadequacy. Whenever there is mass starvation there is apt to be a breakdown in sanitary and public health control with the consequent danger of widespread infections and epidemics. Programmes for the prevention or amelioration of the ill effects of famine must, then, give prominence to other public-health measures as well as the basic matter of nutrition... Vaccinations, anticholera inoculations, malaria control, purification of drinking water, and similar measures must be pursued with vigour from the start of any programme for the control and relief of famine.[27]

Treatment had to be adjusted to the social situation, as well as to each patient. In a catastrophic situation in which large numbers of patients must be treated, complete diagnosis and evaluation for each individual might be impossible, but there could be segregation into groups sharing common nutritional patterns of prescription. To this end, it was useful to classify several varieties of starvation and malnutrition, and to consider several influencing factors too.

The *Duration* of malnourishment was important for both treatment and prognosis. A certain degree of cachexia could be the result of a few weeks of fasting or of many months of undernourishment. Complete return to health was best when inanition had been short, and therefore the length of the treatment was directly related to the period of malnutrition. Concerning duration, starvation and severe malnutrition was classified as: brief, when it lasted less than one month; moderately prolonged, when it affected the population from one month to one year; and very prolonged and chronic or extremely prolonged, when it starved people for more than one year. A different category, namely *lifelong malnutrition*, was applied to those suffering since early infancy.

A rough classification of varieties of starvation was proposed by Keys in terms of the most important deficiencies:

a) *Simple starvation* and *simple undernutrition* occurs when the calorie deficiency is of major importance, a condition that could be recognised by the presence of emaciation, bradycardia and other clinical signs derived from the physio-pathological consequence of calorie under-nutrition, such as polyuria, weakness, depression, hypotension, hypothermia. This clinical picture shows the absence of polyneuritis,

---

27 *Ibidem*, p. 17.

glossitis, extreme oedema, definite night-blindness and severe gingivitis. "Slight to moderate anaemia and dependent oedema were common; tendon reflexes may be reduced, senses and the intellect were usually unimpaired, but prevailing lethargy and apathy gave the impression of dullness or even stupidity. Major complaints were hunger, weakness, fatigue, dizziness, irritability and cold sensitivity".

b) A second variety, which Keys called *primary protein deficiency*, appeared when the total protein content or quality constituted the most serious defect in the diet. Oedema, liver and kidney disease, and little appetite were common signs of primary protein deficiency.

c) A third category was *primary B-complex deficiency*, characterised by cutaneous, mucous-membrane, neurological and sensorial complaints.

d) Other *classical deficiency diseases* encompassed different categories such as beriberi, scurvy, pellagra and vitamin-A deficiency.

e) However, *mixed deficiencies* were common wherever there was malnutrition and, in case of doubt, all severely starved or malnourished patients would be treated as though they had a mixture of nutritional deficiencies.

f) Finally, *nutritional deficiency plus trauma or disease* was a typified condition, taking place when malnutrition or starvation was accompanied by serious injuries or complicated by serious disease, the treatment of the nutritional state being essential as part of the global treatment.[28]

From a purely quantitative perspective, Keys proposed the establishment of several degrees of nutritional deficiency. Based on his clinical experience and the conclusions drawn from his experimental research, this was particularly helpful for large-scale treatment. The categories proposed were:

a) *Mild deficiency:* characterised by a body weight under 15 per cent, mild primary protein deficiency and a moderate degree of oedema and other signs of vitamin deficiencies: gingivitis, follicular keratitis, glossitis, cheilosis, appetite loss, paresthesia, conjunctivitis, muscular weakness, mild polyneuritis…

---

[28] *Ibidem*, p. 19.

b) *Moderate deficiency:* implied a loss of weight from 15 to 20 per cent, moderate oedema, alteration of total plasma protein concentration and decrease in haemoglobin below standards.

c) *Severe deficiency:* implied more than 20 per cent of weight deficit, oedema, mild anaemia and other clinical signs pointing to a state of semi-starvation. A severe deficiency of proteins and vitamins resulted in pronounced signs of deficiency diseases such as scurvy, beriberi, pellagra, rickets…

d) *Extreme deficiencies:* might be diagnosed when the clinical picture indicated imminent danger of death from starvation or malnutrition and major signs and symptoms were present to a very high degree, which used to appear when the body weight was only 60 per cent of the ideal weight.

> The typical severely starved person, without other complications, is emaciated, with a pallid, greyish visage and apathetic, depressed expression. Neglect of personal appearance, indifference to the impression of stupidity. Blotchy, pigmentation on the face or elsewhere may be mistaken for simple dirt. This pigmentation sometimes may be ascribed erroneously to pellagra.[29]

Those and other physical signs were described in Ancel Keys' report, showing the physical impairment induced by under-nutrition, describing in a detailed way the clinical signs identified by medical examination. A physio-pathological description of functional alterations was also described: muscular weakness, rapid movement impairment, visual and hearing difficulties, changes in respiratory, digestive and circulatory function, heart weakness, oedema in knee joints, and many other signs.

> The foregoing descriptions apply to uncomplicated starvation and are accompanied by complaints, more or less in proportion to the degree of starvation, of weakness, hunger, fatigue, sensitivity to cold, depression, dizziness on arising, a sense of being old, and polyuria. Substantial deviations from this picture, including other signs or symptoms than those mentioned, indicate other complications –specific nutritional deficiencies, infection, or other concomitant disease. Paresthesias may suggest thiamine and possibly other B-vitamin deficiencies but the possible role of circulatory factors must not be neglected. Great oedema suggests specific protein deficiency, liver disease, heart failure from causes other than simple starvation, or renal disease. Pain referable to the bones with complaints usually centred in the pelvis and the spine indicates the possibility of nutritional osteopathology, which can be checked by x-ray examination. Visual or auditory defects may be ascribed to vitamin deficiencies. Extreme

29 *Ibidem*, p. 22.

> anaemia suggests the presence of blood-destructive infection, specific blood diseases, or iron deficiency; the latter may be indicated by hypochromia. Severe gingivitis, with bleeding, may indicate ascorbic-acid deficiency which should be confirmed by a search for other diagnostic features. There is an increased incidence of hernias and of thrombophlebitis.[30]

Thanks to his clinical experiments, Keys showed in his report his vast experience in the sequencing and recognition of the clinical signs caused by starvation. In addition, severe starvation could conceal the presence of serious infection, as the normal febrile response to the infection could be diminished or absent, particularly in cold weather. The diagnosis of tuberculosis, for example, could be delayed or missed on this account. The starved person seemed to be relatively unresponsive. Starvation produced changes in muscular and psychological characteristics. Early in the course of starvation there was a loss of muscular endurance with a relatively low loss of fine coordination and muscular strength. The reduction in the ability to make small rapid movements was not marked until the more extreme stages of starvation appeared. A reduction in cardio-circulatory function was large and progressive, but not greatly disproportionate to the basal metabolic demand. Changes in purely respiratory function were not of critical importance in simple starvation, and the same was true for digestive, excretory and renal function. The thermoregulatory function was disturbed in starvation and the limited circulation became increasingly restricted to the more vital organs.

From a purely medical perspective, the psychological influence of severe malnutrition and starvation was conditioned by the somatic impairment that especially affected the person's emotional balance. But the more severe the picture, the more consistent the psychological deterioration pattern, which ended in delirium prior to the comatose state. The most outstanding emotional characteristic was depression and apathy, which took the patient to a state of mindlessness, irritability, weakness and fatigability, all this resulting in very slow movements and quietness. Social kindness and politeness disappeared and moral patterns were altered. Mutual self-help became difficult to maintain without strong leadership from non-starving persons. Neurotic tendencies were exacerbated, but, according to Keys' report, few of them turned into psychosis or psychotic behaviour, suicide being uncommon. The basic intellective abilities were not deeply altered, except for the most extreme starvation cases. But intellective activity was reduced as a result of physical deterioration. When feeding was resumed, the return of

---

30 *Ibidem*, p. 23.

strength made up for the accumulated damage and irritation. At this stage, doctors noticed that the patient was far more troublesome than before starving. When severe deficiencies of vitamin B complex occurred, the psychological picture became altered, producing violent personality changes, which explains why pellagra was also associated to dementia.[31]

The extremely starved person was incapable of any useful work and of taking care of themselves. In less extreme states, starved people could work in line with their limitations, "but constant stimulation and supervision may be necessary". The moderately starved person showed little endurance for heavy manual work, but was still able to do jobs that required little muscular effort or prolonged standing. Obviously, under famine conditions, mortality rates would frequently rise due to several causes leading to direct starvation deaths and fatalities by infection or other causes. However, general mortality did not necessarily rise in times of famine, as it reduced the prevalence of certain diseases. Diabetes mellitus, for instance, was notably reduced; coronary diseases and hypertension also tended to decrease and available data suggested that no rise and possibly a slight fall in deaths from neoplastic diseases took place. On the contrary, under famine conditions, a marked increase in the number of deaths attributed to respiratory and gastro-intestinal diseases, senile decay and violence was observed, with tuberculosis being a major threat.[32] A general pattern of behaviour was recommended from a medical point of view:

> Where there is a mass-starvation problem a single agency or organisation should be in charge of the treatment of starved persons in the area involved and the effective direction must be given to experts in medical nutrition. This agency must have responsibility and authority over the selection of patients and hospitals or treatment centres, over the recruitment, assignment and direction of professional, nursing, and other personnel, over the requisitioning and allocation of supplies and equipment, and over the general policies and methods of treatment. In a city where several hospitals, hotels and other structures or areas are designated as starvation-treatment centres, a single body, agency or board must have authority over all these facilities. Such centralisation of power was essential both for efficiency and to prevent large discrepancies in the aid given to patients in equal need. All food gifts and food distribution by welfare agencies must be rigorously

31 *Ibidem*, p. 23.

32 *Ibidem*, p. 26.

> controlled for the protection of the patients themselves, who may be seriously harmed by over-zealous feeding.[33]

Arrangements for starved patients were to be made by fully acknowledging the special situation of the patients, who were weak, fatigued and frequently troubled with polyuria and diarrhoea. Famine victims were almost universally careless and untidy, which often made sanitation hard to maintain. Under those difficult circumstances, the major risks were tuberculosis, typhus and all forms of sewage and food-borne infections. Experienced doctors and nurses were considered to be essential for efficient health care. Ancel Keys' technical report made reference to the most convenient technical facilities and equipment for the exploration of patients: X-ray, fluoroscopic units, blood analysis and other instruments. However, food was the essential problem:

> The number of patients to be treated and the efficacy of their treatment are strictly dependent upon the food and feeding supplies of the centre for the treatment of starvation. Though some semi-starved adults may demand, and may eat when offered, as much as 5,000 or 6,000 calories a day, calculations as to the real needs for starved patients under treatment can be made at a far more modest level. For a mixed population of ambulatory patients of both sexes and all ages, none of whom is doing heavy work, a supply level of 3,500 cal. should be ample, unless there is excessive waste, and 3,000 cal. should suffice to allow fairly rapid rehabilitation if the distribution is properly adjusted to the size, age, sex, and activity of the patients. These figures cover estimated waste not exceeding 10% and are proposed for a temperate climate and people of the size of ordinary north Europeans.[34]

The actual food items to be supplied had to be selected by taking account of the nutritional characteristics of the diet, acceptability by the patient, cooking and feeding facilities at hand and foods available. The general character of the diet had to be aimed at a high-protein and low-residue level, and be as high in vitamins and minerals as possible. The treatment schedule proposed was as follows: firstly, the patient had to be classified according to the degree of medical urgency; then supportive treatment would be initiated for critical cases; and a diagnosis would then be made. To start with, moderation was the rule and any patients looking moribund would be treated as a medical emergency. In any case, Keys' report recommended that the first feeding underestimated rather than overestimated the capacity of the patient to assimilate food. Patients who were ambulatory and not very emaciated could be put directly on any available diet that was readily digestible and nutritious,

33 *Ibidem*, p. 28.

34 *Ibidem*, p. 31.

but in no case was it recommended to exceed 2,000 cal. on the first day or to exceed 3,000 cal. in any day of the first week. The best guide to the feeding programme for the first few days was considered to be the estimate of the dietary intake of the preceding few days. If this was considered to be of the order of 1,000 to 1,500 cal. it was safe to increase this by 50 per cent. If the patient was extremely cachectic, even this modest amount had to be provided in five or more daily feedings of highly digestive foods, chiefly liquid.

> The whole feeding programme should be devised to increase the nutrient intake as rapidly as is consistent with safety and comfort to reach the maximal rate at which the body can really utilize the food. Surpassing this rate means at best either gastro-intestinal problems or excessive fat deposition or both. Unlimited crowding of either calories or proteins in the diet into the body does not mean necessarily any gain in tissues rebuilt or strength restored. The dietary supply should be reduced with the appearance of any sign of indigestion, cardio-circulatory embarrassment, or appetite surfeit.[35]

After the first few days of dietary treatment many immediate dangers and problems would be overcome, but the succeeding few weeks also brought difficulties. The feeding programme for the first few weeks continued to be conservative. For a severely starved man whose normal body-weight was 65 kg, and who was ambulatory but not labouring or continuously active, an average intake of 3,000 cal. daily for the first month was considered ample and anything over 3,500 cal. Excessive. These amounts were lower for women and older men. When possible, it was considered desirable to divide the daily diet into more than three meals. After one or two weeks, it was time to institute a cautious programme of mild exercise for all patients for whom it would seem appropriate.

But feeding was not deemed to be enough to restore strength and wasted muscles could not be rebuilt without exercise. After a month the most severely starved patients would still be extremely weak, definitely anaemic and in no condition to do without external care. The less severely starved patients could be ready to care for themselves on an outpatient basis, but would still receive dietary and medical guidance and be protected from heavy work or exposure to inclement weather. As a matter of fact, Keys argued that starved patients would not be fully recovered for many months to come. "If the normal body weight of an adult is regained in less than five or six months the body composition will be excessively high in fat and in no case can one expect complete

---

35 *Ibidem*, p. 36.

restoration of proper body composition and function in less than this time or indeed short of eight or ten months. During all this time a relatively high intake of proteins, vitamins, and minerals is advisable".[36]

From a community perspective, the provision of relief could be organised as follows:

1. A public health office to direct all operations and keep records.
2. An emergency hospital, which could serve as a central storehouse of medical supplies and special foods.
3. A nutritional and medical survey team.
4. A chief sanitary officer and assistants.
5. A community kitchen that has medical supervision.
6. An isolation hospital for communicable diseases.
7. An outpatient clinic.
8. A special clinic for pregnant women, nursing mothers and infants.
9. A transport section to move patients, supplies and facilities.[37]

A specific section was to be devoted to parenteral therapy, commonly used in modern hospitals, including intravenous infusions and transfusions. In 1951 the nutrition experts considered these new technologies very useful in the treatment of severely starved persons, where the primary needs were to give the tissues an ample supply of nutrients and to support circulation. But in any other cases "parenteral feeding is an expedient to be resorted to only when other methods of feeding are clearly inadequate or inapplicable. Intravenous infusions always entail some risk and this is much increased when applied under conditions other than those of a good modern hospital.[38] Specific recommendations about the content of intravenous alimentation were detailed in the report.

A section of the clinical report was devoted to the special problems of infants and children, and considered the nutritional requirements for growth and the formation of milk by the nursing woman. The protein requirement for growth was high and, in a situation of shortage, dietary proteins tend to be used for energy purposes only. This leads to a serious protein deficiency in diets poor in calories, even when the protein intake is reasonably high. Moreover, for new tissue to be formed, the

---

36 *Ibidem*, p. 38.

37 *Ibidem*, p. 40.

38 *Ibidem*, p. 41.

incorporation of appropriate vitamins and minerals is necessary, so the amounts of these nutrients must be directly related to the rate of growth. Body size, muscle condition and organic impairment must be explored. The experts believed that infants and young children were best taken care of by their mothers or relatives, wherever possible. In large camps and hospitals, efforts were made to provide separate quarters for family groups or for women with young children. Emergency feeding stations for infants and young children, and pregnant and nursing women, were considered of great value for providing direct nutritional aid to those vulnerable members of the community. Such stations would provide medical help, health education and instruction in the feeding of infants. For school-age children, school canteens were most convenient. Visiting nurses and social workers could be assigned to assessing social conditions that influence malnutrition. Special management for diarrhoeal disease was also included.

After the clinical approach to starvation by Ancel Keys, the last part of the technical report published by the Joint Committee was devoted to the organisation of general relief activities in relation to nutrition when famine conditions prevailed. In the immediate post-war period a lot of experience of organised relief feeding was gained, with some evident examples mentioned: the United Nations Relief and Rehabilitation Administration (UNRRA); UNICEF; the International Red Cross; the League of Red Cross Societies; and the Society of Friends. When the emergency was formidable and needs were great, national action alone was insufficient and relief was regarded on large-scale and food shortages as an international responsibility. The agencies concerned with relief had to be ready to move in supplies and personnel at the right moment.

> Distribution centres, mobile canteens, field kitchens, etc. must be set up without delay in the affected area. Equipment that will provide some means of cooking within the homes may be necessary. It is important to consider also supply of water and fuel needed for cooking. In arranging the provision of food the local dietary habits and patterns of the people to be relieved should be taken into account, as far as this is possible.[39]

The first task was to make surveys of small samples of the population to discover the level of feeding during the famine period and the current state of nutrition. This was intended to show to what extent people were suffering from specific food-deficiency states, as well as from generalised deficient nutrition. Also, it would indicate both the level of relief required and the need for foods rich in particular nutrients

---

39 *Ibidem*, p. 53.

to overcome specific food deficiencies. Under the living circumstances of Western Europe, where famine conditions were not superimposed on chronic deficient nutrition, relief could be needed by three broad categories: a) the normal underfed population; b) ambulant close to starvation cases, affected by 25 per cent body-weight loss; and c) acute starvation cases provoking cachexia, oedema and other clinical signs. To deal with this situation three types of feeding teams were considered necessary: medical selection teams, distribution teams and clinical teams. The types of personnel required were physicians, nurses, nutritionists, distribution officers, cooks and kitchen staff.

Experiments on Fermented Food

Before the Joint FAO/WHO Expert Committee met in Fajara, Gambia, in a long meeting from late November until early December 1952, Paul György (1893-1976), the renowned specialist in the physiology of nutrition who isolated riboflavin and discovered vitamin B6, wrote some comments on the provisional agenda regarding malnutrition and protein consumption in mothers, infants and children.[40] György was at this time professor at the University of Pennsylvania in Philadelphia. He stressed how clinical and experimental studies had made it clear that protein deficiency was the most prominent factor in malnutrition, with *kwashiorkor* and related conditions a notable example in poor countries. However, he considered that protein deficiency was not the only factor and argued that increased protein intake could not be the only possible health measure in preventing or treating those forms of malnutrition. He compiled experimental research carried out with laboratory animals between 1950-52, and after a detailed review of the latest historiography, he concluded that the fermentation of food might, under special circumstances, increase the biological value of foodstuffs, even of a low protein diet. Studies conducted in Jamaica and Guatemala showed that rats fed with fermented mixtures had statistically significant weight gain compared to animals kept on the corresponding unfermented diet. Thiamine, pyridoxine, riboflavin and pantothenic acid supplements had no effect on the growth of either of the two groups of rats used in the experiments. Fermented food was used practically everywhere in the Tropics, and György cited "fermented fish" and "fermented beans" as foodstuffs used for research on the action of fermentation on protein metabolism. Neither the nitrogen nor the vitamin B12 contents of the food mixtures were found to be

---

40 György, P., *Comments on the Provisional Agenda with special reference to items Nos. 5 and 6*, Joint FAO/WHO Nutrition Committee, 1952.

substantially different in the unfermented and fermented mixtures, and thus this could not explain the difference in growth promotion by the two food mixtures.

In the course of the animal experiments, the *choline equivalent* was determined in various samples by using them to supplement a high fat and low protein diet. Together with studies using food mixtures of "authentic" composition in unfermented and fermented states, this research was supposed to illustrate one of the possible directions in which animal experimentation was oriented at that time. The overall problem was indeed malnutrition associated with protein deficiency, and the question of the possible contribution of the FAO and other organisations to the study of and fight against malnutrition in mothers and children throughout the world.

Paul György requested that the Expert Committee take up and put those experiments into a working scheme, forming a permanent working group that not only had to convene once a year but had to remain in constant close contact, under the auspices and with the assistance of the FAO and the WHO. Younger staff, not yet members of the Expert Committee working in those fields were called on to become attached to the Expert Committee by contributing scientific research and reports covering the subject. Such reports would help not only to maintain contact among the researchers, but might also act as an incentive and stimulus.

> The problem of how to secure the necessary financial resources for an ambitious world-wide research program dealing with the problems of malnutrition in mothers and children throughout the world appears to be of secondary importance. It is more pressing to formulate first a workable plan. It may be rightly anticipated that financial support will then become available without great difficulty through foundations, research councils and perhaps through the Technical assistance Program. Clinical, public health and experimental problems have to be dovetailed and coordinated throughout the whole world. I offer the enthusiastic cooperation of our own laboratory, with special reference to animal experimentation.[41]

[41] *Ibidem.*

CHAPTER 10

Nutrition, Public Health and Education

In the opening lecture of the National Vitamin Foundation Conference held in 1957, John Boyd Orr, the first Director-General of the FAO, talked about *Nutrition in programming for public health.*[1] He started his speech by directly recognizing "scientists who have made such a great contribution to the New Science of Nutrition". He told the story of how ten years earlier, when feeling ill, he met the chairman of the conference, Russell Wilder, for the first time: "He told me – *me* – who had devoted the best part of my life to research in nutrition, that I was suffering from vitamin deficiency. He prescribed vitamin capsules made by one of the Companies which give financial support to this Foundation".[2] He introduced himself, therefore, as "an ambulatory advertisement of the value of a generous intake of vitamins for warding off the premature onset of senile decay and maintaining, in old age, the vigor and sprit of youth".[3]

At the time of the economic crisis that was punishing the world in the 1930s, when the governments of industrialised countries were battling with the problem of large-scale unemployment, John Boyd Orr was a colleague of Boudreau, Sebrell and Hazel Stiebeling in the League of Nations Committee of Experts on Nutrition. He summarised the origin of the political economy of nutrition in those years perfectly:

> The idea was that, as there are more people in the world engaged in the production and distribution of food than in all other industries, a market for the great amount of additional food needed to provide a diet adequate for health for the whole human family would bring prosperity to agriculture which would flow into other industries and so help to solve the problem of the economic crisis. That movement, which was approved by 22 nations, was brought to a halt by the outbreak of the Second World War. It was revived by the Hot Springs Conference. When the world becomes sane, that

---

1 Orr, J.B., *Nutrition in programming for public health. Address delivered before the National Vitamin Foundation, March 6, 1957*, National Vitamin Foundation Report to the Board of Governors by Scientific Director for the period Jan. 1, 1956-Dec. 31, 1956, New York, National Vitamin Foundation. 1957.

2 *Ibidem*, p. 11.

3 *Ibidem*, pp. 11-12.

> great ideal of adjusting the production and distribution of food to human needs will be realized, and the promotion of economic prosperity will coincide partly at least with the promotion of human welfare.[4]

Orr situates the time when research first got an inkling of the cause of nutritional deficiency diseases in the second decade of the 20th century. The first discovery, he said, was made when diets assumed to be adequate by chemical analyses were tried out on animals and found to be inadequate. Physics and chemistry in research in nutrition then began to be superseded by biological tests and clinical examinations. Vitamins, minerals and other nutrients emerged as essential elements for health; nevertheless, during the inter-war period, there was great difficulty in getting this new scientific knowledge on nutrition applied, because it was not easy to change the prevailing mentality, convincing senior public health officers and authorities of the key idea: controlling infectious diseases and improving the population's health came through providing a healthy diet to the whole population. The old *medical style of thinking* changed after the results of combined dietary and clinical surveys and feeding experiments with large groups of children carried out in several countries. Experimental and clinical research, as well as social surveys, showed that freedom from deficiency diseases and better health and physical condition were correlated with the level of income. This was one of Boyd Orr's first major contributions.[5] The incidence of food deficiencies increased in times of crisis, particularly because the poor were unable to afford the more expensive vitamin and mineral rich foods. Malnutrition was largely a disease of poverty, and Boyd Orr was convinced that the challenge to combat poverty was a political issue. The fight was therefore carried into the arena of politics and ideological debate:

> The old politicians were honestly confused. They thought that malnutrition was just a new fancy word for hunger and, as bread was so cheap, that hunger, which was the food problem of the nineteenth century, had been almost completely eliminated; the agitation about malnutrition was the work of food faddists. Some even took the view that the high death rate among the poor was due to the beneficent natural law of the elimination of the unfit, their poor physique being evidence of their unfitness, and to interfere with this law would be unwise. Further, public health measures to improve the diet of the poor would involve a good deal of government expenditure, and a demand for higher wages for the worst paid workers. These objections

4 *Ibidem*, p. 12.

5 Orr, J.B., *Food, Health & Income: Report on a Survey of Adequacy of Diet in Relation to Income*, London, Macmillan & Co, 1936.

had to be overcome before nutrition became an important part of public health work.

When there was ample evidence that the children of the poor, when they received a diet as good as the children of the well-to-do, grew at the same rate and were as healthy and vigorous, some research workers and public health officials in Western countries applied a lot of high-pressure salesmanship to sell the idea that, as a Belgian public health officer put it, life and health could be bought, or in the words of a great American, Dr. Hermann Biggs, that public health was "purchasable". Then the advertising appeared. The attractive advertisements of companies selling vitamin preparations or vitamin-rich food, occasionally making exaggerated claims, and popular articles by journalists, sometimes a little inaccurate, made the public food-conscious. The mysterious "magic vitamin" caught the imagination. The new science of nutrition became popular and strong public opinion arose in favour of its application.[6]

The drive to get the new knowledge on nutrition applied to improve the diet and health of the population coincided with the 1930 slump in food in Western countries, so it was relatively easy to persuade governments to use any surplus food to palliate the hunger of the poor and unemployed for the mutual benefit of health, agriculture and trade, although at the taxpayer's expense. Boyd Orr recognised that the increase in unemployment benefits and family allowance for the children of the unemployed had enabled poor children to be better fed. These extensions of public health and social services were followed by the inspection of school children, prenatal care of mothers and education about the value of food. These measures provided awareness about the social dimension of deficiency diseases and contributed to the elimination of acute forms "which had affected more than 50 per cent of the children in industrial towns, of nutritional anaemia and other forms of malnutrition not acute enough to be called diseases. Pellagra in the Southern States of America and in Eastern European countries and beriberi in the East almost disappeared, and the control of these diseases was accompanied by improved health and vigour".[7]

In most European countries, the expansion of industrial areas caused malnutrition to become prevalent among lower social groups, a situation seriously impaired by wars and economic crises. Food rationing became an essential policy, giving priority to mothers and children for milk and fresh fruit, and allowing them a minimum intake of proteins, cod liver oil and cereals; this policy made them available for all children,

---

6 Orr, J.B., 1957, pp. 16-17.

7 *Ibidem*, p. 18.

independently of their social level, with the result that the health and organic condition of children continued to improve even in times of food shortage. All branches of experimental medicine had contributed towards greatly improving the health of the population, but Orr estimated that "none in the last 30 years has made a greater contribution than nutrition, with its elimination of deficiency diseases and its promotion of positive health".[8]

Medical authorities recognised that the new science of nutrition had made a great contribution to public health, occupying a central place in social medicine and politics. It required financial support to ensure that every family needing attention could receive the necessary advice and assistance. The emphasis was initially on the more vulnerable groups, mothers and children, but more attention was paid to the increasingly large number of elderly couples, whose diet in many cases degenerated to no more than bread and other cheap foods.

Burnet and Aykroyd – Nutrition in Public Health

Twenty years earlier, the technical report presented by E. Burnet and W.R. Aykroyd to the League of Nations proposed a programme of education in nutrition as a means for hastening the practical application of scientific knowledge on nutrition to public health.[9]

> It is the task of central and local public health services, the medical profession and its ancillaries (nurses, dieticians, social workers, etc.), to instruct the public, but this cannot teach unless they have the requisite knowledge and enthusiasm. There are, therefore, two aspects of the subject: the education of those responsible for educating the public and the education of the public itself.[10]

During the early years in their curriculum, medical students received information about the physiology of nutrition, sometimes including practical laboratory training, but the subject was presented as a chapter of physiology and not as part of public health and preventive medicine. In practical terms, this implied that a medical practitioner learned how to manage nutritional diseases but ignored the preventive and public health dimension of nutrition. The experts demanded that nutrition be included in the curriculum of post-graduate medical schools, as scientific knowledge on diet appeared to be an important branch of public health, and therefore health administrations and public health organisations had

---

8 *Ibidem*, p. 19.

9 Burnet, E., Aykroyd, W.R., 'Nutrition and Public Health", *League of Nations Quarterly Bulletin of the Health Organisation*, 1935, Vol. 4, No. 2, pp. 323-474.

10 *Ibidem*, p. 386.

to employ specialised experts and develop mechanisms for furthering work in the field. Nutrition specialists, acquainted with the latest developments in research, and capable of formulating and carrying out schemes for their practical application, were considered to be a valuable addition to the personnel of public health organisations.

Advisory committees on nutrition, made up of physiologists, practical cookery experts, medical officers and social workers, were called to work together to fulfill a useful role. Burnet and Aykroyd suggested that these committees should be attached to central public health authorities, assuming the issue of sound educational material and advising other State Departments on matters connected with nutrition among their primary duties. In most Western countries, as well as in Japan and the Soviet Union, national institutes of nutrition – or departments of nutrition in institutes of hygiene – had been created, connecting public health authorities, universities and the general population. "An ideal institute of nutrition would include laboratories, a statistical department, lecture rooms for students and the public, a cookery department, an educational department containing models, posters, diagrams etc. Such institutions or departments would obviously play a prominent part in educating nutrition workers and the public".[11] Educational material issued by responsible authorities, and containing acceptable dietary standards, were of particular value as a basis for practical action. In some cases, museums of public health took over the task of spreading knowledge and popularising new concepts, assisting the National Schools of Hygiene during the inter-war years.

While state and local authorities, expert committees and medical professionals were responsible for the initiation and support of public health nutritional work, to a large degree this was social work requiring the assistance of nutritionists, dieticians, nurses, social workers, school teachers, cooks, etc., working in private and public institutions (schools, dispensaries, prisons, hospitals, industrial canteens, etc.). Within the framework of this collaborative work the figure of the nutritionist emerged, associated with the female sex.

> The nutritionist is not a scientific worker, though she often takes part in scientific enquiries. She must know how to make reliable dietary surveys. She is, in general, expected to keep up with the latest developments of her subject. Although she deals largely in matters closely associated with medicine and often works in close contact with the medical profession, she has had, as a rule, little medical or nursing training. It is only to be expected that there should be members of the medical profession who resent the

---

[11] *Ibidem*, p. 388.

> intrusion of a non-medical worker into medical fields; such critics complain, rightly or wrongly, that the training and knowledge of the nutritionist is too academic, that she lacks the background necessary for the application of laboratory results to human beings. It is to be noted that the inspiration of the "nutrition" movement in the United States of America has come from distinguished scientists who are not members of the medical profession. In general, however, medical men feel that the nutritionist is a useful assistant in hospital, in the out-patient department, and in public health work of all kinds.[12]

A discussion was opened about the professional profile of nutritionists, particularly on whether a nurse who had received post-graduate instruction in dietetics in addition to her ordinary hospital training could successfully fulfill most of the functions of the nutritionist, and be able to deal with deficiency diseases and malnutrition. Their contribution, as well as that of health visitors, in improving dietary habits in the home was widely recognised. All those professionals were able to provide valuable assistance in campaigns against rickets, dental caries, infantile scurvy and other deficiency diseases, and supervising the diets of infants and pregnant and nursing women. Schoolteachers and social workers of all types were also able to help in the campaign against malnutrition.

Education in Nutrition in Schools

Schoolchildren in Western countries received simple instruction at school on the rules of health, and it seemed to be essential that such teaching had to include instruction on diet, a variable subject closely dependent on cultural habits, which differed from country to country. Therefore no general rules were able to be adopted regarding the type and amount of instruction in nutrition, nor which schoolchildren should receive it. Simplicity was considered a good principle, in order to avoid the impression that correct feeding was a difficult problem. The main advice was that elementary principles were transmitted about the composition of the diet (such as green vegetables are healthy foods). School meals were an excellent opportunity to instruct children in the principles of the new science of nutrition. The supplying of milk was also able to help teachers inform children and parents about its nutritional value.

The *nutrition class* was also conceived for malnourished children. Work with outpatient children gave evidence of the existence of a large number of delicate children, belonging to all social classes, who

12 *Ibidem*, p. 393.

appeared to derive little benefit from ordinary medical treatment.[13] Dr. Emerson, working in a clinic in Boston, confirmed this impression by studying 5,000 children attending the clinic. He chose 15 children who showed marked evidence of debility and malnutrition, and put them together in a class for treatment by education in nutrition. Children attending this nutrition class were given a notebook in which to record the nature of meals and their duration, hours of sleep, and the amount of time spent playing in the open air. At the same time, a nurse or social worker visited their homes and surveyed the hygiene conditions in which each child lived.

Similar to other school cards used by medical inspectors to record physical features and clinical examinations, each child was presented with a chart bearing its name, on which two curves were inscribed, one representing the child's actual weight curve and the other an ideal weight curve. The children themselves recorded their weight week by week on the chart, and their parents were invited to attend the class in order to share and assume the content of the programme. Some sort of reward was given to children who made the best progress. If a child was not progressing favourably, an attempt was made to discover the reason: lack of sufficient food, too easy and rapid meals, faulty hygiene or infectious conditions. The parents were informed of the cause of the child's lack of progress. Initially, nutrition classes were attached to clinics, but they were subsequently developed in schools as an activity associated with medical school officers. They were sometimes supplemented by open-air "nutrition camps". "The nutrition class involves an abridgment of school-hours. The program includes a rest and a meal at 10:30, half an hour's rest before the midday meal, and a small meal in the middle of the afternoon".[14]

The results obtained were apparently very positive. Burnet and Aykroyd cited some reports assessing the result of nutrition classes during the period 1921-26, stating that 80 per cent of children attending the class regained average weight, while only 35 per cent of poorly nourished children outside the classes made similar gains during a similar period. It was claimed that the beneficial effects of the nutrition class extended to children not actually enrolled and to the children's homes. Similarly, the London County Council Education Committee established five nutrition clinics in London at the end of the 1930s. Medical intervention was widened and suitable cases were referred to those clinics by school doctors, teachers and child care committees.

---

13 *Ibidem*, p. 395.

14 *Ibidem*, p. 396.

Each child underwent a medical examination to ascertain whether he or she was suffering from a nutritional deficiency. If that were the case, advice was given to the parents and, when necessary, treatment was provided in the form of a specific diet rich in cod-liver oil, iron, proteins, etc.[15]

Home Economics and Schools of Domestic Science

In order to spread scientific knowledge about nutrition and diet, and to change the dietary habits of the population, so-called domestic science or home economics schools, largely attended by young women, provided an excellent opportunity for teaching dietetics. In many European countries, *home economics* were included in general education schemes. Since the school curriculum was separated according to sex, girls were the targets of these new courses, which contained information about food and diet and also household economy and cooking.

> The pupil, in learning how to purchase and prepare attractive meals for her future family, can also be taught the elements of nutritional science, with particular reference to the relative price and nutritive value of foodstuffs. It is often said that maternal ignorance is the main cause of malnutrition in children.[16]

In their approach to the subject, Burnet and Aykroyd considered that it was not strictly true, for no amount of knowledge and skill on the part of housewives made it possible to purchase a satisfactory diet when income was insufficient. However, they assumed that the inefficiency of housewives was an important contributing factor in producing malnutrition in the children of the very poor and unemployed. Therefore, the satisfactory education of women in *domestic science*, including dietetics, cooking and marketing was considered an important public health activity.

Educational Work among Rural Populations

An example of energetic educational work in the field of nutrition was provided by a *Cooperative Extension Service in Agriculture and Home Economics* in the United States of America. These types of agencies extended to most European countries in order to improve agriculture through instruction, technical help and advice to peasants and farmers. Their function was to apply the results of scientific research in agriculture and nutrition to the local problems of the farm and the rural community, particularly knowledge regarding home

---

15 *Ibidem*.

16 *Ibidem*.

economics, such as research into the vitamin and mineral content of foodstuffs, the effects of cooking on the nutritional value and the best methods for food preservation. In the USA, the *Bureau of Home Economics* carried out family budget enquiries and surveys on food consumption trends, devising adequate diets at minimum cost. In order to spread the benefits of such research, an *Extension Service* employed more than 60 extension nutritionists in 1934 in 45 States of the Union. These workers were all college graduates and a considerable number of them had taken advanced degrees and accumulated experience as high school or university teachers, hospital dieticians and county home demonstration agents.

Although rural communities were reached by ordinary publicity methods, the heads of the campaigns were the *home demonstration agents*, who achieved direct contact with the population through cooperatives and other local organisations, or through volunteer leaders chosen from rural communities. Malnutrition was attacked in a number of ways. For example, growing vegetables for home consumption was taught and encouraged, something especially important in the pellagra-affected areas. Methods of preserving meat, vegetables, fruit and other foods were taught, with the object of assisting the small farmer to eliminate waste and make full use of the potential wealth at his disposal. Education programmes also included food values, wise purchasing of foodstuffs, cooking, menu planning, food economy, dietary requirements, school lunches and so on. These activities were focused on preventing the lowering of health standards in critical years, and particularly on improving the diet of rural populations, taking into account that, contrary to popular belief, malnutrition was as common among the poorest people in the countryside as in the major cities.[17] Therefore, educational work in nutrition among rural populations was considered a promising field, since the peasant community rarely made full use of the possibilities at their disposal for obtaining a varied, nutritious and attractive diet.[18] Even in the absence of poverty, it was monotonous and badly cooked. "Cooking-classes in rural communities, at which some instruction in the principles of diet is given, have been organized in a number of European countries. Housewives, as a rule, are eager to attend such classes, to the great benefit of themselves and their families".[19]

---

17 *Ibidem*, p. 397

18 *Ibidem*, p. 398.

19 *Ibidem*, pp. 398-399.

In their report, Burnet and Aykroyd considered that useful dietary knowledge had several possible channels of distribution. It could be transmitted directly to individuals by means of infant and mother welfare dispensaries, nutrition clinics, visiting nurses and social workers, and disseminated through schools as part of health education programmes. It could also use the new methods offered by publicity and propaganda: pamphlets, lectures, exhibitions, cinema, radio, posters, daily press, journals and women's magazines. However, nutrition experts warned of an increasing danger: educational materials about diet and nutrition could be parodied by commercial advertisements, resulting in the population finding it difficult to distinguish ingenious advertising from genuine health information.

> During recent years, there has been, in many countries, a tightening-up of regulations designed to ensure that food preparations, advertised as being rich in this or that food factor, do, in fact, possess the quality stated: preparations alleged to contain vitamins, for example, may be subject to official approval and control on the basis of the standards and units established by the League of Nations. But there is, as yet, no machinery for controlling advertising which is false, no verbally, but by implication such advertising, for example, as attempts to give mothers the idea that, if they do not buy the article in question, their children's health will suffer. Those engaged in teaching dietetics to the public find that the ingenuity of the modern advertisement adds greatly to their difficulties".[20]

New regulations and strict control of advertising were crucial aspects demanded by health authorities. The results of education in nutrition were still hard to assess. During the economic crisis in the 1930s vigorous attempts were made in many European countries to disseminate dietary knowledge, but there was not enough perspective to estimate their effectiveness. However, the experts considered some indirect indicators as positive; the fact that infant and child mortality rates, as well as the death rate from tuberculosis, had not stopped falling, suggested that better nutrition could be involved and that educational campaigns had some influence. It was not only the poorer classes that required dietary education, but since it was the poor who suffered from malnutrition, much of the public health nutrition work was concerned with those social groups. One very valuable strategy, especially under critical circumstances, was spreading knowledge and possibilities of how an adequate diet might be obtained at very low cost. However, a wider goal was to attain the best diet, regarding both nutritive value and palatability, from the vast resources that the modern world can produce.

---

20 *Ibidem*, p. 399.

> In a world suffering from over-production of foodstuffs, emphasis should be placed on the *optimum*, rather than on the minimum... In education the public in nutrition, the simplicity of the principles involved should be emphasized: it should be made clear that it usually requires a little more knowledge, but no more effort and anxiety, to prepare and consume a well-balanced diet than a defective one.[21]

Public health administrations, seconded by private institutions, started different forms of intervention to improve diet and health conditions during the 1930s. Nutrition in childhood, food deficiency diseases and collective feeding were the main fields of action. From a nutritional perspective, the prenatal period is one of the most important in human life. The supervision of a woman's diet during pregnancy was included among the duties of maternal and child welfare services. The diet of pregnant women required regulation in many respects, such as the vitamin D, calcium and iron content, essential factors for the prevention of rickets and anaemia. Most paediatricians agreed with the idea that breastfeeding was the ideal method of nourishing an infant, with particular advantages for poorer classes, which could not easily afford the better grades of fresh cow's milk or dried milk preparations.

The principal aim of public health nutritional work was to raise dietary and health standards, which implied the elimination of food deficiency diseases. Dealing with malnutrition also meant an improvement in the rate of these diseases, although each could be regarded as representing a public health problem in itself, calling for special treatment and prevention measures. Several nutritional deficiency diseases became social problems and received a great deal of attention from the experts and authorities. *Chlorosis*, for instance, was a disease confined to the female sex, mostly affecting the working class (waitresses, shop assistants, domestic servants) and young women between 15 and 25 years old. Initially, the origin of the disease was ascribed to many causes, mostly to a psychological origin, but finally a diet deficient in iron was recognised as the fundamental cause, as a result of a diet composed of white bread, margarine, potatoes and tea. The disappearance of chlorosis in the space of a few years was attributed to the raising of living standards and the dissemination of knowledge about nutrition.

At the same time, nursing women suffering from *hypochromic microcytic anaemia* – as a result of blood loss during delivery and in the post-natal period, and to menorrhagia between pregnancies – consumed a diet low in iron. Many considered their condition of chronic ill-health

---

[21] *Ibidem*, p. 400.

and wretchedness as a natural state and accepted it with resignation. Nevertheless, this type of anaemia could immediately be treated by iron medication or by a rational improvement in diet. There appears to be at least one type of microcytic hyperchromic anaemia, which may justifiably be described as a disease due to dietary deficiency – pernicious anaemia of pregnancy. "Pernicious anaemia, as it occurs in Western civilisation, has been shown to be due to defective production of a specific enzyme, an 'intrinsic factor' in gastric juice, which interacts with an 'extrinsic factor' in food to produce the specific "anti-anaemic principle". Treatment in this disease consisted of supplying either the "anti-anaemic principle" (by liver therapy) or giving gastric tissue products, which supply the intrinsic factor and enable the patient to manufacture the anti-anaemic principle for herself.[22] This was the starting point of the discovery of the important physiological function of folic acid, particularly for pregnant women and especially for the normal development of the foetus.

Another major deficiency disease was rickets, associated with a deficit in vitamin D. The enrichment of artificial milk with vitamin D was widely extended in Europe during the 1930s and there was a tendency to promote fluid milk "as the most valuable anti-rachitic agent", from a public health perspective. As a result of the practical application of scientific discoveries, severe rickets was greatly reduced in Europe and North America as a public health problem, although it was not fully solved.

Dental caries, pellagra and beriberi were also persistent problems associated with deficient nutrition, mostly notable in Western countries and among lower social groups. Collective feeding, public canteens or *meals in common* overseen by experts could avoid many of these problems. During the inter-war years there were primarily three kinds of collective feeding initiatives:

a) Collective feeding in residential institutions, public or private, civil or religious, in armies and navies, in establishments such as hospitals, sanatoria, homes for the aged, asylums, prisons, and educational establishments.

b) Meals given as a relief in times of unemployment and economic distress to the unemployed, or to impoverished students and artists, needy intellectual workers and others.

c) Mass feeding organised by industry or the State in accordance with economic and physiological principles.

22 *Ibidem*, p. 420.

Nutrition in Public Health Programmes

A couple of decades after the publication of Burnet and Aykroyd's report on nutrition in public health, José María Bengoa, a Spanish expert in nutritional policy who worked for the Pan American Health Organization and the WHO during his exile from Franco's dictatorship, published a report on nutritional programmes from a public health perspective. He started by expressing the difficulties in setting the specific targets a public health service had to assume in the field of nutrition.[23] In many countries, nutrition programmes were included in general public health strategies, except in cases such as goitre and rickets.[24]

Public health was defined as the art of scientifically organising and orienting collective efforts in order to safeguard, improve and restore health among populations. The second session of the Joint FAO/WHO Expert Committee on Nutrition established certain regulations for the instruction of nutritionists from a public health perspective. At the end of the 1950s there were institutions in many countries devoted to the protection of specific population groups, such as children. When challenging the introduction of more rational feeding habits in one country, experts often created laboratories to analyse foodstuffs. But this was not considered by Bengoa as a public health measure in itself. Food composition tables from neighbouring countries of similar agricultural characteristics could be enough to improve the nutritional state of a population, although it was obviously not sufficient.[25] To assess the results of nutritional programmes, it was essential to have certain indices, in order to compare the initial situation before, during and after the campaign, as well as calculating the budget required to assess efficiency.

Indices used to assess nutritional problems belonged to two different categories: first, the general indices contained demographic, economic and social items, including food consumption in a specific country, and constituted an excellent description of the state of a certain population; second, specific indices regarding more concrete nutritional problems

---

[23] Bengoa, J.M., *Les programmes de nutrition envisages sous l'angle de la sante publique*, FAO Nutrition Meetings Report Series No. 20, Rome, FAO, 1957; Molina, G., *Organization and Intergration of Public Health Services. First Inter-American Congress of Public Health*, La Havana, WHO Document C.I.H./3, 1952.

[24] "Nutrition Surveys. Their techniques and value", *Bull. Nat. Res. Coun*, No. 117, 1949.

[25] Chatfield, Ch., *Tables de composition des aliments pour l'usage international*, Rome, FAO, 1954;

were necessary to evaluate the actual state of nutrition of a population and to subsequently programme adequate measures. Demographic indicators included birth rates, maternal mortality, rate of stillbirths, infant and child mortality, tuberculosis mortality, as well as mortality due to other diseases considered to be influenced by malnutrition and general mortality. Economic indices included: national income per caput; the cost of living; the proportion of the population working in agriculture and industry; the average salary by categories of occupation; the rapport between agriculture and industrial workers; the percentage of the salary devoted to food expenditure; the cost of a standard diet in a working class family; the cost of 100 g of proteins in different foodstuffs; the cost of 100 g of calories in a standard diet; and the cost of workers housing.

Social indices included: the rate of illiteracy; the number of schools per 1,000 children aged seven to 14; the number of play groups and other institutions for pre-school children; the number of newspapers, journals and other information media per 100,000 inhabitants; the number of hospital beds per 1,000 inhabitants; the ratio of doctors with respect to the whole population; and the proportion of unemployed, alcoholics, abandoned and adopted children, etc.

The establishment of indices showing food availability was promoted by FAO experts in order to demonstrate the importance of planning food production, agriculture and commerce, and to determine the proportion of agricultural products used for feeding animals and human consumption. Although these indices did not express the way in which available food was distributed among different social groups, they were considered a good source of information about the conditions that represented the basis of the nutritional problems in a country, although they were not as specific as food surveys. It was difficult to establish exact figures in many countries lacking good national agriculture statistics, but in those cases general indices could provide useful information about the general conditions. They also allowed calorie intake, animal proteins and fats to be calculated, as well as determine milk consumption, proteins per 100 calories, etc.[26]

Specific epidemiological indices contained records on pellagra, beriberi, scurvy, rickets and other forms of avitaminoses, as well as food deficiencies and malnutrition. Clinical surveys,[27] anthropometric surveys

[26] Bengoa, J.M., *Les programmes de nutrition*, 1957, p. 1866.

[27] Jolliffe, W., "Clinical examination. Methods for evaluation of nutritional adequacy and status", *Bull. Nat. Res.Coun*, Washington.

and food consumption surveys were essential to assess the nutritional state of a population.

Once again, *kwashiorkor*, endemic goitre and pellagra were identified as the main social diseases related to food deficiencies, which required specific public health interventions in many African, American and Asian countries. Food supplementation appeared as the main option, but it required detailed expertise to determine the type, definition, doses and legal regulations. Nutrition experts distinguished between several concepts expressing different methods of intervention in foodstuffs: *reconstitution*, *reinforcement*, *surcharge* and *equivalence.* A foodstuff becomes *reconstituted* when it is subjected to a process of restitution of its original nutritional elements lost during the production process. *Reinforcement* meant adding nutrients in a higher degree than in natural conditions and *surcharge* involved the addition of nutrients over the daily nutritional needs. *Equivalence* was applied to the process of restoring the equivalent nutritional value to similar foodstuffs, e.g. margarine and butter. It is easy to understand how food industrialisation was influencing the management of foodstuffs.

One of the most urgent targets was the supplementary nutrition programmes applied to special groups: pregnant and nursing women, pre-school children, schoolchildren; other population groups such as industrial workers and the elderly; and other vulnerable groups especially sensitive to the consequences of inadequate nutrition. Once again in public health nutrition, education of the public and open information appeared as a cornerstone. The way in which information campaigns and education to specific groups should be implemented was a major concern of FAO and WHO experts, giving rise to a series of publications on the subject.[28]

Education and Training in Nutrition

In December 1959 a symposium on education and training in nutrition in Europe organised by the FAO and the WHO was held in Bad Homburg (German Federal Republic). European experts in nutrition presented a series of papers on complementary aspects of the general subject. C. de Hartog, director of the Nutrition Bureau in The Hague, and A.M. Copping, senior lecturer in nutrition at the Queen Elizabeth College, University of London, presented a paper on "The nutritional

[28] Ritchie, J.A.S., "Pour une alimentation meilleure", *Études de nutrition de la FAO*, No. 6, 1950; *Organisation Mondiale de la Santé. Comité Mixte FAO/OMS d'experts de la Nutrition*, Geneva, OMS, 1954.

state of Europe and the need for education and training in nutrition".[29] They emphasised that, although the relationships between nutrition and health were widely recognised, reports from different countries to the FAO Nutrition Meeting for Europe in June 1958 indicated that varying degrees of malnutrition still existed in European countries in 1959.

Over a long period of increasing industrial development, changes in traditional food patterns were taking place in Europe in many population groups, related to changes in agricultural and economic conditions. New foodstuffs had been introduced, which were cheaper and more easily prepared, but sometimes "of unknown quality" from a nutritional point of view. The upheaval of the war and post-war conditions influenced eating habits in areas where tradition was previously prevalent. One issue of the *Bulletin of Agricultural and Food Statistics* (1959) published by the OEEC showed that a meaningful change had occurred from 1948-49 in the general pattern of European food consumption.[30] The most notable trends were increased consumption of fruit and protein-rich foods such as meat, eggs, cheese and milk, and a simultaneous decrease in the consumption of potatoes and cereals. An increase in the consumption of sugar and fats was noted and a decrease in that of fish. These trends arose from social and economic changes in post-war Europe. "While on the one hand they have led to increase in the consumption of valuable foods, on the other they have been associated with over-nutrition and its probably harmful results. Examples of this tendency will be found in the reports of Denmark, Norway, Sweden, the Netherlands, the United Kingdom, Belgium, Austria, Switzerland".[31]

The overall European consumption records and average food consumption figures for specific countries did not give a picture of family and individual consumption, which varied widely within countries according to income groups, the urban/rural divide and cultural traditions. The Bad Homburg conference aimed to analyse how the available food was used, and the participants were concerned with the question of whether those responsible for food policy fully appreciated the need for education in nutrition. Unbalanced diets and their harmful effects upon health were frequently attributed to lack of nutritional knowledge and to ignorance of the special needs of

---

29 Hartog, C. den, Copping, A.M., "The nutritional state of Europe and the need for education and training in nutrition", FAO/WHO Symposium on Education and Training in Nutrition in Europe, Bad Homburg, December 2-11, 1959, FAO D. Lubin Mem. Library, 060275, NU, FAO/59/10/7588.

30 Hartog, C. den, Copping, A.M., "The nutritional state of Europe", 1959, p. 1.

31 *Ibidem*, p. 2.

vulnerable groups such as pregnant women and young children. It was often observed that in families that had only a limited budget available for the purchase of food, a better diet could have been chosen if the housewife had had more knowledge of nutrition and correct feeding. Once again, the experts insisted on the fact that ill-balanced diets were consumed not only by lower income groups, but also by higher ones in which ignorance might affect the choice. Therefore, nutrition education was called upon to do more than teach good eating habits – it was also expected to develop public awareness of the importance of good nutrition and food policies for health and social stability. Employers were to appreciate how good nutrition increased work efficiency and cut down on absenteeism, and taxpayers were expected to realise that good nutrition decreased public expenditure for medical care. Through proper education and training of public health officers, doctors, teachers and social workers in nutrition, greater awareness of the need for knowledge of good food in the whole population was able to be created. This started with the instruction of pregnant and nursing women.

While rickets was no longer a serious problem in most European countries, reports from Norway, Finland and Denmark indicated that it still existed in advanced countries where preventive programmes were in operation and it was common in Poland. Improving the diets of mothers and their children led to a positive change, and if knowledge of the relationship between diet and rickets were to be spread, rickets would disappear completely in Europe. The same could be said of other deficiency diseases and malnutrition cases. Nutritional training of those responsible for the care of young children from weaning to school age was essential; this age-group was particularly vulnerable as this is a period of rapid growth and mental development, an age at which good or bad habits might be learned and the nutritional pattern for their entire life set. Physicians, public health nurses, social workers and teachers were expected to have solid training in nutrition.

> In many countries measures are now taken to protect the health and nutrition of the school children. There is increasingly well-organized medical inspection and knowledge of the relation between good feeding and mental ability and general well-being has been put into practice. Effective school feeding programs benefiting large numbers of children are in operation in a number of European countries. School feeding is particularly valuable in schools in which there are long morning school hours and free afternoon hours. Children often do not have a good breakfast before coming to school in the morning. Teachers are sometimes unaware that their pupils would be less tired and uninterested and would learn better and perhaps behave better, if they were allowed a short break during which food was provided. More knowledge of nutrition on the part of educational authorities and the

> teachers themselves would favor the development and expansion of school feeding programs.[32]

The school meal was considered to have a direct value from a health and nutritional point of view, but was also of great value for educational purposes. School feeding programmes could become an excellent means of providing education in nutrition as well as of supplying additional nutritious food to scholars. Adolescents were also an important target group, since it was demonstrated that failure of normal physical development and susceptibility to disease in adolescents might be related to an unbalanced diet. Physical examination and biological tests indicated that the whole biological stability might be disturbed if the diet was inadequate. The experts proposed educating housewives in nutrition through information given by public services. It was even more important to provide education in nutrition at an earlier stage in life, by teaching the future housewives in school the value of food, so that when feeding her family she would have the ability to choose and prepare food efficiently.

Hartog and Copping denounced the fact that people were continually bombarded with publicity, advertisements, manufacturers' recommend-dations and other people's opinion, lacking any reference about the legitimacy and reliability of nutritional information. Therefore, the housewife had to be helped to develop her power of discrimination about the information she received on food and nutrition.

The problem of malnutrition in the elderly required greater attention. Malnutrition frequently occurred as the result of low protein intake and vitamin deficiency. Long-term and continual poor nutrition might be cumulative and find clinical expression because the older body adapts less easily to injury and infection, and poor nutrition contributed to this negative situation. The need for changing food habits was seldom recognised by old people or those taking care of them. Education in nutrition was called to find a place among gerontologists, making an important contribution to community welfare.[33]

> In view of reports from European countries indicating that unsatisfactory nutrition still exists, the problem arises of finding a solution for nutritional inadequacies. The problem differs from that in developing countries in that most European countries have a good educational system, though education in the principles of nutrition may be lacking. We must investigate the extent and nature of the teaching of nutrition to members of those professions who may in turn pass on their knowledge to the whole population. We must

[32] *Ibidem*, 1959, p. 3.

[33] *Ibidem*, 1959, p. 6.

> consider not only formal training in the science and application of nutrition, but also training in connection with food policies, food supplies, cultural backgrounds and food habits. In general when the existence of nutritional inadequacy is established it must be attacked by improvement in food supplies to the needy groups as well as by nutrition education based on the principle of modifying nutritionally unsound customs or habits. The social and economic condition must be fully understood in order to attack the nutrition problem effectively. Thus, in the training of any specialist in nutrition, social science is an important subject. Without the appreciation of the influence of socio-economic factors on food habits and dietary patterns it is impossible to teach the use of food to the best advantage or to train nutritionists who can assist the community by passing on their knowledge.[34]

Professional groups meant to have responsibility for teaching nutrition and influencing people as part of their professional activities included nutritionists and dieticians, medical doctors, health workers, nurses, midwives, home economists, agricultural extension workers, social workers and school teachers. These groups all required specific education and training in nutrition in order to serve as a bridge to the general population. The Bad Homburg conference concentrated on the training of professional workers at universities in applied nutrition and dietetics, medicine and public health, home economics, agronomy and school teaching. Nutrition education programmes were in action in some European countries, but criticism was expressed at the results obtained before 1960:

> Some countries have fairly developed programs of training. For instance, in the United Kingdom, there are at present an undergraduate university course in nutrition, graduate courses in dietetics, special training courses in public health and tropical nutrition and a diversity of contributions to teaching nutrition in medical studies and in courses in physiology or in biochemistry. Outside the universities there are various courses in dietetics providing for full qualification in the profession of therapeutic dietitian and courses in nutrition in colleges of domestic science where training is given to teachers of domestic subjects. Refresher courses are provided from time to time both for dietitians and for teachers of domestic science.
>
> In other countries such as Poland and Turkey the problem is beginning to be tackled by the institution of new courses in nutrition in training of public health officers. In the Netherlands and in Finland more fully developed training up to university level is available. In Denmark, Norway and Sweden, studies in household science and in nursing provide good background work in nutrition. In some countries almost no general instruction in nutrition comes into the picture. It is probably true of all

[34] *Ibidem*, 1959, pp. 6-7.

> countries in Europe that the extent of training and education in nutrition is limited by availability of suitable teachers. Recommended reading and study courses are an essential part of keeping teachers up-to-date in their knowledge and unless these are provided work can soon fall below a desirable standard.[35]

The main concern was to investigate how the education and training programmes available in European countries could be designed to be fully effective in training the types of workers for whom they were intended, and whether trained nutritionists were employed to the best advantage in the health and welfare, agriculture and education services.

Gino Bergami, professor of human physiology at the University of Naples, presented a paper on "The Problems of Nutrition in Europe from the Public Health Standpoint".[36] He started by classifying the factors that influenced adequacy of diet, since from the public health standpoint, this was the main problem in preventing malnutrition and deficiency diseases. Two main factors were said to determine the individual choice of foods: availability and dietary habits. According to Bergami, these could be summarised as follows: availability depended on seasonal variations in agricultural production, food imports, existence of subsidised foods and taxes; dietary habits were related to national traditions, religious norms, climatic conditions, taste and nutritional information. The latter was based on knowledge of the nutritional properties of foods, knowledge of some principles of nutrition, nutritional advice obtained from the media and specific nutritional advice given by competent experts. Both factors could be influenced differently; while dietary habits could be directly influenced by physicians, nurses, health staff, home economists, schoolteachers and social workers, the availability of food was outside the range of intervention of nutrition experts.[37] Availability depended upon agricultural planning, government economic decisions and national and international trade.

> The problem is one of increasing magnitude, because food technology today is introducing so many new chemical entities, is modifying so deeply the physical and chemical properties of natural foods, and so easily transforms inedible food into apparently attractive food, that a great effort is needed, at

35 *Ibidem*, p. 7-8.

36 Bergami, G., "The Problems of Nutrition in Europe from the Public Health Standpoint", FAO/WHO Symposium on Education and Training in Nutrition in Europe, Bad Homburg, 2-11 December, 1959, FAO D. Lubin Mem. Library, 060275, NU, FAO/59/10/7588.

37 *Ibidem*, p. 2.

a high level, to ensure that the nutritional properties of these kinds of semi-artificial food are scientifically determined.[38]

Bergami considered the existence of two different types of nutrition problems in Europe. One was quantitative (calorie intake) and the second was qualitative, linked to the composition of the diet. The quantitative problem, following the economic recovery of European countries and the gradual extension of the production of foodstuffs, was regarded as minimal and restricted to the extent that poverty still existed in some countries. However, he also testified to the growing risk of obesity derived from the nutritional transition. He stressed the wide differences in dietary habits existing among northern European and Mediterranean countries, and the risk of industrialisation in impairing the nutritional quality of food.

A more pedagogical approach was taken by B. Markovic, chief of the Department of Health Education at the Central Institute of Hygiene in Zagreb. He described his experience working with group methods as a useful approach for nutrition education. The principles of the group decision method were to avoid any criticism and to present the problem to the group so that its members realised that they were invited to express their own viewpoint. Field trips were another option that increased understanding and knowledge of food processing and distribution, leading to the establishment of good human relations with those experts and professional groups working on food and nutrition. Lectures were another option, although their impact was considered to be temporary and superficial, limitations that the author remarked upon, since the training systems at many European universities were based on this method of teaching.

Markovic recommended opening the doors to small group discussions and role-playing as a spontaneous acting out of a situation. Feeding experiments and audiovisual materials were also mentioned. As nutrition was an essential element for the population, he recommended that prominent persons – respectable people who had a marked influence on the community – were contacted to participate in planning nutrition education. In any case, nutrition education programmes had to be evaluated and the progress assessed in order to determine the effectiveness of teaching methods, the extent of the improvement and the changes in attitudes and behaviour they had brought about. Questionnaires were the most common method of evaluation, complemented by clinical examination, surveys on food consumption,

38 *Ibidem*, p. 3.

analysis of epidemiological changes and other modifications in food intake and eating habits.

Joachim Kühnau, professor of biochemistry at the University of Hamburg, presented a paper on the problems of nutrition in Europe from a medical viewpoint.[39] He considered that the basic character of the nutritional situation in the highly industrialised European countries in 1959 was determined by the fact that, although a general food shortage no longer existed and the requirements of all essential nutrients could be met without difficulties, as the statistics showed, people were looking with suspicion and distrust at their food, which had undergone transformations due to industrial and technological processing. This general feeling of uncertainty about the quality and health risk of many foodstuffs that had undergone extensive changes from their natural origin to consumption was likely to have been intensified by alarming articles in journals, magazines and newspapers. Sensationalist information was not a good element to challenge the threat. This probably influenced the housewife's fear of being poisoned by ordinary food. The worst consequence of this widespread apprehension was the fact that people became attracted to food reformers and faddists who had no scientific training, which could lead to pathogenic food patterns. Kühnau demanded public information and education by any possible means such as lectures, radio and television, giving details on food additives and their legislative control, contamination of food by pesticides and residues, insecticides, antibiotics and fertilisers.

> Action will have to be based on studies and experience in social psychology and in traditional food patterns as well as on an exact and objective analysis of the numerous forms of food faddism. Much work has to be done in this respect in order to avoid the failure of efforts to improve knowledge of nutrition among the public. These efforts must also be extended to inmates of hospitals, children's and maternity homes, and old pensioners institutions.
>
> The basic fact of industrialization and rationalization of food production is an unavoidable step in the irreversible process of modern civilization and has created new patterns of nutrition, which have to be accepted as part of present-day life. If the average man is harassed by the fear of being poisoned by his food, he must be in a position to obtain reliable evidence that his fear is unjustified, and that modern trends in nutrition cannot be

39 Kühnau, J., "The Problems of Nutrition in Europe from a medical standpoint", FAO/WHO Symposium on Education and Training in Nutrition in Europe, Bad Homburg, December 2-11, 1959, FAO D. Lubin Mem. Library, 060275, NU; FAO/59/10/7588.

arrested by any unrealistic attempt to "return to Nature" or by other sectarian programs.[40]

Nutritional disorders of childhood might be avoided by proper instruction and training of mothers, nurses, school teachers and managers in nursing homes. Catering staff also had to be trained in order to ensure the sound nutrition of workmen in large industrial plants, employees in public services, soldiers and prison inmates. However, Kühnau considered that the most urgent need was the education of physicians in nutritional sciences. Doctors represented the ultimate authority in questions of nutrition, and had to take over full responsibility for educating all personnel required to disseminate practical nutritional knowledge among the public.

Education in nutrition could not be separated from food policy directed at the most vulnerable groups, such as pregnant and nursing women, children and convalescents, while the specific requirements of the increasing number of elderly people in the community had to be considered. Food policy meant finding a balance between the diet most desirable under existing conditions and the economically justified or practicable diet. This applied to the government when it concerned a population, and it equally applied to the individual when it concerned personal nutrition. To a great extent the success of a food policy was dependent upon the cooperation of the people.[41]

Undoubtedly, social and cultural factors influenced diets and the state of nutrition of the European population. "It is most important that a nutritionist should bear continuously in mind the concept that the diet of man is determined, not only by economics, but also by a non-finite set of factors, described under the general and rather vague term of *food habits*".[42]

J. Claudian, a member of the nutrition department at the *Institut National d'Hygiène* in Paris, reviewed cultural and social factors influencing the state of nutrition in Europe. He defined human behaviour with regard to food not as an individual function, but bound

---

40 *Ibidem*, p. 4.

41 Dols, M.J.L., "Food policy, its application and impact on nutrition in Europe", FAO/WHO Symposium on Education and Training in Nutrition in Europe, Bad Homburg, 2-11 December, 1959, FAO D. Lubin Mem. Library, 060275, NU, FAO/59/10/7588.

42 Claudian, J., "A review of the cultural and social factors which influence diets and the state of nutrition in Europe, FAO/WHO Symposium on Education and Training in Nutrition in Europe, Bad Homburg, 2-11 December, 1959, FAO D. Lubin Mem. Library, 060275, NU, FAO/59/10/7588.

to the social environment: an organised body of individuals following a given way of life. Nutrition has to be considered as an integral part of the set of rules that govern the way in which a human group sharing a long common history lives and thinks, that is to say, as an essential part of *culture.* Tastes and preferences in choosing food, cooking techniques, rules governing the rhythm and make-up of meals are to a very large extent shared by the community. "A *food pattern*, a term commonly used to designate this whole *attitude to food*, is therefore seen to be the expression of a culture or a given social environment".[43] Food consumption and the level of nutrition could be expressed numerically and correspond with exact biological and economic criteria; on the contrary, the *food pattern* represented a very complex concept determined by factors connected with the way of life, habits and psychological factors.

The concept of *way of life* was proposed by ethnologists and geographers to express all the human activities focused on providing for people's needs. Claudian considered that it was essentially concerned with job, profession and working activities, which determine the nutritional needs according to their more or less strenuous nature. In this sense, the division of work among the sexes and the role of women in society and in the different branches of housekeeping should be taken into account, "determined as it is by *technical* and *economic* standards, the way of life represents the particular method of a human group of adapting itself to the material environment; it is therefore clearly oriented towards the satisfaction of physiological needs".[44]

Habits represent the automatic behaviour, of a partly ritual kind, which a social and cultural group has adopted and follows implicitly. Habits are the result of collective experience transmitted from generation to generation, constituting a sort of implicit norm controlling all aspects of human life: the way the population thinks, ways of acting, and, obviously, also of eating. Traditional customs, the legacy of the past, but also recently acquired habits are involved, and Claudian considered that habits do not necessarily have an *adaptive character.*[45]

Anthropologists tend to assume that at the root of each mode of behaviour there is always a sense, a mode of thought, which can be considered as determining or guiding it. However, regarding nutrition and dietary habits, it is not what man knows, thinks or believes that determines what he eats, but more particularly what he *likes*, and the

43 *Ibidem*, p. 1.

44 *Ibidem*, p. 2.

45 *Ibidem*.

emotional attitude to food is far from being simple. Cultural studies have shown that in addition to the sensory value of food, there is also a *symbolic value*, subconsciously determined, complex and full of many nuances. Certain foodstuffs, like meat, white bread, sweets, pastries and certain fats have a long-standing prestige value in most cultural areas of Europe, while other products have a negative perception associated with poverty and scarcity.

The act of eating is intimately bound up with cultural habits and a collective way of organising community life. It is not the same in Northern, Central and Mediterranean countries in Europe. The pleasure of eating is not only the satisfaction of a basic instinct or simple enjoyment, but also a pleasure derived from common fruition. Meals taken in company also represent a social function that no one neglects, and the act of drinking in a group occupies an important place in the rituals of friendship and hospitality. The feast, in its nutritional connotations, plays an important role in human behaviour. Side by side with rational behaviour, and more or less subconscious attitudes, food habits include an amount of automatic behaviour and reactions such as taste or disgust, which are rarely a matter of conscious thought.

Claudian demanded a certain distance and prevention when interpreting the results of psychological surveys, taking into consideration the opinions of people on the benefits obtained from eating different foods, or on the food preferences of social groups, stating that "the *motivation* which we obtain by this type of research often represents an attempt of justification of a rationalistic king, of affective or purely automatic behaviour".[46] A complete dichotomy usually takes place between theoretical knowledge of food values and normal behaviour. As an example, Claudian cited research carried out by the *Institut National d'Hygiène* of Paris that showed that some people who drank minimal quantities of milk were nevertheless fully aware of the value of this foodstuff.

> The *ideas* which the average European has about food are an incongruous mixture of subjective "impressions", of ancestral beliefs and of scientific notions which have been more or less well understood. Their relative proportions naturally vary with the amount of education, which makes a man more or less receptive to scientific ideas (or ideas considered to be scientific), and also to the ideas disseminated by commercial publicity.[47]

Depending on the way of life, food habits, mode of thought, and also collective and individual emotional attitudes to food, each human being

---

[46] *Ibidem*, p. 3.

[47] *Ibidem*.

and each human group has a more or less specific food pattern. Claudian noted that the concept of *food pattern*, which stresses the diversity of human behaviour in the realm of food, and on what might be called the *different food habits* of human groups, is not a part of the science of nutrition. It is indeed a concept shared by a whole range of disciplines that study humans in their social environment from slightly different perspectives. By considering data from the anthropological sciences, human geography, ethnology, cultural sciences and sociology, the nutritionist is prompted to take into consideration the plurality of *food patterns* in Europe, putting them in relation to a few main *human environments:* cultural and historical traditions; the two big ecological divisions: towns and countryside (the rural/urban divide); and the social and professional groups, a specificity characteristic of the urban environment.

When bearing these contexts in mind in order to understand the influence of social and cultural factors on the food habits of the various groups, according to Claudian, a major difficulty arose: the instability of European food patterns, which had been changing continuously throughout the previous century. Under the pressure of the technical and industrial revolution, the social, economic and demographic structure of Europe, nutrition patterns and food habits had been extensively transformed. The raising of standards of living and lifestyle changes had brought about considerable modifications in eating habits. Anthropological research had shown that the very unequal spread of the benefits of the new era on the whole continent resulted in a *new geography of food* in accordance with differences in economic and technical levels of development. This new geography of food was superimposed on the traditional cultural geography.

In the western countries where the industrial revolution had expanded strongly, traditional food habits were disappearing or were being relegated to the *folklore* of the culture. The differences between the urban food pattern and the rural food pattern were also in the process of being swept away. In a modern town, which is the off-shoot of an industrial civilisation, new social classes tended to build up new eating habits and new food patterns. While nutritionists, nutritional physiologists and public health authorities talked about a more or less standard European food pattern, corresponding to a European or Western civilisation, already foreseen by certain sociologists, Claudian expressed his scepticism. He noted that in 1960 there were only *transitional food patterns* in Europe, which were considerably influenced by developments in technical and economic conditions. The point that differentiated food patterns in particular was the proportion of traditional social and cultural factors and new components that went into their respective structures.

He considered it relevant in this respect that the factors that determined human feeding behaviour did not reach the same dynamic values. Closely linked to economic and technical conditions – as the way of life itself – it undergoes the first changes, whilst the psychological factors undergo a slower and more incomplete transformation and therefore *food habits* are most resistant to change. A traditional food pattern represents an adaptation to a given environment; a new food pattern requires a re-adaptation involving a new apprenticeship. This involves a transitional phase, which is always critical, so that certainly some of the nutritional problems observed in Europe after the post-war years, according to Claudian, were the consequence of the rapid development of European society.[48]

Claudian discussed a few examples, as case studies, to show the role of social and cultural factors in the genesis of certain food patterns, as well as their influence on the nutritional state of certain European populations. The first case discussed relates to the tradition of cereal porridge and the occurrence of pellagra in Central Europe. It was in the central and eastern areas of Europe where Claudian found the clearest survival of certain long-standing food habits. Indeed, in vast areas of the Danubian countries, porridge with flour or semolina made from cereals unsuitable for breadmaking, and no longer used on the rest of the continent, was still the basic foodstuff. Even if maize, the cereal used in those days, was a recent innovation, the consumption of porridge was a long-standing tradition in those countries. In the 17th century cereals from America merely replaced another cereal unsuitable for breadmaking which had been cultivated in those regions traditionally: millet.

Compared with the old *panicium milliaceum*, maize presented clear advantages in yield, but the fact that it was accepted without hesitation by populations that did not easily change their habits also had another explanation: the new plant did not change the traditional cooking methods to which the population was particularly attached in any way. This *attachment* of Danubian peasants to their polenta was very special. Besides bread, which was a food for festive occasions, maize porridge was the main item of daily food and all cooking was based on it. Replacing porridge with bread would have required a complete remodelling of their food techniques and even to some extent the whole economic system. However, if the substitution of maize had some

---

48 *Ibidem*, p. 5.

evident economic advantages for the population, it also concealed a serious danger, which the Danubian peasants could not foresee: pellagra.

In Romania, pellagra appeared around a century after maize came into general use, at the exact time when the amount of milk available to the rural population was drastically reduced as a consequence of a change in economic policy. Cheese and milk represented the traditional supplement of these age-old cereal preparations, and without these supplements maize porridge turned out to be a *pellagrogenic food.*[49]

The Italian pellagra endemic that had already been overcome was particularly instructive, furnishing a double example: a deficiency disease with a long-standing food behaviour that did not keep pace with the economic conditions of that time as its basis, and the danger that the introduction of a new food that had not been tested previously might present for a traditional food pattern.

The second case discussed by Claudian regarded the geography of fats in Western Europe, closely connected with the survival of old food patterns. Fairly well-defined boundaries separated the zone of Nordic countries where butter is eaten and the Mediterranean countries where the consumption of vegetable oil is prevalent. The geography of lard and other fats of animal origin were lot as well defined, with lard being the main fat used in cooking in Central and Eastern Europe, but also playing an important role in certain Mediterranean and Nordic areas. Therefore, a clear contrast could be established between two civilisations that had been opposed to each other since ancient times, in spite of the economic changes: the butter civilisation and the olive oil civilization. "This contrast of tastes, of cravings and of exclusive feelings of repulsion for fats which the European has more than for other foods is easy to explain. Fats play a very special part in man's food behavior: they are intimately linked with the ways of preparing food. The type of fat used is characteristic of the type of cooking".[50]

During the war and post-war years the traditional fats of Europe were replaced by less expensive synthetic substitutes made from foreign fats of vegetable or animal origin. In the Nordic countries, margarine increasingly replaced butter; in the Southern countries arachis oil gradually replaced olive oil. These substitute fats were accepted insofar as they reproduced the physical and sensory qualities of the traditional fats. Anthropologists noticed that the replacement of a new food product was accepted when offering economic advantages, but only on condition

---

[49] *Ibidem*.

[50] *Ibidem*, p. 6.

that the new food fitted in with food preparation habits and previous experience.

Habits connected with the choice of fats brought Claudian to an important and much debated subject: the role of food in increasing the incidence of degenerative vascular diseases observed in Northern European countries.[51] Statistical and clinical research indicated that in general the Mediterranean food pattern produced less cholesterol and was less liable to generate infarcts than the butter-margarine type of the Northern countries. This statement was discussed in the early 1960s, required qualification and was the origin of the prestige obtained by the so-called *Mediterranean diet*, a concept proposed initially and defended by Ancel Keys. However, Claudian recognised that the consumption of lipids is closely linked with the availability of food and the living standards of the population. Surveys on food consumption indicated that as soon as economic conditions evolved, the European citizen increases the total consumption of fats, particularly fats of animal origin such as meat, milk, eggs and fish. As the butter- and margarine-consuming countries are also rich countries, the population easily consumed large quantities of fats and animal products. Consequently, the geographical distribution of heart and vascular diseases in Europe were conditioned by a cultural factor: traditional habits connected with the type of fat and an economic factor related to the standard of living.[52]

The third case discussed by Claudian regarded the different food patterns in the rural environments in France. In contrast to the trend towards uniformity, which urban districts seemed to impose on eating habits, in rural areas large regional differences were preserved. "The food patterns which we find today in France in the countryside are not completely explicable by the natural or economic conditions and clearly show the survival of traditional cultural factors".[53]

Indeed, from the perspective of fat consumption, several fairly well-defined zones could be distinguished in France. The north-western regions represented the butter zone, with butter the only fat used in cooking; in the south-western area the traditional fat was lard and melted goose fat; the south, which had always been the traditional olive oil area, still used vegetable oils; and finally, in the central and eastern areas, the population was less selective, and different fats were consumed in varying proportions. This geography of fats also

---

51 *Ibidem*.

52 *Ibidem*, p. 7

53 *Ibidem*.

corresponds with regional food patterns and helped determine them to a great extent.

In the overall nutrition picture, surveys showed difficulties in these regions in meeting the animal protein, calcium and vitamin B2 needs, despite the fairly high consumption of meat in urban areas. In the less rich regions in the south and south-west, where butter was practically non-existent, deficiencies in fat-soluble vitamins were sometimes found as well as a shortage of animal products and calcium. On the contrary, in the areas where mixed fats were eaten and a satisfactory balance between milk, cheese and butter was struck, nutritional problems did not arise.

The fourth case study regarded the nature of urban life and its effect on eating. The time the housewife had available for preparing food, and the time given to meals, undoubtedly represented a determining factor in the food pattern of social groups. In this respect, conditions were very different in the rural and urban areas. In towns, a housewife working outside the home had to very considerably reduce the time she could spend on cooking and preparing meals. In French towns, the average duration of activities related to food procedures in families of workers and minor staff per 24 hours, calculated by Claudian after some studies carried out by the Nutrition Section of the *Institut National d'Hygiène* in Paris, were as follows:[54]

	Housewife only in the home	Housewife working outside
Shopping time	1 hour	45 minutes
Preparation of food	3 hours 30 minutes	2 hours 30 minutes
Duration of meal	1 hour 15 minutes	45 minutes
Washing up	2 hours	1 hour 30 minutes

This time distribution implies a tendency to prepare simple dishes that require less work and a shorter cooking time instead of time-consuming cooked dishes. Therefore, the use of manufactured foods, more or less "ready to serve", was rising. In addition, the accelerated tempo of the urban way of life cut down the time available for the midday meal. These two factors, imposed by the *way of life* in modern towns, were partly responsible for giving the urban food pattern its particular trend and shape.

---

[54] *Ibidem*, p. 8.

The last case discussed by Claudian related to food trends of different professional groups in the town. In a series of studies carried out in several large French towns by the Nutrition Section of the *Institut National d'Hygiène* in Paris, staff and industrial workers showed rather different tendencies in their food habits. Considering the consumption of certain foodstuffs among professional groups spending the same amount of money on food, around 200 Francs per person per day, in 1950-51 the distribution of food consumption was as follows:[55]

Type of foodstuff	Office workers (in grammes)	Industrial workers (in grammes)
Bread	268	347
Meat	118	144
Butter	20	16
Eggs	20	15
Fruit	206	141
Drink during meals (wine & beer)	196	366

These differences enabled Claudian to distinguish two food patterns, one followed by the sedentary citizen, the other by the urban manual worker. These two patterns could only be explained by the way of life, mentality and specific lifestyle habits of the two groups of workers. The higher consumption of bread among manual workers could be related to the greater calorific output required by their work. The greater tendency of workers to drink alcoholic beverages, a phenomenon found in all countries of the world, was related by anthropologists to the monotonous and depressing nature of work in the factories. On the other hand, psychological factors presumably explain the peculiar craving of workers for meat, as well as their relative indifference to fruit.

Opinion surveys carried out in the same environment show that among certain groups of workers, *red meat* has a special nutritional prestige (not shared by fruit and milk) and that manual workers consider alcoholic drinks to be far more stimulating than coffee (which on the contrary is appreciated by workers in sedentary professions).

These factors, which are undoubtedly important, should not make us forget the important role of *food habits* which a social group preserves and consolidates over many generations. A recent survey on the

55 *Ibidem*, p. 9.

consumption of alcoholic drinks in France shows that the "highest consumption is found in manual workers, who are sons of manual workers, and who have not changed their environment".[56]

Nevertheless, differences in consumption between manual and office workers with equal incomes considerably diminished as the standard of living increased, and above a certain level the food pattern of the manual workers disappeared. Claudian considered this was due to a phenomenon of imitation. Humans show a tendency to imitate the behaviour of social groups that have a certain prestige. Country dwellers forsook their food and other customs to conform to those of the town. In an urban environment the workers adopted the *bourgeois* food habits as soon as they could. This double tendency was found at every stage of human behaviour regarding food: zealously maintaining their own tradition and the constant need for change, something that Claudian considered was not the only paradox of human culture.

[56] *Ibidem*, p. 10.

Conclusion

During the first half of the 20th century a significant transition from hunger to malnutrition took place. The great international crisis experienced by Europe between 1914 and 1960 gave political, economic and social priority to food availability and the problems of hunger and diet. As a consequence of the crisis caused by the First World War, the end of the European empires, international conflicts and the 1929 stock market crash, food production and consumption became the responsibility of the State. The role of experimental science not only influenced knowledge, it also inspired agricultural and health policies and had effects on the economy, education and cultural habits. Hunger was the traditional demographic regulator, associated with poverty and exclusion. However, food and nutrition reached a qualitatively different dimension when they became transformed by Western *civilised societies*, being the subject of scientific analysis, the central issue of international economic policy and an instrument in the context of war conflicts.

In this particular context, international experts became the principal agents for the development of public health and social welfare policies. Hunger and poverty became an economic and political issue and a problem affecting human rights and health. Consequently, international organisations, in collaboration with states and philanthropic associations, pushed for experimental research and launched field studies on the diet, as well as campaigns to coordinate food production with trade demands, according to the principles of the new science of nutrition. Hunger was transformed and classified: nutritional deficiency, under-nutrition, malnutrition and starvation.

The League of Nations, the International Labour Office, the International Institute of Agriculture, the Rockefeller Foundation, the Food and Agriculture Organization and the World Health Organization all became major agents. Between 1918 and 1960 diet and nutrition became the best argument for historical research that aimed to explore the relationships between the genesis of scientific knowledge, political and commercial uses, its economic dimensions and the associated social and political practices. Researching the plural factors involved allowed the mechanisms behind the origin and circulation of scientific knowledge, as well as its political uses and social reactions, to be analysed.

The great upheaval experienced by European societies during the three decades from 1914 to 1945 prompted the State to act as an element of social stabilisation in national and international conflicts, and accentuated its regulatory role concerning the economy and citizens' health. This function achieved even more importance during the Cold War, with the spread of social-democratic policies based on the *Keynesian paradigm.* The international sphere, identified by the United Nations organisations and other international agencies involved, played an essential role as a reference point for national politics. During the process of hunger becoming malnutrition – the *medicalisation*, *politicisation* and *economisation* of hunger – an immense amount of knowledge was generated and a great deal of political action and economic organisation was deployed.

Nevertheless, policies on diet and nutrition implemented between 1920 and 1950 were a great failure in general. The transfer of scientific knowledge as a pattern of production and consumption for a new economy required a difficult adaptation and the most radical proposals, such as the creation of a World Food Board, were immediately dismissed. Global regulation of food markets interfered with the interests of the big powers. On the other hand, the scientific approach to hunger and its transformation into a plurality of medical conditions revealed an overwhelming presence of nutritional deficiencies, famine and malnutrition. Experimental science was an excellent instrument to diagnose the problem but not a political tool to fight against social exclusion.

Europe went through an exceptional crisis between the Great War and 1960. Although the situation had a global dimension, what currently matters is to emphasise the emergence of hunger and malnutrition as an economic, political and medical issue that transformed the European population into a vast laboratory. The new science of nutrition, which won international support, analysed the effects of nutritional deficiencies on human health, established levels of malnutrition, classified nutritional deficiencies and defined the parameters of a balanced diet and the concept of *optimum diet.* The new experimental science of nutrition was the background for rationing policies in times of crisis and the guarantee of the *minimum diet*, conceived as a political expression of human rights. In many European countries, the nutritional situation even improved as a consequence of rationing in times of crisis.

In addition, the European population (mainly children and pregnant women, but also workers and at-risk groups) was subjected to a massive clinical examination to detect malnutrition and other associated clinical entities. Production, trade and consumption were readapted for health, economic and political reasons, as the essential starting point of new social development.

Indeed, the physiology of nutrition received a strong stimulus due to a social interest in evaluating the impact of the international crisis on health. A balanced diet came to be considered essential for the establishment of optimum health, which was needed to fight off infectious diseases. It was considered to be the basis of organic energy. Conversely, *consumption* levels were too low among the European population, compared with scientific standards of calorie intake. Increasing levels of consumption and changing dietary habits were considered to be the essential goal. School canteens, collective meals for industrial workers, mothers and poor people constituted a field where social policies had a clear international dimension.

The close interaction between the international context and national politics was evident in the case of agricultural policies, food production, food availability and experimental research on nutrition and diet. The League of Nations played a coordinating role through a Technical Commission on Nutrition, which conducted not only experimental research but also clinical and somatometric tests to identify deficiency diseases and prevent malnutrition during the Inter-war years. A similar function was developed by the FAO and the WHO after World War II through world food surveys, reports on the nutritional state of the population and other more specific studies devoted to population groups, education in nutrition, clinical definitions of malnutrition, regulations on food quality, household consumption, food composition tables, standards of rationing and many other related issues.

International groups of experts supported by world organisations worked together to establish a powerful reference for nutritional politics, the instruction of experts and health standards. Expert committees, international conferences, food surveys and technical reports encouraged experimental research, to ascertain optimum standards for each country; they tried to ensure that medical students, medical officers, district nurses, teachers and civil servants received the latest nutritional knowledge and they encouraged a vigorous policy of education for the general public.

Pregnant and nursing women, infants and children, peasants, farmers, industrial workers and rural populations all became the main target of an internationally connected policy that included laboratory research, clinical screening, dietary standards for low incomes and previously defined social groups at risk. Food and diet were not only a matter of economy, physiology and survival – new trends in community nutrition became crucial for social stability and social change, a political tool to overcome crisis and civilise people according to scientific patterns and liberal values.

Technical reports discussed dietary standards, especially concerning infants and low-income families, criteria for an optimum diet, the nutritive value of foodstuffs, as well as methods of screening the nutritional state of the population to detect and correct deficiencies. Dieticians, nutritionists, experts in nutritional physiology and public health officers achieved legitimacy in the eyes of political authorities as a reference for food production. They also imparted knowledge about popular habits at a time when the food industry gained momentum. National policies received legitimisation from international experts on nutritional science and community initiatives were reinforced by the international context. As a consequence, the new science of nutrition became a political tool and one of the main focal points of action in the big programme of civilisation developed in Western countries during the first half of the 20th century. It was a field of knowledge and action to overcome famine, malnutrition and deficiencies, outlining a global governance of the food economy and changing traditional dietary habits.

The political economy of scientific knowledge constructed around hunger and malnutrition during the period 1918-1960 constituted a powerful instrument for international stabilisation. In fact, it contributed concepts and instruments towards the drafting of a cartography of nutritional deficiencies. However, once the big picture of nutritional problems had been outlined, the political action and economic governance that was required failed under the pressure of national interests and the free market. Thus, in the 1940s, deficiency illnesses were identified and evaluated by the technically and conceptually solid science of nutrition. However, the political economy was shown to be unable to alleviate the underlying nutritional problem. Internment camps were the most dramatic research laboratory for extreme, seriously impaired conditions. The experimental and clinical screening of inmates in internment camps, used as an argument for health and charitable intervention, exceeded all limits of respect for human dignity and civil rights. Other experiments with humans followed similar patterns, without any international restriction. The Declaration of Helsinki, which set the ethical principles of experimentation on humans, was first adopted as a global regulation by the World Medical Association in 1964. The intervention of experimental science and clinical examination led to the analysis, identification and classification of famine and a variety of forms of malnutrition, under-nutrition and specific nutritional deficiencies. While the newest knowledge was neither able to provoke a global political response nor change the dynamics of the food market, it did nevertheless stimulate the emergence of a powerful food industry and the pharmaceutical production of nutrients and vitamins. Nutrition entered the big market and included publicity, advertising and marketing campaigns.

The new approach to a global food policy, promoted by the FAO and other international organisations, was driven hand in hand with the development of what has been more recently called global civil society, a less developed face of globalisation. The significance of cooperatives for mutual aid and democratic culture, as well as for agricultural production and distribution, had been stressed by the FAO since its inception at the Hot Springs conference in May 1943. Yet today's global market, based on exploitation and not on equity, still lacks the instruments and capacity for regulation that are needed to fight global hunger. Hunger and malnutrition are not a major matter of concern for European citizens. Conversely, during the summer of 2011, Somalia became the tragic image of the failure of the global political economy to coordinate food production, trade, prices, the control of basic foodstuffs and consumption. The incapacity of capitalism as a global system, and the limited influence of international/national and public/private initiatives to challenge the problem of food availability and nutrition by means of a wise combination of science, production, the market and politics, means the problem today remains unsolved.

References

Archival Sources

Documents and Technical Reports

Ad Hoc Committee on Nutrition. Nu Report 5/add 1, February 27th-March 1st, 1946, FAOArchives.

Aykroyd, Wallace R., Personal History Card, FAO Archives.

Aykroyd, W.R., Vergara, A., Nutrition in Central America. Nutrition Division FAO, May 14, 1947, FAO Archives.

Bergami, G. "The Problems of Nutrition in Europe from the Public Health Standpoint", FAO/WHO Symposium on Education and Training in Nutrition in Europe, Bad Homburg, 2-11 December, 1959, FAO D. Lubin Mem. Library, 060275, NU, FAO/59/10/7588.

Chairman's report of the meeting of the Ad Hoc Nutrition Committee. February 27th-March 1st, 1946, FAO Archives, Nu.Report 5/Rev.1.

Claudian, J., "A review of the cultural and social factors which influence diets and the state of nutrition in Europe, FAO/WHO Symposium on Education and Training in Nutrition in Europe, Bad Homburg, 2-11 December, 1959, FAO D. Lubin Mem. Library, 060275, NU, FAO/59/10/7588.

Conférence Européenne sur Hygiène Rurale (29 juin-7 juillet 1931), Recommandations sur les Principes directeurs de l'organisation de l'Assistance médicale, des Services d'hygiène et de l'Assainissement dans les districts ruraux, Organisation d'Hygiene, Société des Nations, Geneva, C.473.M.202.1931.III, FAO Archives.

Conférence Européenne sur Hygiène Rurale (29 juin-7 juillet 1931), Vol. II, Proces-Verbaux, Organisation d'Hygiene, Société des Nations, Geneva, C.473.M.202.1931.III (Vol. II), FAO Archives.

Conférence Européenne de la Vie Rurale, Rapport présenté par les deuxième et septième Commissions à l'Assemblée, Genève, 24 septembre, 1938, FAO Archives.

Dols, M.J.L., "Food policy, its application and impact on nutrition in Europe", FAO/WHO Symposium on Education and Training in Nutrition in Europe, Bad Homburg, 2-11 December, 1959, FAO D. Lubin Mem. Library, 060275, NU, FAO/59/10/7588.

Données sur la FAO, Organisation des Nations Unies pour l'Agriculture et l'Alimentation, Washington, 1947[BGE Zt 2598/12].

Enquête Mondiale sur l'Alimentation, Washington, Rome, Organisation des Nations Unies pour l'Agriculture et l'Alimentation, 1946-1953 [Cote QU 146.1 53OR HIST].

Étude de l'état alimentaire, LNA, R.5936, 1932-1933.

Études sur la meilleure utilisation, pour l'alimentation des budgets réduits, LNA, R.5936, 1932-1933.

FAO Questionnaires to Governments, November, 1946, FAO Archives.

Food Supplies: reparation and distribution, LNA, R.5910, 1929.

Food Supplies: Preparations alleged to contain vitamins, LNA, R.5910, 1929-1932.

Food Supplies: Standardisation of vitamins, LNA, R.5921 and R.6078-79, 1930-32.

Food Supplies: Distribution of vitamin standards, LNA, R.5935 and R.6009, 1932.

György, P. Comments on the Provisional Agenda with special reference to ítems Nos. 5 and 6. Joint FAO/WHO Nutrition Committee, 1952.

Hartog, C. den, Copping, A.M., "The nutritional state of Europe and the need for education and training in nutrition", FAO/WHO Symposium on Education and Training in Nutrition in Europe, Bad Homburg, 2-11 December, 1959, FAO D. Lubin Mem. Library, 060275, NU, FAO/59/10/7588.

Introductory note on the work accomplished (History and method) by the League of Nations up to October 1935 (Nutrition), 1935, 12 p. [C.H.1194].

Joint FAO/WHO Expert Committee on Nutrition 1949, 24-29 October, Geneva, Palais des Nations, WHO Nutrition Programme, 1950, Provisional Agenda, Standing Advisory Committee on Nutrition Provisional Agenda, Washington DC, 29 November-7 December, 1948, FAO Archives WHO/NUT/1 Add.

Joint FAO/WHO Expert Committee on Nutrition, Report on the first session, Geneva, World Health organisation, 1950.

Joint FAO/WHO Expert Committee on Nutrition, Prevention and treatment of severe malnutrition in times of disaster. Presented to World Health Assembly, Geneva, World Health Organisation, 1951.

Joint FAO/WHO Expert Committee on Nutrition, Rome April 10th – 17th 1951. Past activities and future program. FAO Archives.

Joint FAO/WHO Expert Committee 1952. Presented by Paul Gyorgy, Treatment and Prevention of Malnutrition Associated with Protein Deficiency, FAO Archives, 1376157.OI7.

Kühnau, J. "The Problems of Nutrition in Europe from a medical standpoint", FAO/WHO Symposium on Education and Training in Nutrition in Europe, Bad Homburg, 2-11 December, 1959, FAO D. Lubin Mem. Library, 060275, NU, FAO/59/10/7588.

League of Nations Health Organisation, Technical Commission on Nutrition, *On the Food Problem of the Civil Population of Madrid*, August 1938. [C.H./Com.Exp.Alim./57] R.6135/8A/23831/20883.

League of Nations Health Organisation, Technical Commission on Nutrition, "Report by a Special Committee which met in Geneva… 1938", *League of Nations Bulletin of the Health Organisation*, No. 7, 1938, 666-678 [C.H.1355, 10p.M.].

Markovic, B., *Health education and nutrition. Education sanitaire et nutrition*, FAO/WHO 1959, FAO/WHO Symposium on Education and Training in Nutrition in Europe, Bad Homburg, Fed. Rep. of Germany, 2-11 December, 1959, Rome, FAO Nutrition Meetings Report Series, No. 26, 1960.

Mayer, J., Letter to DM Lubbok, on "Questionnaire on Nutrition organization..." October 7, 1948, FAO Archives 57.OC2.

Meeting on Food Technology, Friday April 14, 1950. FAO Archives.

Memorandum on nutrition and health, prepared by the Health Section for the Mixed Committee on the problem of Nutriton, 1936, 30 p. [C.H.1204].

Milk and Milk Products in Sweden (Studies on nutrition), 1926, [C.H./Com.Exp.Alim./5: Divers/I].

Nolte, A.J., Letter to Dr. Aykroyd on "Hungarian Experiment on Wheat Germ Oil", July 17, 1947, FAO Archives, 57.0C2.

Norris, Thema J., "Report of the Committee on Calorie Requirements", FAO Archives, 57.OC2.

[Note on] The Conference on Rural Life and the Problem of Nutrition, 1938, 4 p. [C.H./Com.Exp.Alim./44].

Nutrition, LNA, R.990, 1926.

Nutrition: general, LNA, R.5865-5866, 1928-1935.

Nutrition, WHO/NUT/1 Add.2, FAO Archives.

Nutritional state of Europe and the need for education and training in nutrition, FAO/WHO Symposium on Education and Training in Nutrition in Europe, Bad Homburg, Fed. Rep. of Germany, 2-11 December, 1959, Rome, FAO, 1960.

Office Memorandum, Nutrition Program in Greece, From Miss Tsongas to Dr. Aykroyd, April 16, 1947, FAO Archives.

Office Memorandum from Nutrition Division to Mr. Lubbock, "Proposed Questionnaire on Nutrition Institutions and Workers", October 29, 1947, FAO Archives 57.OC2.

Organization for European Economic Cooperation, Food and Agriculture Committee. Food consumption levels in OEEC countries, Report of the working group on food consumption levels, Paris, OEEC Document AG(50)35.

Problem of nutrition with special reference to rural districts, Geneva, 1935, 4 p. [C.H./Hyg.rur./E.H./3].

Rapport au Conseil sur les travaux de la vingt-cinquième session du Comité d'Hygiène (Genève, 26 avril-1 mai 1937), Organisation d'Hygiene, Société des Nations. Geneva C.219.M.159.1937.III, FAO Archives

Rapport de la Réunion de la FAO sur la Nutrition en Europe, Rome, Food and Agriculture Organisation, 1958, 28 p. [QU 146. GA1 58OR HIST].

Relation of Nutrition to Health, Agriculture and Economy Policy, Final report of the mixed Committee of the League of Nations, Geneva, 1937, 340 p. A.13.1937, 1937.II.A.10.

Report on the Physiological Basis of Nutrition drawn up by the Technical Commission of the Health Committee at the meeting held in London

(November 25th-29th, 1935) (C.H.1197), revised and amplifies at the meeting held at Geneva (June 4th-8th, 1936) Geneva, 1936, A.12(1).1936.II.B.

Report of the Sub-Committee on Nutrition (Meeting of the Directors of National Schools and Institutes of Hygiene in Europe), Geneva, 1937, 6 p. [C.H.1298].

Report on the health situation in Spain, Rockefeller Foundation, 20 August, 1939, Rockefeller Archive Centre, New York, 1939.

Report to Ad Hoc Committee on Nutrition, FAO Nu Report 2. February 27, 1946, FAO Archives.

Report Ad Hoc Committee on Nutrition, Nu 5/add 1, February 27th-March 1st, 1946, FAO Archives.

Ritchie, Jean, Letter to Dr. Aykroyd onNutrition Education, 18 November 1947, FAO Archives 57.OC2.

Saiki, T., Progress of the Science of Nutrition in Japan, Geneva, 1926 [C.H.523].

Saiki, T., Necessity of the study of nutrition, Geneva, [1927], 8p. [Doc. C.H. 558].

Standing Advisory Committee on Nutrition and Food Management, Copenhaguen, August, 1946, FAO Archives, 57.OI3.

Standing Advisory Committee on Nutrition, First report to the Director-General, Copenhaguen, 31 August, 1946, FAO Archives Con 2/Nu 1.

Standing Advisory Committee on Nutrition, 2nd meeting, Geneva, September 11-19, 1947, Second report to the Director-General, Washington DC, USA, 24 October 1947.

Standing Advisory Committee on Nutrition Provisional Agenda, Washington DC, 29 November-7 December, 1948, FAO Archives N/N3/1.

Standing Advisory Committee on Nutrition Third Meeting, Washington DC, 29 November-7 December, 1948, FAO Archives N/N3/10.

Statement on Nutrition Services in Belgium, April 1949, Standing Advisory Committee on Nutrition Provisional Agenda, Washington DC, 29 November-7 December, 1948, FAO Archives.

Statistics of food production, consumption and prices, Documentation prepared by the International Institute of Agriculture, presented to the Mixed Committee on the Problem of Nutrition at its second session, June 4th, 1936, [A.12(c).1936.II.B].

Stiebeling, H.K., The State of the L.O.N. in investigations of problems of food and nutrition, Geneva, [1938], 21 p. [C.H./Com.Exp.Alim/51].

Technical Commission on Nutrition, Documentation, League of Nations Health organisation, 3rd session, London, 15th November, 1937. [R.6134, 8a, 23831, 20883: Docs: C.H./Com.Exp.Alim/33, C.H./Com.Exp.Alim/26, C.H./Com.Exp.Alim/27, C.H./Com.Exp.Alim/28, C.H./Com.Exp.Alim/12, C.H./Com.Exp.Alim/13, C.H./Com.Exp.Alim/15, C.H./Com.Exp.Alim/16, C.H./Com.Exp.Alim/18, C.H./Com.Exp.Alim/19, C.H./Com.Exp.Alim/30, C.H./Com.Exp.Alim/32, C.H./Com.Exp.Alim/35, C.H. 1261, C.H., 1216]

The state of food and agriculture, 1948, A survey of world conditions and prospects, FAO Economic Analysis Division, FAO, Washington, DC, USA, 1948, 219 p.

The state of food and agriculture, 1949, A survey of world conditions and prospects. FAO Economic Analysis Division, FAO, Washington, DC, USA, 1949, 140 p.

Tsongas, A., Letter to A. van Houtte on FAO mission in Greece, No. 3, February, 1948, FAO Archives, 57.OC2.

Tsurumi, M., Notes communiquées par le Dr... à la 22e session du Comité Hygiène (7-16.10.1935), Sur l'alimentation, 6 p. [C.H. 1173].

World Food Survey [1st], Washington, Food and Agriculture Organisation, 1946, 39 p.
[QU 146.1 46FO HIST].

World Food Survey [2nd], Rome, Food and Agriculture Organisation, 1952, 59 p.
[QU 146.1 52FO HIST].

Printed Sources

Agricultural Production in Continental Europe during the 1914-1918 War and the Reconstruction Period, Geneva, League of Nations, 1943.

Aldecoa y Juarista, J.L., "Contribución al estudio de la lactancia materna (experiencias de guerra en Bilbao)", *Revista de Sanidad e Higiene Pública*, Vol. 1, 1938/1939, pp. 241-245.

Alimentación de Europa, La, Traducido del alemán, Madrid, Ed. Blass, 1942.

Alvarado, C., Pastor, M.A., "Estudio de la composición química de algunos alimentos españoles", *Revista de Sanidad e Higiene Pública*, Vol. 8, No. 4, 1933, pp. 366-370.

American Medical Association, *Handbook of nutrition*, Chicago, *1951.*

Anguera A., "Servicios sanitarios con motivo de la inmigración durante la guerra", *Revista de Sanidad e Higiene Pública*, Vol. 1, 1938/1939, pp. 25-42.

Annual report of the Chief Medical Officer of the Ministry of Health for the year 1933, Geneva, League of Nations, 1934.

Apfelbaum, E. (ed.), *Maladie de famine. Recherches cliniques sur la famine executes dans le Ghetto de Varsovie en 1942*, Warsaw, 1942.

Arias Vallejo, E., "Dietas fisiológicas, máxima y mínima en el régimen de alimentación del hombre adulto", *Revista de Sanidad e Higiene Pública*, Vol. 8, 1943, pp. 290-304.

Arias Vallejo, E., *Alimentación y síndromes carenciales*, Madrid, Ediciones Morata, 1943.

Aykroyd, W.R., "Diet in relation to small incomes", *League of Nations Quarterly Bulletin of the Health Organisation*, 1933, Vol. 1, pp.130-153.

Aykroyd, W.R., "The poor rice-eater's diet", *League of Nations Bulletin of the Health organisation*, 1940, Vol. 10, pp. 342-356.

Bachet, M., *Études des troubles causes par la dénutrition dans un asile d'aliénés*, Paris, 1943.

Bengoa, J.M., *Les programmes de nutrition envisages sous l'angle de la sante publique*, FAO Nutrition Meetings Report Series No. 20, Rome, FAO, 1957.

"Bibliography of the Technical Work of the Health Organisation of the League of Nations, 1920-1945", *League of Nations Bulletin of the Health Organisation*, 1945, Vol. 11.

Bigwood, E.J., Roost, G., *L'alimentation rationnelle et les besoins énergétiques d'une population ouvrière*, Bruxelles, Université Libre de Bruxelles, Institute Solvay, 1934.

Bigwood E.J., *L'alimentation rationnelle de l'homme normale en Belgique*, Bruxelles, Ministère de la Santé publique, 1938.

Bigwood E.J., 'Le problème de l'alimentation rationnelle, ses aspects, ses difficulties', *Revue de l'Institut de Sociologie*, No. 16, 1939, pp. 535-83.

Bigwood, E.J., *Guiding Principles for Studies On the Nutrition of Populations. Technical Commission on Nutrition*, Health Organisation of the League of Nations Geneva, 1939 [C.H.1401; C.H./Com.Exp.Alim./50(2)].

Bigwood, E.J. (ed.), *Enseignements de la guerre 1939-1945 dans le domaine de la nutrition*, Liège/ Paris, 1947.

Brull, L. (ed.), *Les états de carence en Belgique pendant lóccupation allemande 1940-1944*, Liège/ Paris, 1945.

Biraud, M., "Health in Europe. A Survey of the Epidemic and Nutritional Situation", *League of Nations Bulletin of the Health Organisation*, 1943-1944, Vol. 10, pp. 557-699.

Blankenstein H. van, *L'Organisation d'Hygiène de la Société des Nations*, Purmerend, J. Musses, 1934.

Bootello, A., "Nuestros primeros resultados en la determinación del yodo en los alimentos y aguas de España", *Contribución al I Congreso Nacional de Sanidad del laboratorio de Higiene de la Alimentación y de la Nutrición y Técnica Bromatológica*, Madrid, Escuela Nacional de Sanidad, 1934, pp. 87-94.

Bourne, G.H., *Starvation in Europe*, London, Allen & Unwin, 1943.

Burnet, E., Aykroyd, W.R., 'Nutrition and Public Health", *League of Nations Quarterly Bulletin of the Health Organisation*, Vol. 4, No 2, 1935, pp. 323-474.

Calderón, A.M., "Vitaminas y sordera. Experiencia carencial del Madrid rojo: julio de 1936-marzo de 1939", *Revista de Sanidad e Higiene Pública*, Vol. 2, 1940, pp. 420-445.

Calleja, C., *Guía para individualizar el régimen alimenticio con especial referencia a la edad y a la crasis o constitución*, Madrid, Administración de la Revista de Medicina y Cirugía Prácticas, 1911.

Carrasco Cadenas, E., *Ni gordos, ni flacos. Lo que se debe comer*, Madrid, Diana, 1935.

Carrasco Cadenas, E., "Escuela Nacional de Sanidad. Sección de Higienede la Alimentación y de la Nutrición y Técnica Bromatológica. Su orientación yprograma de trabajo al año y medio de su organización", *Revista de Sanidad e Higiene Pública*, Vol. 8, 1933, pp. 258-260.

Carrasco Cadenas, E., "Lo que se come en España. Interés sanitario de este problema", *Contribución al I Congreso Nacional de Sanidad del laboratorio deHigiene de la Alimentación y de la Nutrición y Técnica Bromatológica*, Madrid, Escuela Nacional de Sanidad, 1934a, pp. 5-24.

Carrasco Cadenas, E., "Lo que se come en España. Interés sanitario de este problema", *Archivos de Medicina, Cirugía y Especialidades*, Vol. 37, No. 25, 1934b, pp. 669-675.

Carrasco Cadenas, E., "Alteraciones oculares, dentarias, de crecimiento y desarrollo general en relación con el insuficiente aporte proteínico, de minerales y vitaminas, *Progresos de la Clínica*, Vol. 42, 1934c, pp. 563-571.

Carrasco Cadenas, E., "Datos para suponer una carencia general vitamínica en algunas regiones españolas", *Contribución al I Congreso Nacional de Sanidad del laboratorio de Higiene de la Alimentación y de la Nutrición y Técnica Bromatológica*, Madrid, Escuela Nacional de Sanidad, 1934d, pp. 95-104.

Carrasco Cadenas, E., "Datos para suponer una carencia general vitamínica en algunas regiones españolas", *Archivos de Medicina, Cirugía y Especialidades*, Vol. 37, No 19, 1934e, pp. 501-503.

Carrasco Cadenas, E., *Sobre las necesidades alimenticias de la mujer. Elproblema de las vitaminas en la alimentación doméstica*, Madrid, Aguilar, 1934f.

Carrasco Cadenas, E., *Temas de higiene alimenticia de urgente atenciónsanitaria*, Madrid, Escuela Nacional de Sanidad, 1934g.

Carrasco Cadenas, E., Piñoles, L., "La riqueza vitamínica de algunos alimentos españoles. Primeros resultados obtenidos para el tomate valenciano y aceite de oliva andaluz", *Revista de Sanidad e Higiene Pública*, Vol 8, No. 1, 1933, pp. 1-22.

Carrasco Cadenas, E., Jiménez, F., Bootello, A., Alvarado, C., "La eliminación de yodo por la orina en los individuos normales sometidos a la sal yodada", *Contribución al I Congreso Nacional de Sanidad del laboratorio de Higiene de la Alimentación y de la Nutrición y Técnica Bromatológica*, Madrid, Escuela Nacional de Sanidad, 1934, pp. 75-86.

Carrasco Cadenas, E., Olmeda, C., "Contribución al estudio de la riqueza vitamínica de los alimentos españoles", *Contribución al I Congreso Nacional de Sanidad del Laboratorio de Higiene de la Alimentación y de la Nutrición y Técnica Bromatológica*, Madrid, Escuela Nacional de Sanidad, 1934, pp. 105- 133.

Chatfield, Ch., *Tables de composition des aliments pour l'usage international, Rome*, FAO, 1954.

Chodzko W., *The Rural Centre for Public Health and Social Welfare and the Improvement of Rural Health Conditions, Sixteenth Session of the Health Committee*, Geneva, League of Nations, 1930.

Comenge, M., *Análisis de Alimentos*, Toledo, Anastasio Medina, 1934.

Comenge, M., *Principios bioquímicos de Dietética Normal y Tabla de composición de los alimentos españoles*, Madrid, 1948, 206 p.

Committee on Calorie Requirements. *Report of the Committee on the Clorie Requirements*, Washington, FAO Nutritional Studies No. 5, 1950.

"Conference of Experts for the Standardisation of Certain Methods used in making Dietary Studies. Held in Rome on September 2nd and 3rd, 1932", *League of Nations Quarterly Bulletin of the Health Organisation*, Vol. 1, No. 1, 1932, pp. 477-483.

Cosin, J., *Estado actual de los standard internacionales de hormonas y vitaminas*, Madrid, Imprenta de J. Cosano, 1941.

Coward, K.H., "The relative antirachitic potencies of vitamin D2 (calciferol from irradiated ergosterol) and of vitamin D3 (from irradiated 7-dehydrocholesterol). A summary of experiments organised for the Accesory Food Factors Committee (Lister Institute and Medical Research Council), *League of Nations Bulletin of the Health organisation*, 1940/41, Vol. 9, pp. 425-435.

"Cuadro de las vitaminas y distribución de las más importantes. Instituto Nacional de Higiene de la Alimentación", *La voz de la Sanidad*, Vol. 1, 1938, 5 p.

Conferencias sobre alimentación, Madrid, Publicaciones de la Comisaría General de Abastecimientos y Transportes, 1944, 199 p.

"Current Notes on the Work of the Health Organisation. Conference on Nutrition", *League of Nations Quarterly Bulletin of the Health Organisation*, Vol. 1, No. 1, 1932, p. 311.

Dantín Cereceda J., *La alimentación española. Sus diferentes tipos.* Introducción, edición e índice onomástico de Juan Riera, Valladolid, Acta Histórico-Médica Vallisoletana, 1934.

Dietary Surveys: their technique and interpretation, Rome, FAO, 1949.

Dols, M.J.L., "Food policy, its application and impact on nutrition in Europe", FAO/WHO Symposium on Education and Training in Nutrition in Europe, Bad Homburg, Fed. Rep. of Germany, 2-11 December, 1959, Rome, FAO Nutrition Meetings Report Series No. 26, 1960.

Données sur la FAO, Washington, Organisation des Nations Unies pour l'Agriculture et l'Alimentation, 1947.

"Economic Depression and Public Health, Memorandum prepared by the Health. Section III. The Nutrition of the Unemployed", *League of Nations Quarterly Bulletin of the Health Organisation*, Vol. 1, 1932, pp. 443-457.

Economic Stability in the Post-War World, Report of the Delegation on Economic Depressions, Geneva, League of Nations, 1945.

Enquête Mondiale sur l'Alimentation, Washington/Rome, Organisation des Nations Unies pour l'Agriculture et l'Alimentation, 1946-1953.

"Famine Disease and its Treatment in Internment Camps", *League of Nations Bulletin of the Health Organisation*, Vol. 10, 1943-1944, pp. 722-772.

FAO, *Standing advisory comité on nutrition, First report to the director-general. Nutrition Division*, Copenhague, 23-31 August, 1946, Washington, FAO, 1946.

FAO, *Report of the special meeting on urgent food problems*, Washington, FAO, 1946.

FAO, *World Food Survey. Monograph living worldwide nutrition statistics and food production statistics by continent and country. Figures and proteins from pre-war food supplies and nutritional targets in several areas, pre-war food consumption survey, food production statistics per head of population*, Rome, FAO, 1946.

FAO, *The Nutritive Value of Foods. Conference*, Montevideo, FAO, 1948.

FAO, *Note on Nutrition and Agricultura. Nutrition Conference*, Montevideo, FAO, 1948.

FAO, *Food composition tables. Nutrition Division*, Washington, FAO, 1948.

FAO, *Nutrition education. Third Meeting of the Standing Advisory Comité on Nutrition*, Washington, FAO, 1948.

FAO, *Food composition tables of international use*, Washington, FAO, 1949.

FAO/WHO, *Joint FAO/WHO expert committee on nutrition*, Geneva, FAO/WHO, 1949.

Final Report of the Mixed Committee of the League of Nations on Relation of Nutrition to Health, Agriculture and Economic Policy, Geneva, League of Nations, 1937 [A.13.1937.II.A].

Food and the War, Boston, United States Food Administration, 1918.

Food, Famine and Relief 1940-1946. Economic, Financial and Transit Department, Geneva, League of Nations, 1946, 162 p.

"Food: a first on the agenda for of the postwar world", *Survey Graphic* (USA). Calling America Series (USA. v. 37(3), No. 11, East Stroudsburg, PA (USA), Survey Associates, 1948. 92 p.

Food Rationing and Supply, 1943/44, Geneva, League of Nations, 1942.

García Luquero, "Aspectos sanitarios de la evacuación de refugiados en Santander", *Revista de Sanidad e Higiene Pública*, Vol. 1, 1938-1939, pp. 68-81.

García Triviño F., "Predisposición y tuberculosis", *Revista de Higiene y Tuberculosis*, Vol. 8, 1914, pp. 4-6.

Giral, J., *Ración alimenticia desde los puntos de vista higiénico y social*, Madrid, Adrián Romo Editor, 1914.

Giral, J., "Repercusiones económicas y sociales de la alimentación humana. Conferencia dada en la Escuela Nacional de Sanidad el 24 de mayo de 1934", *Revista de Sanidad e Higiene Pública*, 1934, pp. 121-139.

Godoy Ramírez, J., *Vitaminas y avitaminosis*, Almería, Sempere, 1922.

Gómez Ocaña, J., *Los alimentos minerales. Discurso leído en la solemne sesión inaugural del año de 1914... en la Real Academia de Medicina*, Madrid, Real Academia Nacional de Medicina, 1914.

González Campo, J., *La alimentación de las clases pobres de Madrid como factor etiológico de enfermedades gástricas e intestinales*, Madrid, Estudio Tipográfico Idamor Moreno, 1903.

Gorter, E., De Lange, C., "Nutritive food requirements during the first year of life", *League of Nations Bulletin of the Health Organisation*, Vol. 6, No. 2, 1937, pp. 291-298.

Grande Covián, F., *La alimentación en Madrid durante la Guerra. (Estudio de la dieta suministrada a la población civil madrileña durante diecinueve meses de guerra: Agosto 1937 a Febrero 1939)*, Madrid, Publicación de la Revista de Sanidad e Higiene Pública, 1939.

Grande Covián, F., Jiménez García, F., "Sobre los trastornos carenciales observados en Madrid durante la Guerra. II. Presentación en el tiempo de los distintos cuadros carenciales", *Revista Clínica Española*, Vol. 1, 1940, pp. 318-322.

Grande Covián, F., Jiménez García, F., "Algunas observaciones acerca de la acción del ácido nicotínico sobre la glucemia y la lactacidemia", *Revista Clínica Española*, Vol. 1, 1940, pp. 325-329.

Grande Covián, F., Jiménez García, F., "El contenido en ácido nicotínico de las dietas consumidas en Madrid durante la guerra", *Revista Clínica Española*, Vol. 8, 1943, pp. 28-30.

Grande Covián, F., Jiménez García, F., "El tratamiento de la pelagra por el ácido nicotínico", *Revista Clínica Española*, 1940, Vol. 1, pp. 49-81.

Grande Covián, F., "Sobre el peso de los recién nacidos, durante la guerra en Madrid", *Revista Clínica Española*, 1940, Vol. 1, pp. 501-504.

Grande Covián, F., "La secreción láctea durante la hipoalimentación. (observaciones en las madres lactantes de Madrid durante la guerra)", *Revista Clínica Española*, 1940, Vol. 1, pp. 180-188.

Grande Covián, F., "Dietas fisiológicas, máxima y mínima en el régimen de alimentación del hombre adulto", *Revista de Sanidad e Higiene Pública*, 1943, pp. 115-129.

Grande Covián, F., "L'alimentation et les troubles alimentaires durant la Guerre Civile Espagnole", *Les Vitamines*, Bâle, Roche, 1944.

Grande Covián, F., Peraita, M., *Avitaminosis y Sistema Nervioso*, Barcelona, Miguel Server, 1941a.

Grande Covián, F., *La ciencia de la alimentación*, Madrid, Ediciones Pegaso, 1947.

Grande Covián, F., Peraita, M., "Vitaminas y Sistema Nervioso", *Revista Clínica Española*, Vol. 2, 1941b, pp. 209-232.

Grey, E., *The Food of Japan*, Geneva, League of Nations, 1928.

Guerra y Estapé, J., *Adición de sustancias extrañas a los alimentos*, Barcelona, Academia de Higiene de Cataluña, 1921.

Handbook for the preparation of food balance sheets, Washington, FAO, 1949.

Health Organisation Report, Geneva, League of Nations, 1936, p. 6.

Hindende, M., "The Effect of Food Restriction During War on Mortality in Copenhagen", *Journal of the American Medical Association*, Vol. 74, No. 6, 1920.

"International standards for vitamin E", *League of Nations Bulletin of the Health organisation*, Vol. 9, 1940/41, pp. 436-442.

Jiménez, F., Jiménez, M., "La alimentación en la provincia de Jaén. Deducciones sanitarias", *Contribución al I Congreso Nacional de Sanidad del laboratorio de Higiene de la Alimentación y de la Nutrición y Técnica Bromatológica*, Madrid, Escuela Nacional de Sanidad, 1934, pp. 25-34.

Jiménez, F., "Necesidades energéticas y dietéticas en la zona de Navalmoral de la Mata (Cáceres)", *Revista de Sanidad e Higiene Pública*, 1935, pp. 470-477.

Jiménez García, F., "Estudio clínico de los trastornos carenciales observados en la población civil de Madrid durante la Guerra (1936-1939)", *Revista Clínica Española*, Vol. 1, 1940, pp. 231-237.

Jiménez García, F., Grande Covián, F., "Sobre los trastornos carenciales observados en Madrid durante la Guerra. I. Los cuadros clínicos presentados con más frecuencia y su clasificación", *Revista Clínica Española*, Vol. 1, 1940a, pp. 313-318.

Jiménez García, F., Grande Covián, F., "Algunas observaciones sobre las dietas consumidas por los enfermos carenciales de Madrid", *Revista Clínica Española*, Vol. 1, No. 1, 1940b.

Jiménez García, F., Grande Covián, F., "Sobre los trastornos carenciales observados en Madrid durante la Guerra. III. La presentación de los cuadros carenciales, en relación con la edad y el sexo de los pacientes", *Revista Clínica Española*, Vol. 1, 1940, pp. 323-328.

Jiménez, F., Torres, T., "Las necesidades calóricas alimenticias de los internados en nuestras instituciones benéficas", *Primer Congreso Nacional de Sanidad. Madrid, 6-12 de mayo de 1934*, Madrid, Vol. 4, 1935, pp. 137-142.

Jiménez Díaz, C., *Estudios de nutrición*, Madrid, Instituto de Investigaciones Médicas, 1941-1943.

Jolliffe, W. "Clinical examination. Methods for evaluation of nutritional adequacy and status", *Nat.Res.Coun*, Washington.

Keys, A. *et al.*, *The biology of human starvation*, Minneapolis, 1950.

Kriegsernährungsplan für den Zeitraum 1.10.1938-1.8.1939. Teil I 1938, BBAW, Institut für Ernährung, Historische Abteilung, No. 72.

Kusama, Y., Ochi, T., Higuchi, T., *Studies on the basal metabolism*, Geneva, League of Nations, 1937, 6 p. [C.H. 1256].

Lacaisse R., *L'Organisation d'Hygiene de la Société des Nations*, Société des Nations, Geneva, 1923.

Lacaisse R., *L'Hygiène internationale et la Société des Nations*, Editions du 'Mouvement Sanitaire', Paris, 1926.

Laugier, H., "General Programme of Research into Biological Measurements and Tests for the Definition of States of Malnutrition", *League of Nations*

Quarterly Bulletin of the Health Organisation, Vol. 5, No. 3, 1936, pp. 505-530.

Lesné, E., Dreyfus-Sée, G., "Nutrition in childhood", *League of Nations Quarterly Bulletin of the Health Organisation*, Vol. 5, No. 3, 1936, pp. 531-43.

[Lindberg, J.] *Wartime rationing and consumption*, Geneva, League of Nations Financial Section and Economic Intelligence Service, 1942.

[Lindberg, J.] *Food rationing and supply 1942/43*, Geneva, League of Nations Financial Section and Economic Intelligence Service, 1943.

[Lindberg, J.] *Food, Famine and Relief, 1940-1946*, Geneva, League of Nations Financial Section and Economic Intelligence Service, 1946.

Mackenzie, M.D., "The Administrative Machinery by which the Adequate Nourishment of the Poor is Ensured in Great Britain", *League of Nations Quarterly Bulletin of the Health Organisation*, Vol. 2, 1933, pp. 333-352.

MacRae, T.F., "The adoption of crystalline vitamin B1 Hydrochloride as the new international standards of vitamin B1 and comparison of its potency with that of the former standard. A summary of Co-operative Experiments organised by the Accessory Food Factors Committee (Lister Institute and Medical Research Council)", *League of Nations Bulletin of the Health organisation*, Vol. 9, 1940-1941, pp. 371-424.

Maestre Ibañez, M., *Doce conferencias de análisis de alimentos: guía práctica de* análisis, Madrid, Sucesores de Rivadeneyra, 1926.

Malnutrition and starvation in Western Netherlands, September 1944-July 1945, The Hague, 1948.

Martínez García, F., "Trastornos nutritivos como causa de la mortalidad infantil. Peligros del calor", *Conferencias radiadas por el médico jefe del Servicio Provincial de Puericultura durante el año 1938*, La Coruña, Instituto Provincial de Higiene de la Coruña "Al Servicio de España y del niño español", 1939, p.5-9.

Martínez Vargas, A., "Selección de los niños 'pretuberculosos'. Ponencia al Congreso Nacional de Tuberculosis (Zaragoza, 1908)", *La Salud Pública. Revista de Higiene y Tuberculosis*, 1909, Vol. 5, pp. 6-9.

[McDougall, E.J.] "Rural dietaries in Europe", *Bulletin of the Health Organisation*, Vol. 8, No. 3, 1939, pp. 470-497 [C.H./Com.Exp.Alim./59, 25 p.].

Mejoramiento de la nutrición a través de los servicios de salud pública, Fourth Conference on Nutrition Problems in Latin America – Guatemala City, Guatemala, 23 Sep - 1 Oct 1957, FAO and WHO, 1957.

"Memorandum prepared by the Health Section of the League of Nations: the Economic Depression and Public Health", *League of Nations Quarterly Bulletin of the Health Organisation*, Vol. 1, 1932, pp. 425.

"Memorandum on the International Standard for vitamin E from the Department of Biological Standards, National Institute of Medical Research. (Lister Institute and Medical Research Council)", *League of Nations Quarterly Bulletin of the Health Organisation*, Vol. 9, 1940-1941, pp. 443-446.

Methodology of diet surveys, Washington, FAO, 1948.

"Milk Problem, The", *League of Nations Bulletin of the Health Organisation*, Vol. 6, No. 2, 1937, pp. 371-504.

Milk Problem. A Critical Study of its Nutritional, Hygienic, Economic and Social Aspects by HC Bendixen, GJ Blink, JC Drummond, AM Leroy, GS Wilson, Geneva, League of Nations, 1937.

Moerkeberg, H.C., *Meat Inspection in Denmark and Inspection of Milk in Denmark*, Geneva, League of Nations, 1924 [C.H./E.P.S./49].

Molina, G. *Organization and Intergration of Public Health Services. First Inter-American Congress of Public Health*, La Havana, WHO Document C.I.H./3, 1952.

Moreno Luque, J., *Algunas normas sobre alimentación humana y sobre Economía, Agrícola, Ganadera y Forestal estudiadas durante su cautiverio en Madrid*, Prólogo de José Mª Fernández-Ladreda, Madrid, 1939.

Moroder, J., "Los puntos de vista sanitarios de la alimentación humana", *Revista de Sanidad e Higiene Pública*, 1934, pp. 167-175.

"Most Suitable Methods of Detecting Malnutrition Due to the Economic Depression, The. Conference held at Berlin from December 5th to 7th, 1932", *League of Nations Quarterly Bulletin of the Health Organisation*, Vol. 1, 1933, pp. 116-129.

Muehel, W., "Ill effects of food restrictions in Europe, 1940-1944", *League of Nations Bulletin of the Health Organisation*, Vol. 12, 1945-1946.

Nobécourt, P., Vitry, G., "Clinical methods for determining the state of nutrition in school children", *League of Nations Quarterly Bulletin of the Health Organisation*, Vol. 5, No.3, 1936, pp. 544-48.

Noguer-Moré, J., *Nuestra alimentación en tiempos de* escasez, Barcelona, Biblioteca Hygia, 1937

Nutrition: the newer diagnostic methods. Proceedings of the round table on nutrition and public health, New York, Milbank Memorial Fund, 1938.

Nutrition in various countries, Series of League of Nations Publications, Geneva, 1936. [Technical Report A.12(b).1936.II.B]

Nutrition programs in public health departments, Nutrition Conference, Rio De Janeiro, Brazil, 5-13 Jun 1950, WHO/FAO, Rome, FAO, 1952.

"Nutrition Surveys. Their techniques and value", *Bull. Nat. Res. Coun*, No. 117, 1949.

Olmeda Viorreta, C., "Contribución al estudio vitamínico de los alimentos españoles. Experiencias llevadas a cabo entre 1934 y 1935", *Revista de Sanidad e Higiene Pública*, Vol. 11, No. 3, 1936, pp. 205-231.

Orr J.B., *The Influence of Nutrition on the Incidence of Disease*, London, Hudson and Son, 1925.

Orr, J.B., *Minerals in Pastures and Their Relation to Animal Nutrition*, London, Lewis, 1929.

Orr, J.B., *The National Food Supply and Its Influence on National Health*, London, King, 1934.

Orr J.B., *Food, Health & Income: Report on a Survey of Adequacy of Diet in Relation to Income*, London, Macmillan & Co, 1936.

Orr, J.B., "Nutritional Science and State Planning", *What Science Stands For*, in John Boyd Orr (eds.), *What Science Stands For*, London, Allen & Unwin, 1937.

Orr, J.B., Lubbock, D., *Feeding the People in Wartime*, London, Macmillan, 1940.

Orr, J.B., *Fighting for What?*, London, Macmillan, 1942.

Orr, J.B., *Food and the People*, London, Pilot Press, 1943.

Orr J.B., *The Role of Food in Post-war Reconstruction*, Geneva, International Labour Organisation, 1943.

Orr, J.B., *Food: The Foundation of World Unity*, London, National Peace Council, 1948.

Orr, J.B. "Can mankind make good? Food: a first on the agenda for of the postwar world", *Survey Graphic* (USA), East Stroudsburg, PA (USA), Survey Associates, 1948, pp. 97-98.

Orr, J.B., *International Liaison Committee of Organisations for Peace: A New Strategy of Peace*, London, National Peace Council, 1950.

Orr, J.B., *The White Man's Dilemma: Food and the Future* (with the cooperation of David Lubbock), London, Allen & Unwin, 1953.

Orr, J.B., *Nutrition in programming for public health. Address delivered before the National Vitamin Foundation, March 6, 1957*, National Vitamin Foundation Report to the Board of Governors by Scientific Director for the period Jan. 1, 1956-Dec. 31, 1956, New York, National Vitamin Foundation, 1957.

Orr, J.B., *The Wonderful World of Food: The Substance of Life*, Garden City, New York, Garden City Books, 1958.

Palanca y Martínez Fortún, J.A., "Rapport sur la situation epidemiologique de l'Espagne pendant l'année 1939", Genève, Société des Nations, 1939, pp. 40-52.

Palanca y Martínez Fortún, J.A., *Les services sanitaires espagnols pendant la guerre civile*, Genève, Société des Nations, 1939.

Peraita, M., "Sobre el tratamiento por el ácido nicotínico de los síntomas nerviosos y mentales de los pelagrosos", *Revista de Sanidad e Higiene Pública*, 1940, pp. 482-503.

Pi i Sunyer, A., *El hambre de los pueblos.* Conferencia dada por el Doctor d. Augusto Pi i Sunyer en la Academia de Medicina en 29 de enero de 1922, Asociación instructiva de obreros y empleados municipales, Barcelona, 1922.

Pi i Sunyer Bayo, J., *Principis generals de dietética*, Barcelona, Monografies Mèdiques, 1930.

Pittaluga, G., *El problema de las vitaminas y la alimentación del obrero*, Madrid, Sociedad Española de Higiene, 1917.

Pittaluga, G., *La constitución de la Escuela Nacional de Sanidad de Madrid (España)*, Madrid, Escuela Nacional de Sanidad, 1930.

Prescott, S.C., Proctor, B.E., *Food Technology*, New York, 1937.

Prevention and Treatment of Severe Malnutrition in Times of Disaster, Report approved by the Joint FAO/WHO Expert Committee on Nurrition and presented to the Fourth Health Assembly, Geneva, World Health Organization, 1951.

The Problem of Nutrition. Interim Report of the Mixed Committee on the Problem of Nutrition, 3 vols., Geneva, Series of League of Nations Publications, 1936 [Technical Report A.12.1936.II.B].

Proposals for a world food board and world food survey.World Food Program, 1946, World Food Program, Washington, FAO, 1946.

Pulido, A., "Prólogo", Úbeda y Correal, J. (ed.), *El presupuesto de la familia obrera*, Dirección General de Sanidad (Monografías), Madrid, 1902, pp. 7-8.

Puche Alvarez, J., "El hambre en Europa", *Ciencia (México)*, Vol. 1, 1940, 6 p.

Randoin, L., "On the necessity for a biological supervisión of food (with Special Reference to its Vitamin Content)", *League of Nations Quarterly Bulletin of the Health Organisation*, Vol. 5, No.3, 1936, pp. 493-504.

Rapport sur la mission sanitaire en Espagne (28 decembre 1936-15 janvier 1937), Genève, Société des Nations, 1937, 62 p.

Rapport de la Réunion de la FAO sur la Nutrition en Europe, Rome, Food and Agriculture Organisation, 1958, 28 p.

Rationement alimentaire et ravitaillement 1943-1944, Genève, Société des Nations, 1944.

Raventós, J., *L'Alimentació humana*, Mancomunitat de Catalunya (Publicacions divulgadores dels Serveis Tècnics d'Agricultura, núm. 8), Barcelona, 1923.

Raw Materials and Foodstuffs: Production by Countries, 1935 and 1938, Geneva, League of Nations, 1939.

Relief Deliveries and Relief Loans, Geneva, League of Nations, 1943.

Relation of Nutrition to Health, Agriculture and Economy Policy, The Final Report of the Mixed Committee of the League of Nations, Geneva, League of Nations, 1937.

Report on the food requirements of man, Food war committee, London, Royal Society, 1919.

"Report on the Best Methods of Safeguarding the Public Health during the Depression", *League of Nations Quarterly Bulletin of the Health Organisation*, Vol. 2, 1933, pp. 286-332.

"Report on the Physiological Bases of Nutrition by the Technical Commission of the Health Committee in the meeting held in London 25-29 November 1935", *League of Nations Quarterly Bulletin of the Health Organisation*, Vol. 5, No. 3, 1936, pp. 391-415.

"Report of the Health Organisation for the Period October 1932 to September 1933. IV. Economic Depression and Public Health", *League of Nations Quarterly Bulletin of the Health Organisation*, Vol. 2, 1933, pp. 529-535.

"Report by the Technical Commission on Nutrition on the work of its second session held in Geneva, June 4th to 8th, 1936", *League of Nations Quarterly Bulletin of the Health Organisation*, Vol. 5, No. 3, 1936, pp. 416-426.

"Report on the work of the group of experts appointed to study methods of assessiong the state of nutrition in infants and adolescents", *League of Nations Bulletin of the Health Organisation*, Vol. 6, No 2, 1937, pp. 129-204.

"Report by the Technical Commission on Nutrition on the Work of its third session, held in London from November 15th to 20th, 1937", *Bulletin of the Health Organisation*, Vol. 7, 1938, pp. 460-502.

"Report on the Meeting of Directors of Institutes and Schools of Hygiene held in Geneva from November 22nd to 27th, 1937. F. Nutrition", *League of Nations Bulletin of the Health Organisation*, Vol. 7, 1938, pp. 186-190.

"Report on the work of the Health Organisation between June 1937 and May 1938, and on its 1938 Programme. 4. Nutrition", *League of Nations Bulletin of the Health Organisation*, Vol. 7, 1938, pp. 642-647.

"Report on the work of the Health Organisation between June 1938 and April 1939 and on its 1939 programme. B. Nutrition", *League of Nations Bulletin of the Health Organisation*, Vol. 8, 1939, pp. 27-32.

"Report on Bread in several European Countries", *League of Nations Bulletin of the Health organisation*, Vol. 8, 1939, pp.498-550.

Report to the Board of Governors by the Scientific Director for the period January 1, 1956 - December 31, 1956. With the address of Nobel Laureate, Lord John Boyd Orr: *Nutrition in Programming for Public Health*, delivered before the National Vitamin Foundation, March 6, 1957, New York, National Vitamin Foundation, 1957.

Report of the FAO nutrition meeting for Europe – Rome, Italy 23-28 June 1958, Rome, FAO, Nutrition Meetings Report Series No. 21, 32 p., 1958.

Report of the symposium on the nutritional state of Europe and the need for education and training in nutrition, FAO/WHO Symposium on Education and Training in Nutrition in Europe, Bad Homburg, Fed. Rep. of Germany, 2-11 December, 1959, Rome, FAO Nutrition Meetings Report Series No. 26, 1960.

Richet, Ch., "The nutritional requirements of puberty", *League of Nations Quarterly Bulletin of the Health Organisation*, Vol. 5, No. 3, 1936, pp. 549-553.

Richet, Ch., *Alimentación y regímenes alimentarios*, Madrid, Espasa-Calpe, 1942.

Robinson, W.D., Janney, J.H., Grande (Covián), F., "An Evaluation of the Nutritional Status of a Population Group in Madrid, Spain, during the Summer of 1941", *Journal of Nutrition*, Vol. 24, No. 6, 1942, pp. 557-584.

Rockefeller Foundation, *Report on the health situation in Spain*, New York, Rockefeller Archive Centre, 20 August, 1939.

Rodríguez Abaytúa, R., *Bioenergética y termoquímica alimenticia: estudio razonado para la alimentación del adulto*, Madrid, Nicolás Moya, 1921.

Rof Carballo, J., Grande Covián, F., "Calambres musculares como síntomas carenciales", *Revista Clínica Española*, Vol. 8, 1943.

Rosell, J.M., *Los actuales conocimientos del metabolismo mineral: la importancia fisiológica, patológica, terapéutica e higiénica de los elementos minerales contenidos en los alimentos y en el agua*, Barcelona, 1927.

Rosen, J., *Wartime food developments in Switzerland*, Stanford, Cal., Stanford University, 1947.

Ruiz Gijón, J., *El diagnóstico de la pelagra por el laboratorio*, Madrid, J. Cosano, 1941.

Ruiz Gijón, J., *Estudio de las relaciones entre el metabolismo de la creatina y el de los hidratos de carbono*, Madrid, J. Cosano, 1942.

Saiki, T., *Progress of the Science of Nutrition in Japan*, Geneva, League of Nations, 1926.

Saiki, T., *Necessity of the Study of Nutrition*, Geneva, League of Nations, 1927.

Sanidad Nacional. Disposiciones oficiales emanadas del Ministerio de la Gobernación (Dirección General de Sanidad), 32 vols., Madrid, Ministerio de la Gobernación, 1903-1935.

"Second Conference on Vitamin Standardisation", *League of Nations Quarterly Bulletin of the Health Organisation*, Vol. 3, 1934, pp. 428-440.

"Second General Report on certain European Schools and Institutes of Hygiene. 5. School of Health and National Institute of Hygiene, Madrid", *League of Nations Bulletin of the Health Organisation*, Vol 7, 1938, pp. 309-312.

Schiötz, C., *Appreciation de l'etat de nutrition des enfants. Remarques préliminaires*, Geneva, League of Nations, 1936.

"Standardisation of certain methods used in making dietary studies. Conference of experts held in Rome", *League of Nations Quarterly Bulletin of the Health Organisation*, Vol. 1, 1932, p. 477.

State of food and agriculture 1948, The. A survey of world conditions and prospects, FAO Economic Analysis Division, Washington, FAO, 1948, 219 p.

State of food and agriculture 1949, The. A survey of world conditions and prospects, FAO Economic Analysis Division, Washington, FAO, 1949, 140 p.

Statistical Year-Book of the League of Nations, 1940/41, Geneva, League of Nations, 1941.

Statistical Year-Book of the League of Nations, 1941/42, Includding addendum 1942/43, Geneva, League of Nations, 1943.

Statistical Year-Book of the League of Nations, 1942/44 (Seventeenth Year), Geneva, League of Nations, 1943.

Tarralluela i Albareda, J., *Higiene de l'alimentació*, Minerva, Diputación de Barcelona, Barcelona, 1919.

Teaching better nutrition. A study of approaches and techniques, Rome, FAO, 1950.

"Technical Commission on Nutrition. Report by a Special Committee which met in Geneva from August 22nd to 24th, 1938", *Bulletin of the Health Organisation*, Vol. 7, 1938, pp. 667-678.

Terroine, E.F., "The Protein Component in the Human Diet", *League of Nations Quarterly Bulletin of the Health Organisation*, Vol. 5, No. 3, 1936, pp. 427-492.

Transition from War to Peace Economy, The. Report of the Delegation on Economic Depressions, Geneva, League of Nations, 1943.

Úbeda y Correal, J., *El presupuesto de la familia obrera*, Dirección General de Sanidad, Madrid, 1902.

Veen, A.G. van, "The rice problem", *League of Nations Bulletin of the Health Organisation*, Vol. 9, 1940, pp. 357-60.

Voit, C. von, *Food and the Principles of Dietetics*, London, 1927.

Wartime rationing and Consumption, Geneva, League of Nations, 1942.

Von Loesecke, H.W., *Outlines of food technology*, New York, 1949.

Worker's nutrition and social policy, League of Nations, Geneva, 1936.

World Economic Survey, 1939/41, Geneva, League of Nations, 1941.

World Economic Survey, 1941/42, Geneva, League of Nations, 1942.

World Economic Survey, 1942/44, Geneva, League of Nations, 1945.

World Food Situation, Geneva, League of Nations, 1946.

World Food Survey [1st], Washington, Food and Agriculture Organisation, 1946, 39 p.

World Food Survey [2nd], Rome, Food and Agriculture Organisation, 1952, 59 p.

Selected Bibliography

A'Hearn, B., "Anthropometric evidence on living standard in Northern Italy, 1730-1860", *Journal of Economic History*, No. 63, 2003, pp. 351-381.

Alexandratos, N., "The Mediterranean diet in a world context", *Public Health Nutrition*. 9, 2006, pp. 111-117.

Anderson, G.H. *et al.*, "Dietary Guidelines: Past experience and New Approaches", *Journal of the American Dietetic Association*, No. 103, Supplement 2, 2003.

Amrith, S., "Development and Disease: Public Health and the United Nations, c. 1945-55", in Daunton, M., Trentmann, F. (eds.), *Worlds of Political Economy. Knowledge and Power in the Nineteenth and Twentieth Centuries*, Basingstoke, Palgrave Macmillan, 2006, pp. 221-50.

Andresen, A., Elvbakken, K.T., Hubbard, W. (eds.), *Public Health and Preventive Medicine 1800-2000*, Bergen, Stein Rokkan Centre for Social Studies, Report 1-2004.

Andresen, A., Grønlie, T., Ryymin, T. (eds.), *Science, Culture and Politics. European Perspectives on Medicine, Sickness and Health*, Bergen, Stein Rokkan Centre for Social Studies, 2006.

Andresen, A., Grønlie, T., Ryymin, T. (eds.), *Transferring Medico-Political Knowledge in Nineteenth- and Twentieth-Century Europe*, Bergen, Rokkan Centre for Social Studies, 2007.

Andresen, A. *et al.* (eds.), *Citizens, Courtrooms, Crossings*, Bergen, Stein Rokkan Centre for Social Studies, 2008.

Andresen, A., Groenlie, T., Hubbard, W., Ryymin, T. (eds.), *Healthcare Systems and Medical Institutions*, Oslo, Novus Press, 2009.

Andresen, A., Hubbard, W., Ryymin, T. (eds.), *International and Local Approaches to Health and Health Care*, Oslo, Novus Press, 2010.

Andresen, A., Barona, J.L., Cherry, S. (eds.), *Making a new countryside? Health Policies and Practices in European History c. 1860-1950*, Frankfurt, Peter Lang, 2010.

Apple, R.D., *Vitamania: Vitamins in American Culture*, New York, New Brunswick, 1996.

Apple, R.D., "Vitamins win the war: nutrition, commerce, and patriotism in the United States during the Second World War", in Smith, D.F., Phillips, J. (eds.), *Food, Science, Policy and Regulation in the Twentieth Century: International and Comparative Perspectives*, London, Routledge, 2000, pp. 135-150.

Aranceta Bartrina, J., *Nutrición comunitaria.* Barcelona, 2001.

Atkins, P., "The Glasgow Case: Meat, Disease and Regulation, 1889 – 1924", *Agricultural History Review*, No. 52, 2004, pp. 161-82.

Atkins, P., "Fattening Children or Fattening Farmers? School Milk in Britain, 1921 – 1941", *Economic History Review*, No. 58, 2005, pp. 57-78.

Atkins, P., "School Milk in Britain, 1900-1934", *Journal of Policy History*, No. 19, 2007, pp. 395-427.

Atkins, P., Lummel, P., Oddy, D. (eds.), *Food and city in Europe since 1800*, Aldershot, Asghate, 2007.

Badger Anthony, J., *The New Deal. The Depression Years 1933-1940*, New York, Hill and Wang, 1989.

Bakker, N., "Fresh Air and Good Food: Children and theAnti-Tuberculosis Campaign in the Netherlands, c. 1900 – 1940", *History of Education*, No. 39, 2010, 343-61.

Baldwin, P., *The Politics of Social Solidarity. Class Bases of the European Welfare State 1875-1975*, Cambridge, Cambridge University Press, 1990.

Barciela López, C., *Ni un español sin pan: la Red Nacional de Silos y Graneros*, Zaragoza, 2007.

Barnes, G.N., *History of the International Labour Office*, London, Williams and Norgate, 1926.

Barnes, D.S., *The Great Stink of Paris and the Nineteenth-Century Struggle against Filth and Germs*, Baltimore, The Johns Hopkins University Press, 2006.

Barona, J.L. (ed.), *Ciencia, salud pública y exilio. España 1875-1939*,Valencia, Publicacions de la Universitat de València, 2003, 284 pp.

Barona, J.L., *Salud, tecnología y saber médico*, Madrid, Ed. Ramón Areces, 2004.

Barona, J.L., "Rural Life and the Problem of Nutrition. Technical Approaches by the Nutrition Committee of the League of Nations", in Andresen, A.,

Grønlie, T., Ryymin, T. (eds.), *Science, Culture and Politics. European Perspectives on Medicine, Sickness and Health*, Bergen, Stein Rokkan Centre for Social Studies, 2006, pp. 201-14.

Barona, J.L., "Nutrition, knowledge, and action. International trends and social policies in Spain, 1931-1944", in Andersen, A., Gronlie, T. (eds.), *Transferring Medico-Political Knowledge in 19th and 20th Century Europe*, Bergen, Stein Rokkan Centre for Social Studies, 2007a, pp. 91-108.

Barona, J.L., "La salud de la población según los informes internacionales", *Actas del Congreso Internacional sobre la Guerra Civil Española*, Madrid, Sociedad Estatal de Conmemoraciones Culturales, 2007b.

Barona, J.L., "Nutrition and Health. The International Context during the Inter-war Crisis", *Social History of Medicine*, Vol. 21, No. 1, 2008a, pp. 87-105.

Barona, J.L., "International Organisations and the Development of a Physiology of Nutrition during the 1930s", *Food & History*, Vol. 6, n° 1, 2008b, pp. 129-162.

Barona, J.L., "Science, Democracy and the Global Market", *Chinese Cross Currents*, No. 7, (2008c), pp. 24-40.

Barona, J.L., Cherry, S. (eds.), *Health and Medicine in Rural Europe (1850-1945)*, València, Seminari d'Estudis sobre la Ciència, Universitat de València, 2005.

Barona, J., Bernabeu-Mestre, J., Perdiguero, E., "Health Problems and Public Policies in Rural Spain (1854-1936)", in Barona, J.L., Cherry S. (eds.), *Health and Medicine in Rural Europe (1850-1945)*, València, Seminari d'Estudis sobre la Ciència, Universitat de València, 2005, pp. 63-82.

Barona, J.L., Perdiguero E., "Health and the War. Changing schemes and health conditions during the Spanish Civil War", *Dynamis*, No. 28, 2008, pp. 103-123.

Barona, J.L., *The problem of nutrition. Experimental science, public health and economy in Europe 1914-1945*, Brussels, P.I.E. Peter Lang, 2010.

Barona, J.L., "Nutrición y salud. De la génesis del conocimiento experimental a las prácticas sociales (1918-1950)", in Bernabeu-Mestre, J., Barona, J.L. (eds.), *Nutrición, salud y Sociedad. España y Europa en los siglos XIX-X*, Valencia, SEC/PUV, 2011.

Barona, J.L., "Los Organismos Internacionales y la fisiologia de la nutrición durante los años 1930", in Bernabeu-Mestre, J., Barona, J.L. (eds.), *Nutrición, salud y Sociedad. España y Europa en los siglos XIX-X*, Valencia, SEC/PUV, 2011.

Barry, A., *Political machines: governing a technological society*, London, The Athalone Press, 2001.

Basch, P.F., *Textbook of Internacional Health*, New York/Oxford, Oxford University Press, 1999.

Baum, Warren C., *Partners Against Hunger*, Washington, DC, The World Bank, 1986.

Bauman, Z., *Globalization. The Human consequences*, Cambridge, Polity Press, 1998.

Beck, U., *Risk Society: Towards a New Modernity*, Newbury Park, CA, Sage, 1992.

Beck, U., "From industrial Society to the Risk Society: Questions of Survival, Social Structure and Ecological Enlightenenment", *Theory, Culture and Society*, No. 9, 1992, 97-123.

Beck, U., *What is Globalisation?*, Cambridge, Polity Press, 2000.

Belasco, W., *Food*, Oxford/New York, Berg, 2008.

Belasco, W., Horowitz, R. (eds.), *Food Chains: from Farmyard to Shopping Cart*, Philadelphia, Univerity of Pennsylvania Press, 2010.

Beneito, A., Puche Gil, J., "Creixement econòmic i desenvolupament fabril en Alcoi, 1840-1915: Misèria fisiològica sota l'esplendor industrial?", *La societat industrial al País Valencià*, Alcoi, 2008.

Bengoa Lecanda, J.M., *Tras la ruta del hambre. Nutrición y salud pública en el siglo XX*, Alicante, Publicaciones Universidad de Alicante, 2007.

Bengoa Lecanda, J.M., "Historia de la nutrición en salud pública", in Serra Majem, L., Aranceta Bartrina, J. (eds.), *Nutrición y salud pública. Métodos, bases científicas y aplicaciones*, Barcelona, Elsevier & Mason, 2006, pp. 52-61.

Bengtsson, T., Saito, O. (eds.), *Population and economy. From hunger to modern economic growth*, Oxford, Oxford University Press, 2000.

Bennett, J., *The Hunger Machine: The Politics of Food*, Cambridge, Politi, 1987.

Benner, M., Löfgren, H., "The Bio-economy and the Competition State: Transcending the Dichotomy between Coordinated and Liberal Market Economies", *New Political Science*, No. 29, 2007, pp. 77-95.

Bentley, A., *Eating for victory. Food rationing and the politics of domesticity*, Champaign, University of Illinois Press, 1998.

Berkov, R., *The World Health organisation: A Study in Decentralised Internacional Administration*, Geneva, Librarie E. Droz, 1957.

Bernabeu-Mestre, J. *et al.*, "La alimentación como problema sanitario: nutrición y salud pública en la España de la primera mitad del siglo XX", *VIII Congreso de la ADEH*, Maó, 2007, 63 p.

Bernabeu-Mestre, J. *et al.*, *Investigación e innovación tecnológica en la ciencia de la nutrición. El abordaje de la malnutrición en el contexto de la cultura científica*, Alicante, Editorial Club Universitario, 2008.

Bernabeu-Mestre, J. *et al.*, "Nutrition and public health in the contemporary Spain, 1900-1936", *Food and History*, Vol. 6, No. 1, 2008.

Bernabeu-Mestre, J., Galiana, M.E., Esplugues, J.X., and Cid, P., "Overexploitation, malnutrition and stigma in a women's illness: chlorosis in contemporary Spanish medicine (1877-1936)", in Harris, B., Gálvez, L., Machado, E. (eds.), *Gender and wellbeing in Europe: historical and contemporary perspectives*, Ashgate, Hampshire, 2009, pp. 154-171.

Bernabeu-Mestre, J., "Notas para una historia de la desnutrición en la Iberoamérica del siglo XX, *Nutr Hosp*, 25 (supl. 3), 2010, pp. 10-17.

Bernabeu-Mestre, J., Barona, J.L. (eds.), *Nutrición, Salud y Sociedad. España y Europa en los siglos XIX-XX*, Valencia, SEC/PUV, 2011.

Bernabeu-Mestre, J., "El contexto histórico de la transición nutricional en España", in Bernabeu-Mestre, J., Barona, J.L. (eds.), *Nutrición, salud y Sociedad. España y Europa en los siglos XIX-XX*, Valencia, SEC/PUV, 2011.

Bernabeu-Mestre, J., Esplugues, J.X., Galiana, M.E., Moncho, J., "Nutrición y salud pública en España, 1900-1936", in Bernabeu-Mestre, J., Barona, J.L. (eds.), *Nutrición, salud y Sociedad. España y Europa en los siglos XIX-XX*, Valencia, SEC/PUV, 2011.

Bhargava, A., *Food, economics, and health*, Oxford, Oxford University Press, 2008.

Blecourt, W., Usbourne, C. (eds.), *Cultural Approaches to the History of Medicine. Mediating Medicine in Early Modern and Modern Europe*, Basingstoke, Palgrave, 2004.

Blaxter, K., Waterlow, J.C. (eds.), *Nutritional adaptation in man*, London, John Libbey, 1985.

Bonzon, T., "Consumption and total Warfare in Paris (1914-1918)", in Trentmann F., Just, F. (eds.), *Food and Conflict in Europe in the Age of the Two World Wars*, Palgrave, New York, 2006, pp. 49-64.

Borowy, I., Grüner, W.D. (eds.), *Facing Illness in Troubled Times. Health in Europe in the Interwar Years 1918-1939*, Frankfurt, Peter Lang, 2005.

Borowy, I., "Crisis as opportunity: International health work during the economic depression", *Dynamis*, No. 28, 2008, pp. 29-51.

Borowy, I., *Coming to terms with world health*, Frankfurt, Peter Lang, 2009.

Boudia, S., Jas, N., "Introduction: Risk and 'Risk Society' in Historical Perspective", *History and Technology*, Vol. 23, No. 4, December 2007, pp. 317-331.

Boudia, S., "Global Regulation: Controlling and Accepting Radioactivity Risks", *History and Technology*, Vol. 23, No. 4, December 2007, pp. 389-406.

Boyce, R., *The Great Interwar Crisis and the Collapse of Globalization*, London, Palgrave Macmillan, 2009.

Brassley, P., Potter, A., "A view From the Top: Social Elites and Food Consumption in Britain, 1930s-1940s", in Trentmann F., Just, F. (eds.), *Food and Conflict in Europe in the Age of the Two World Wars*, Palgrave, New York, 2006, pp. 223-242.

Brown, W., *Edgework: Essays on Knowledge and Politics*, Princeton, Perinceton University Press, 2005.

Brunton, D. (ed.), *Medicine Transformed: Health, Disease and Society in Europe 1800-1930*, Manchester, Manchester University/Open University Press, 2004.

Burnett, J., *Plenty and Want. A Social History of Food in England from 1815 to the Present Day*, London, Routledge, 1989.

Butterly, John R., Shepherd, Jack., *Hunger: the biology and politics of starvation*, Hanover, N.H. Dartmouth College Press: Published by University Press of New England, 2010.

Caballero, B., Popkin, B.M. (eds.), *The nutrition transition: Diet and Disease in the Developing World*, London, Academic Press, 2002.

Cannon, G., *The Politics of Food*, London, 1988.

Caplan, P. (ed.), *Food, Health and Identity*, London, Routledge, 1997.

Carpenter, K.J., A Short History of Nutritional Science, *The Journal of Nutrition*, No. 133, 2003, pp. 638-45, 975-84, 3023-32, 3331-42.

Carpenter, K.J., Nutritional Studies in Victorian Prisons, *The Journal of Nutrition*, No. 136, 2006, pp. 1-8.

Castejón-Bolea, R., Perdiguero-Gil, E., "The closest thing to a mother's milk": the introduction of 'formula milk' and bottle feeding and their medical regulation in Spain (1926-1936)", *Food & History*, Vol. 6, n° 1 (2008), pp. 247-276.

Castejón Bolea, R., Perdiguero Gil, E., "Médicos, regulación estatal y empresas alimentarias en la introducción y consumo de las fórmulas infantiles en España (1900-1936)", in Bernabeu-Mestre, J., Barona, J.L. (eds.), *Nutrición, salud y Sociedad. España y Europa en los siglos XIX-X*, Valencia, SEC/PUV, 2011.

Christensen, T., Lægreid, P., *New Public Management. The transformation of ideas and practice*, Aldershot, Ashgate 2001.

Cinnirella, F., "Optimists or pessimists? A reconsideration of nutritional status in Britain, 1740-1865", *European Review of Economic History*, 2008, No. 12, pp. 325-354.

Cinnirella, F., "On the road to industrialization: nutritional status in Saxony, 1690-1850", *Cliometrica*, No. 2, 2008b, pp. 229-257.

Como vivíamos: alimentos y alimentación en la España del siglo XX, Madrid, 2007.

Contreras Hernández, J., Gracia Arnáiz, M., *Alimentación y cultura. Perspectivas antropológicas*, Ariel, Barcelona, 2005.

Cooter, R., Pickstone, J. (eds.), *Companion to Medicine in the Twentieth Century*, London/New York, Routledge, 2003.

Corni, G., Horst, G., *Brot – Butter- Kanonen. Die Ernährungswirtschaft in Deutschland unter der Diktatur Hitlers*, Berlin, 1994.

Counihan, C., Van Esterik, P. (eds.), *Food and Culture. A Reader*, London/New York, Routledge, 2008.

Crawford, E., *Nationalism and Internationalism in Science, 1880-1939*, Cambridge, Cambridge University Press, 1992.

Cueto, M., *Historia de la Oficina Panamericana de Salud*, Washington, Oficina Panamericana de Salud (OPS), 2005.

Cullather, N., "The Foreign Policy of the Calorie", *The American Historical Review*, Vol. 112, 2007, pp. 337-64.

Cussó Segura, X., "Estado nutritivo de la población española, 1900-1970: análisis de las necesidades y disponibilidades de nutrientes", *Revista de Agricultura e Historia Rural*, Vol. 36, 2005, pp. 329-358.

Cussó Segura, X., Garrobou, R., "La transición nutricional en la España contemporánea: las variaciones en el consumo de pan, patatas y legumbres", *Investigaciones de Historia Económica*, Vol. 7, 2007, pp. 69-100.

Cussó Segura, X., "Transición nutricional y globalización de la dieta en España en los siglos XIX y XX. Un análisis comparado con el caso francés", in Chastagnaret, G. *et al.* (eds.), *Los niveles de vida en España y Francia (Siglos XVIII-XX)*, Alicante, Universidad de Alicante, 2010, pp. 105-128.

Cwiertka, K., "Propagation of Nutritional Knowledge in Poland, 1863 – 1939", in Fenton, A. (ed.), *Order and Disorder: the Health Implications of Eating and Drinking in 19th and 20th Centuries*. East Linton, Tuckwell Press, pp. 96-111, 2000.

Daunton, M., Hilton, M. (eds.), *The Politics of Consumption: Material Culture and Citizenship in Europe and America*, Oxford, Oxford University Press, 2001.

Daunton, M., Trentmann, F. (eds.), *Worlds of Political Economy. Knowledge and Power in the Nineteenth and Twentieth Centuries*, Basingstoke, Palgrave Macmillan, 2006.

Davis, B.J., *Home Fires Burning: Food, Politics and Everyday Life in World War I Berlin*, NC, Chapel Hill, 2000.

Davis, R., Wheatcroft, S., *The Years of Hunger*, Palgrave, Basingstoke, 2004.

De Jonge, J. *et al.*, "How trust in institutions and organizations builds general consumer confidence in the safety of food", *Appetite*, No. 51, 2008, No. 2, 311-7.

De Lavergnée, M., "Alimentation populaire et secours charitables. L'example Parisien, 1840 – 1870", *Food & History*, 5 (2), 2007, pp. 95-127.

De Knecht-Van Eekelen, A., Van Otterloo, A.H., "What the body needs: developments in medical advice, nutritional science an industrial production in thetwentieth century", in Fenton, A. (ed.), *Order and disorder. The health implications ofeating and drinking in the nineteenth and twentieth centuries*, East Linton, Tuckwell Press, 2000, pp. 112-144.

De Onís, M., Blössner, M., "The World Health Organization Global Database on Child Growth and Malnutrition: methodology and applications", *International Journal of Epidemiology*, No. 32, 2003, pp. 518-526.

Del Cura, M.I., Huertas, R., *Alimentación y enfermedad en tiempos de hambre. España, 1937-1947*, Madrid, Consejo Superior de Investigaciones Científicas, 2007.

Del Cura, I., Huertas, R., "The siege of Madrid (1937-1939). Nutritional and clinical studies during theSpanish civil war", *Food & History*, Vol. 6, n° 1, 2008, pp. 193-214.

Del Cura, I., Huertas, R., "Estudios nutricionales en Madrid durante la Guerra Civil espanyola", in Bernabeu-Mestre, J., Barona, J.L. (eds.), *Nutrición, salud y Sociedad. España y Europa en los siglos XIX-XX*, Valencia, SEC/PUV, 2011.

Den Hartog, A., "The Role of Nutrition in Food Advertisements: the Case of the Netherlands", in Den Hartog, A. (ed.), *Food Technology, Science and Marketing. European Diet in the 20th Century*, East Linton, Tuckwell Press, 1995, pp. 268-80.

Den Hartog, A., "The Diffusion of Nutritional Knowledge: Public Health, the Food Industry and Scientific Evidence in the Netherlands in the 19th and 20th centuries", Oddy, D., Petranova, L. (eds.), *The Diffusion of Food Culture in Europe from the Late 18th Century to the Present Day*, Prague, Academia, 2005, pp. 282-94.

De Vries, J., *The Industrious Revolution,* New York/Cambridge, Cambridge University Press, 2008.

De Vooght, D., *The King Invites. Performing Power at a Courtly Dining Table*, Brussels, P.I.E. Peter Lang, 2011.

Dinter, A., *Berlin in Trümmern. Ernährungslage und medizinische Versorgung der Bevölkerung Berlins nach dem II. Weltkrieg*, Berlin, 1999.

Dolowitz, D.P. *et al.*, *Policy Transfer and British Social Policy. Learning from the USA?*, Buckingham-Philadelphia, Open University Press, 2000.

Drèze, J., Sen, A., *The Political Economy of Hunger*, Oxford/New York, Clarendon Press, Oxford University Press, 1990-1991.

Dubin, M., "The League of Nations Health Organization", in Weindling, P. (ed.), *International health organisations and movements, 1918-1939*, Cambridge, Cambridge University Press, 1995, pp. 56-80.

Effosse, S., Ferrière le Vayer, M., *Les entreprises de biens de consummation sous l'occupation*, Tours, Presses Universitaires François Rabelais, 2010.

Elias Roel, A., "La historia de la alimentación en la España moderna. Resultados y problemas", *Obradoiro de Historia Moderna*, No. 2, 1993, pp. 35-64.

Elias, N., *Über den Prozeß der Zivilisation. Soziogenetische und psychogenetische Untersuchungen. Erster Band. Wandlungen des Verhaltens in den weltlichen Oberschichten des Abendlandes* and *Zweiter Band. Wandlungen der Gesellschaft. Entwurf einer Theorie der Zivilisation*, Basel, Verlag Haus zum Falken, 1939 (Published in English as *The Civilizing Process, Vol.I. The History of Manners*, Oxford, Blackwell, 1969, and *The Civilizing Process, Vol. II. State Formation and Civilization*, Oxford, Blackwell, 1982.

Elvbakken, K.T., Lægreid, P., Rykkja, L.H., "Regulation for Safe Food; a Comparison of Five European Countries", *Scandinavian Political Studies*, Vol. 31, No.2, 2008, pp. 125-148.

Ensminger, A. *et al.*, "History of Nutrition", in Ensminger, A. *et al.* (eds.), *Food and Nutrition Encyclopedia*, Boca Raton/London (CRC Press), 1994, 1172-84.

FAO, the first 40 years, Rome, Food and Agriculture Organization of the United Nations, 1985.

Farley, J., *The cast out disease: a history of the International Health Division of the Rockefeller Foundation (1913-1951)*, Oxford, Oxford University Press, 2004.

Fenton, A. (ed.), *Order and disorder. The health implications of eating and drinking in the nineteenth and twentieth centuries*, East Linton, Tuckwell Press, 2000, pp. 112-144.

Feuerhahn, W., Rabault-Feuerhahn, P., "La fabrique internationale de la science: les congrès scientifiques de 1865 à 1945, *Revue Germanique Internationale*, No. 10, 2010, Paris, CNRS, 258 p.

Floud, R.C., Watcher, K.W., "Poverty and physical stature", *Social Science History*, No. 6, 1982, pp. 422-452.

Floud, R.C., Watcher, K.W., Gregory, A.S., *Height, health and history: Nutritional status in Britain, 1750-1980*, Cambridge, Cambridge University Press, 1990.

Floud, R., Fogel, R.W., Harris, B., and Chul Hong, *Diet, Health and work intensity in England and Wales, 1700-1914*, Working Paper 15875, Cambridge, National Bureau of Economic Research, 2010.

Floud, R., Fogel, R.W., Harris, B., Chul Hong, *The Changing Body: Health, Nutrition, and Human Development in the Western World since 1700*, Cambridge, Cambridge University Press, 2011.

Fogel, R.W., *Second Thoughts on the European escape from Hunger: famines, price elasticities, entitlements, chronic malnutrition and mortality rates*, Cambridge, NBER, 1989.

Fogel, R.W., "Economic growth, population theory, and physiology: the bearing of long-term processes on the making of economic policy", *American Economic Review*, No. 84, 1994, pp. 369-395.

Fogel, R.W., *The escape from hunger and premature death, 1700-2100: Europe, America, and the Third World*, Cambridge/New York, Cambridge University Press, 2004.

Forman, P., "The Primacy of Science in Modernity, of Technology in Postmodernity, and of Ideology in the History of Technology", *History and Technology*, No. 23, 2007, 1-152.

Frankenburg, F.R., *Vitamin Discoveries and Disasters. History, Science, and Controversies*, Santa Barbara, Greenwood Press, 2009.

French, M., Phillips J., "Compositional food standards in the United Kingdom: the case of the Willis Inquiry, 1929-1934", in Smith, D.F., Phillips J. (eds.), *Food, Science, Policy and Regulation in the Twentieth Century. International and Comparative Perspectives*, London, Routledge, 2000, pp. 17-36.

French, M., Philips, J., *Cheated not poisoned? Food Regulation in the United Kingdom, 1875 – 1938*, Manchester, Manchester University Press, 2000.

Freeman, R., *The Politics of Health in Europe*, Manchester University Press, Manchester, 2000.

Fressoz, J.-B., "Beck Back in the 19th Century: Towards a Genealogy of Risk Society", *History and Technology*, Vol. 23, No. 4, December 2007, pp. 333-350.

Frohlich, X.Z., *Accounting for Taste: Regulating Food Labeling in the Affluent Society, 1945-1995*, Cambridge, Ma., Massachussets Institute of Technology, 2011.

Frohlich, X.Z., "Imaginer des consommateurs, constituer les sujets: l'étiquetage nutritionnel aux États-Unis, 1945-1995", *Science de la Société*, No. 80, 2011, pp. 11-27.

Galius M., Volkmann, H., *Der Kampf um das tägliche Brot: Nahrungsmangel, Versorgungspolitik und Protest, 1770-1990*, Opladen, 1994.

García-Albea Ristol, E., "Las neuropatías carenciales en Madrid durante la Guerra Civil", *Neurología*, Vol. 14, 1999, pp. 122-9.

Gavroglu, K. *et al.*, "Science and Technology in the European Periphery. Historiographical Reflections", *History of Science*, No. 46, 2008, pp. 153-175.

Geyzen, A., Popular Discourse on Nutrition, Health and Indulgence in Flanders, 1845 – 1960, *Appetite*, No. 56 (2), 2011, pp. 278-83.

Gibbons M., Limoges, C., Nowotny, H., Schwartzman, S., Scott, P., Trow, M., *The New Production of Knowledge. The Dynamics of Science and Research in the Contemporary Societies*, London, Sage, 1994.

Gingras, J., "The Educational (Im)possibility for Dietetics: a Post-structural Discourse Analysis", *Learning Inquiry*, No. 3 (3), 2009, 177-91.

Goodman, N.M., *International Health Organisations and Their Work*, London, Churchill, 1952.

Gracia Arnaiz, M., *Somos lo que comemos. Estudios de alimentación y cultura en España*, Ariel Antropología, Barcelona, 2002.

Gracia Arnaiz M., Comelles, J.M., (eds.), *No comerás. Narrativas sobre comida, cuerpo y género en el nuevo milenio*, Icaria, Observatorio de la Alimentación, Barcelona, 2007.

Graciani, A. *et al.*, *Consumo de alimentos en España en el período 1940-1988*, Madrid, 1986.

Gratzer, W., *Terrors of the Table: The Curious History of Nutrition*, Oxford University Press, Oxford, 2005.

Grigg, D., "The nutritional transition in western Europe", *Journal of HistoricalGeography*, Vol. 22, No. 1, 1995, pp. 247-261.

Gries, R., *Die Rationen-Gesellschaft. Versorgungskampf und Vergleichs-mentalität: Leipzig, München und Köln nach dem Kriege*, Münster, 1991.

Guillem-Llobat, X., Perdiguero, E., "Fighting adulteration in early European food industrialisation. The case of Alicante (Spain)", in Vámos, É. (ed.), *History of the Food Chain. From Agriculture to Consumption and Waste*, Budapest, Hungarian Chemical Society, 2006, pp. 33-40.

Guillem-Llobat, X., "Industrialització i alimentació en la societat valenciana. El control de qualitat dels aliments (1850 – 1939)", in Herran, N. *et al* (eds.),

Synergia: Primer Encuentro de Jóvenes Investigadores en Historia de la Ciencia, Consejo Superior de Investigaciones Cientificas, Madrid, 2006.

Guillem-Llobat, X., *El control de la qualitat dels aliments. El cas valencià en el context internacional (1878-1936)*, Valencia, PUV, 2007.

Guillem-Llobat, X., "El control dels aliments. Una perspectiva històrica", *L'Espill*, 2008a, Vol.29, pp. 153-157.

Guillem-Llobat, X., "El establecimiento de nuevos límites de calidad para los alimentos en el cambio de siglo (1880-1936)", in Ortiz Gomez, T. *et al.* (eds.), *La Experiencia de enfermar en perspectiva histórica. Actas XIV Congreso de la Sociedad Española de Historia de la Medicina*, Granada, Editorial Universidad de Granada, 2008b, pp. 271-274.

Guillem-Llobat, X., "El paper dels laboratoris municipals valencians en el control de qualitat dels aliments (1881-1936)", *Actes del Congrès de la Societat Catalana d'Història de la Ciència i de la Tècnica*, Vol 1, 2008c, pp. 293-300.

Guillem-Llobat, X., "Food quality controls in the European Periphery. Valencian scientists and laboratories in the late nineteenth century", in Simon, J. *et al* (eds.), *Beyond Borders: Fresh perspectives in history of science*, Cambridge Scholars Publishing, Cambridge, 2008d, pp. 301-324.

Guillem-Llobat, X., "Losing the global view in the establishmentof new limits to food quality. The regulationof the food market in Spain (1880-1936), *Food & History*, Vol. 6, n° 1, 2008e, pp. 215-246.

Guillem-Llobat, X., *De la cuina a la fàbrica. L'aliment industrial i el frau. El cas valencià en el context internacional (1878-1936)*, Alacant, Publicacions de la Universitat d'Alacant, 2009.

Guillem-Llobat, X., "The Foundation of a New Site for Food Safety Regulation. The Municipal Chemical Laboratory of València (1881-1936)", in Andresen, A., Gronlie, T., Hubbard, W., Ryymin, T. (eds.), *Healthcare Systems and Medical Institutions*, Bergen, Novus Press, 2009, pp. 142_153.

Guillem Llobat, X., "La regulación de la calidad de los alimentos en el mercado español entre los siglos XIX y XX. Actores e intereses que marcaron tendencias", in Bernabeu-Mestre, J., Barona, J.L. (eds.), *Nutrición, salud y Sociedad. España y Europa en los siglos XIX-XX*, Valencia, SEC/PUV, 2011.

Guillem-Llobat, X., "The sugar industry, political authorities, and scientific institutions in the regulation of saccharin: Valencia (1888-1939)", *Annals of Science*, No. 68, 2011, pp. 401-424.

Gulberg, E., "Food for Future Citizens", *Food, Culture & Society*, No. 9, 2006, pp. 337-43.

Harper, A., (2000), "Recommended dietary allowances and dietary guidance", in Kiple, K., Cornée Ornelas, K. (eds.), *The Cambridge World History of Food*, Cambridge, Cambridge University Press, pp. 1606-21.

Haines, M.R., Steckel, R.H., "Childhood mortality & nutritional status as indicators of standard of living: Evidence from World War I recruits in the United States", *Jahrbuch für Wirtschafts Geschichte*, No. 11, 2000, pp. 43-60.

Harrison, M., *Disease and the Modern World*, Cambridge, Polity Press, 2004.

Harrison, M., "Disease, diplomacy and international comerce: the origins of international sanitary regulation in the nineteenth century", *Journal of Global History*, No. 1, 2006, pp. 197-217.

Heim, S., *Kalorien, Kautschuk, Karrieren. Pflanzenzüchtung und landwirtschaftliche Forschung in Kaiser-Wilhelm-Instituten 1933-1945*, Göttingen, 2003.

Hendrick, H., *Child Welfare. Historical Dimension, Contemporary Debate*, Cambridge, Polity Press, 2003.

Hionidou, V., *Famine and death in occupied Greece, 1941-1944*, Cambridge/New York, Cambridge University Press, 2006.

Hobson, Asher, *The International Institute of Agriculture*, Berkeley, University of California Press, 1931.

Hobson, W., *World Health and History*. Bristol, John Wright, 1963.

Hobsbawm, E., *Industry and Empire. The Birth of the Industrial Revolution*, London, Weidenfield & Nicholson, 1968.

Hobsbawn, E., *The Age of Extremes, 1914-1991*, London, Abacus, 1995.

Horrocks, S.M., "Nutrition Science and the Food and Pharmaceutical Industries in Inter-war Britain", in Smith, D.F. (ed.), *Nutrition in Britain. Science, Scientisits and Politics in the Twentieth Century*, London/New York, Routledge, 1997, pp. 53-74.

Huertas, R., Del Cura, I., "Deficiency Neuropathy in Wartime: The"Paraesthetic-Causalgic Syndrome" described byManuel Peraita during the Spanish Civil War", *Journal of the History of the Neurosciences*, No. 19, 2010, pp. 173-181.

Hyldtoft, O., "Food as Social Marker: a Copenhagen Hospital, c. 1800", *Food & History*, 5: 2, 2007, 131 51.

Irwin, A., *Citizen Science. A Study of People, Expertise and Sustainable Development*, London, Routledge, 1995.

Jacobsen, E., "The Rhetoric of Food: Food as Nature, Commodity and Culture", in Lien, M., Nerlich, B. (eds.), *The Politics of Food*, Oxford/New York, Berg, 2004.

Jaime, P.C., Lock, K., Do School Based Food and Nutrition Policies Improve Diet and Reduce Obesity? *Preventive Medicine*, 48 (1), 2009, 45-53.

Jas, N., "Public Health and Pesticide Regulation in France Before and After *Silent Spring*", *History and Technology*, Vol. 23, No. 4, December 2007, pp. 369-388.

Johnston, B.F., Mellor, J.W., "The Role of Agriculture in EconomicDevelopment", *American Economic Review*, 51(4), 1961, pp. 566-593.

Kamminga, H., Cunningham, A., *The Science and Culture of Nutrition (1840-1940)*, Amsterdam, Rodopi, 1997.

Kamminga, H., "Axes to grind": popularising the science of vitamins, 1920s and 1930s", in Smith D.F., Phillips J. (eds.), *Food, Science, Policy and*

Regulation in the Twentieth Century. International and Comparative Perspectives, London, Routledge, 2000, pp. 83-100.

Kates, R., Millman, S., "On Ending Hunger: The Lessons of History", in Newman, L.F. (ed.), Crossgrove, W. *et al.* (ass.ed.), *Hunger in History: food shortage, poverty and deprivation*, Cambridge, Mass., B. Blackwell, 1990, pp. 389-407.

Kjaernes, U., *Consumer Trust in Food under Varying Social and Institutional Conditions. Threats to Food and Water Chain Infrastructure*, NATO Science for Peace and Security Series, C: Environmental Security, Session I, 2010, pp. 75-86.

Knapp, V., "The Democratization of Meat and protein in Late Eighteenth and Nineteenth- century Europe", *The Historian*, No. 59, 1997, pp. 541-551.

Krausmann, F., "Milk, manure and muscular power. Livestockand the industrialization of agriculture, *Human Ecology*, 2004, No. 32, 735-773.

Komlos, J. (ed.), *Stature, Living Standards and Economic Development*, Chicago, University of Chicago Press, 1994.

Komlos, J., Baten, J. (eds.), "Special Issue: Recent research in Anthropometric History", *Social Science History*, 28 (2), 2004, pp. 191-350.

Komlos, J., "Anthropometric history: an overview of a quarter century of research", *Anthropologischer Anzeiger*, No. 67, 4, 2009, pp. 341-356.

Krimsky, S., Golding, D. (eds.), *Social Theories of Risk*, Westport, CT, Praeger, 1992.

Labisch, A., *Homo Hygienicus. Gesundheit und Medezin in der Neuzeit*, Frankfurt, Campus, 1992.

Landau – Czajka, A., Kreczmar, A., "Diet Patterns in 19th and 20th Century School Manuals", *Acta Poloniae Historica*, No. 85, 2010, 265-84.

Langreo, A., Pujol Andreu, J., "Evolución económica agroalimentaria", *Como vivíamos: alimentos y alimentación en la España del siglo XX*, Madrid, Lunwerg, 2007, pp. 41-66.

Latour, B., Essays on Science and Society: From the World of Science to the World of Research?, *Science*, 5361, 1998, pp. 208-9.

Latour, B., Woolgar, S., *La vie de laboratoire: la production des faits scientifiques*, Paris, La Découverte, 1979.

Latour B., *Politiques de la nature. Comment faire entrer les sciences en démocratie*, Paris, La Découverte, 1999.

Lifton, R.J., The *Nazi Doctors. Medical Killing and the Psychology of Genocide*, New York, Basic Books, 1986.

Lindeboom, M., Portrait, F., Van den Berg, G.J., "Long-run effects on longevity of a nutritional shock early in life: the Dutch Potato Famine of 1846-1847", *International Journal of Epidemiology*, 29 (5), 2010, pp. 617-629.

Livi-Bacci, M., *Population and Nutrition: An Essay on European Demographic History*, Cambridge, Cambridge University Press, 1991.

López Núñez, A., *Los inicios de la protección a la infancia en España*, Madrid, 1992.

Löwy, I., Krigge, J. (eds.), *Images of Disease. Science, Public Policy and Health in Post-war Europe*, Luxembourg, Office for Official Publications of the European Communities, 2001.

Ludvigsen, K., Elvbakken, K.T., *The Public, the Mother and the Child. Public Health Initiatives Promoting the Strong and Happy Child—Focusing on Food and Mental Health*, Bergen, Rokkan Centre for Social Studies, 2005.

Lyngo, I.J. "The Oslo Breakfast. An Optimal Diet in One Meal. On the Scientification of Everyday Life as Exemplified by Food", *Etnologia Scandinavica*, No. 28, 1998, pp. 62-76.

Lyngo, I.J., "The National Nutrition Exhibition. A New Nutritional Narrative in Norway in the 1930s", in Scholliers, P. (ed.), *Food, Drink and Identity*, Oxford/New York, Berg, 2001, pp. 141-161.

Marchisio, S., Di Blasé, A., *The Food and Agriculture Organization*, Dordrecht, 1991.

Maier, C.S., "Between Taylorism and Technocracy: European Ideologies and the Vision of Industrial Productivity in the 1920s", *Journal of Contemporary History*, Vol. 5, 1970, pp. 27-61.

Martínez Carrión, J.M., "Biología, historia y medio ambiente: la estatura como espejo del nivel de vida de la sociedad española", *Ayer*, Vol. 46, 2002, pp. 93-122.

Martínez Carrión, J.M., "El nivel de vida en la España rural. Siglos XVIII-XX. Nuevos enfoques, nuevos resultados", in Martínez Carrión, J.M., Pérez Castejón, J.J. (eds.), *El nivel de vida en la España rural, siglos XVIII-XX*, Alicante, Universidad de Alicante, 2002.

Martínez Carrión, J.M., "El estado nutricional en la Europa contemporánea. Una visión desde la historia antropomètrica", in Bernabeu-Mestre, J., Barona, J.L. (eds.), *Nutrición, salud y Sociedad. España y Europa en los siglos XIX-XX*, Valencia, SEC/PUV, 2011.

Maurer, D., Sobal, J. (eds.), *Eating Agendas: Food and Nutrition as Social Problems*, New York, 1995.

McCalla, A.F., Revoredo, C.L., *Prospects for Global Food Security: A Critical Appraisal of Past Projections and Predictions*, Washington, DC, IFPRI, 2001.

McCalla, A.F., *FAO in the Changing Global Landscape. Working Paper No. 07-006*, Davis University of California, Department of Agricultural and Resource Economics, 2007.

Meng, N.Q., *The long term consequences of famine on survivors: evidence from a unique experiment using China's Great Famine*, Cambridge, Mass., National Bureau of Economic Research, 2009.

Miller, J., Deutsch, J., *Food Studies. An Introduction to Research Methods*, Oxford/New York, Berg, 2009.

Millman, S., Kates, R., "Toward Understanding Hunger", in Newman, L.F. (ed.), Crossgrove, W. *et al.* (ass.ed.), *Hunger in History: food shortage, poverty and deprivation*, Cambridge, Mass., B. Blackwell, 1990, pp. 3-24.

Millman, S. *et al.*, "Organization, Information, and Entitlement in the Emerging Global Food System", in Newman, L.F. (ed.), Crossgrove, W. *et al.* (ass.ed.), *Hunger in History: food shortage, poverty and deprivation*, Cambridge, Mass., B. Blackwell, 1990, pp. 307-330.

Milward, A., Saul, S.B., *The Development of the Economies of Continental Europe*, London, Allen and Unwin, 1977.

Milward, A.S., Martin, B. (eds.), *Agriculture and food supply in the Second World War*, Ostfilden, Scripta Mercaturae, 1985.

Mintz, S.W., "Food and eating: some persisting questions", in Belasco, W., Scranton, P. (eds.), *Food nations. Selling taste in consumer societies*, London/New York, Routledge, 2002, pp. 24-32.

Mitscherlich, A., Mielke, F. (eds.), *Medizin ohne Menschlichkeit: Dokumente des Nürnberger Prozesses*, Frankfurt, Fisher Verlag, 1960.

Mokyr, J., Ó Gráda, C., "What do people die of during famines: the Great Irish Famine in comparative perspective", *European Review of Economic History*, No. 6, 2002, pp 339-363.

Moran, B.T., *Patronage and Institutions: Science, Technology and Medicine at the European Court, 1500-1750*, Woodbridge, Suffolk, Boydell Press, 1991.

Moreno, L.A., Sarría, A., Popkin, B.M., "The nutrition transition in Spain: aEuropean Mediterranean country", *European Journal of Clinical Nutrition*, Vol. 56, 2002, pp. 992-1003.

Moskoff, W., *The bread of affliction: the food supply in the USSR during World War II*, Cambridge, Cambridge University Press, 1990.

Murcott, A. (ed.), *The Nation's Diet. The Social Science of Food Choice*, London/New York, Longman, 1998.

Nafziger, E.W., Stewart, F., Väyrynen, R. (eds.), *War, Hunger and Displacement: the origins of humanitarian emergencies*, New York, Oxford University Press, 2000.

Neill, D., "Finding the Ideal Diet: Nutrition, Culture and Dietary Practices in France and the French Equatorial Africa, 1890s to 1920s", *Food and Foodways*, No. 17, 2009, pp. 1-28.

Newman, L.F. (ed.), Crossgrove, W. *et al.* (ass.ed.), *Hunger in History: food shortage, poverty and deprivation*, Cambridge, Mass., B. Blackwell, 1990.

Nicolau Nos, R., Pujol Andreu, J., "El consumo de proteínas animales en Barcelona entre las décadas de 1830 y 1930: evolución y factores condicionantes", *Investigaciones de Historia Económica*, Vol. 3, 2005, pp. 101-134.

Nicolau Nos, R., Pujol Andreu, J., "Variaciones regionales de los precios de consumo y de las dietas en España, en los inicios de la transición demográfica", *Documents de Treball (UAB. Unitat d'Història Econòmica)*, 2005, No. 29.

Nicolau Nos, R., Pujol Andreu, J., "Alimentación, beneficencia y condiciones de vida en la transformación de las zonas rurales durante la industrialización: Olot, siglos XIX-XX", *Documents de Treball (UAB. Unitat d'Història Econòmica)*, 2005, No. 30.

Nicolau Nos, R., Pujol Andreu, J., "Los factores condicionantes de la transición nutricional en la Europa Occidental: Barcelona, 1890-1936", *Scripta Nova: Revista Electrónica de Geografía y Ciencias Sociales*, Vol. 12, 2008, pp. 256-265.

Nicolau, R., Pujol, J., Hernández, I., "Milk, social acceptance of a new food in Europe: Catalonia, 19th-20th centuries", *Dynamis*, No. 30, 2010, pp. 119-141.

Nicolau, R., Pujol-Andreu, J., "Aspectos políticos y científicos del Modelo de la Transición Nutricional: evaluación crítica y nuevas perspectivas", in Bernabeu-Mestre, J., Barona, J.L. (eds.), *Nutrición, salud y Sociedad. España y Europa en los siglos XIX-X*, Valencia, SEC/PUV, 2011.

Nijs, T. de, "Food Retailing in The Hague, 1914-1930", in Trentmann F. and Just, F. (eds.), *Food and Conflict in Europe in the Age of the Two World Wars*, Palgrave, New York, 2006, pp. 65-87.

Nourrisson, D., "Manger à l'école: une histoire morale", *Food & History*, No. 2, 2004, pp. 227-40.

Nowotny, H., Scott, P., Gibbons, M., *Re-thinking Science. Knowledge and the Public in an Age of Insecurity*, Cambridge, Polity Press, 2001.

Nützenadel, A., "Dictating Food: Autarchy, Food Provision, and Consumer Politics in Fascist Italy, 1922-1943", in Trentmann, F., Just, F. (eds.), *Food and Conflict in Europe in the Age of the Two World Wars*, Palgrave, New York, 2006, pp.88-108.

Oddy, D., Petranova, L. (eds.), *The diffusion of food culture in Europe from the late eighteenth century to the present day*, Prague, Academia, 2005, pp. 282-294.

Omran, A.R., "The Epidemiologic Transition. A Theory of the Epidemiology of Population Change", *The Milbank Quarterly*, Vol. 83, nº 4, 1971, pp. 731-757.

Ó Gráda, C., *Famine: A Short History*, Princeton, Princeton University Press, 2009.

Ó Gráda, C., *Ireland's great famine: interdisciplinary perspectives*, Dublin, University College, 2006.

Osokina, E.A., *Our daily bread: socialist distribution and the art of survival in Stalin's Russia, 1927-1941*, Translated and edited by K. Transcheld and G. Bucher, Armonk NY, M.E. Sharpe, 2001.

Paquy, L., "Santé publique, repression des frauds et action municipal à la fin du XIXe siècle: le laboratoire grenoblois d'analyses alimentaires", *Revue d'Histoire Moderne et Contemporaine*, No. 51, 2004, pp. 44-65.

Pasternak, A., *Inhuman Research. Medical Experiments in German Concentration Camps*, Budapest, HUN Akadémiai Kiadí, 2006.

Paul, V.C., *The Politics of Hunger: the allied blockade of Germany, 1915-1919*, Athens, Ohio, Ohio University Press, 1985.

Pemberton, J., White, J. "The Boyd Orr Survey of the Nutrition of Children in Britain, 1937-1939", *History Workshop Journal*, No. 50, 2000, pp. 205-29.

Perdiguero, E., "On Food. The popularization of nutrition in Internar Spain", in Andresen, A., Gronlie, T. (eds.), *Transferring Medico-Political Knowledge in 19thand 20th-Century Europe*, Bergen, Stein Rokkan Centre for Social Studies, 2007.

Perdiguero-Gil, E., Castejón-Bolea, R., "Popularising right food and feedingpractices in Spain (1847-1950). The handbooks of domestic economy", *Dynamis*, No. 30, 2010, pp. 141-165.

Pestre, D., *Science, argent et politique. Un essai d'interprétation*, Paris, INRA Editions, 2003.

Pestre, D. "Postface. The Historical Heritage of the 19th and 20th Centuries: Techno-science, Markets and Regulations in a Long-term Perspective", *History and Technology*, Vol. 23, No. 4, December 2007, pp. 407-420.

Pestre, D., "Challenges for the Democratic Management of Technoscience: Governance, Participation and the Political Today", *Science as Culture*, No. 17, 2008, pp. 101-119.

Philipott, J., "How Healthy are Government Dietary Guidelines? Part 1. Origin and Evolution of Dietary Guidelines", *The Nutrition Practitioner*, Summer, 2009, pp. 1-15.

Phillips, R.W., *FAO, its Origins, Formation and Evolution 1945-1981*, Rome, FAO, 1981.

Popkin, B., *The World Is Fat--The Fads, Trends, Policies, and Products That Are Fattening the Human Race*, New York, Avery-Penguin Press, 2008.

Porter, D. (ed.), *The History of Public Health and the Modern State*, Amsterdam, Rodopi, 1994.

Porter, R. (ed.), *The Popularisation of Medicine 1650-1850*, London, Routledge, 1992.

Power, M. *The Risk Management of Everything*, Londres, Demos, 2004.

Pozzi, L., Breschi, M. (eds.), *Salute, malatia e sopravivenza in Italia fra '800 e '900*, Udine, Editrice Democratica Sarda, 2000.

Pozzi, L., *La lotta per la vita: evoluzione e geografia della sopravvivenza in Italia fra '800 e '900*, Udine, Forum, 2000.

Proctor, R.N., *Racial Hygiene: Medicine under the Nazis*, Cambridge, Mass., Harvard University Press, 1988.

Pujol Andreu, J., Nicolau Nos, J., "El consumo de proteínas animales en Barcelona entre las décadas de 1830 y 1930: evolución y factores condicionantes", *Investigaciones de Historia Económica*, No. 3, 2005, pp. 101-134.

Pujol Andreu, J., Nicolau Nos, J., "El consumo de leche fresca en Cataluña entre mediados del siglo XIX y 1935: la difusión de un nuevo alimento", *Historia Agraria*, No. 42, 2007, pp. 303-326.

Rabier, Ch. (ed.), *Fields of Expertise: A Comparative History of Experts Procedures in Paris and London, 1600 to Present*, Cambridge, Cambridge Scholars Publishing, 2007.

Rasmussen, A., "Les Congrès internationaux liés aux Expositions universelles de Paris (1867-1900)", *Mil neuf cent. Revue d'histoire intellectuelle*, No. 7, 1989, pp. 23-44.

Rawlings, E., "Choosing Health? Exploring Children's Eating Practices at Home and at School", *Antipode*, No. 4, 2009, pp. 1084-109.

Rodríguez Ocaña, E., "La salud pública en España, en el contexto europeo, 1890-1925", *Revista de Sanidad e Higiene Pública*, No. 68, (1994), pp. 11-28.

Rodríguez Ocaña, E., "The making of the Spanish Public Health Administration during the First Third of the Twentieth Century", *Quaderni Internazionali di Storia della Medicina e della Sanità*, No. 3, 1994, pp. 49-65.

Rodríguez Ocaña, E., Bernabeu Mestre, J., Barona, J.L., "La Fundación Rockefeller y España, 1914-1936. Un acuerdo para la modernización científica y sanitaria", in García, J.L., Moreno, J.M., Ruiz, G. (eds.), *Estudios de historia de las técnicas, la arqueología industrial y las ciencias*, Vol. 2, Salamanca, Junta de Castilla y León, 1998, pp. 531-9.

Rodríguez Ocaña, E., "Foreign Expertise, Political Pragmatism and Professional Elite: The Rockefeller Foundation in Spain, 1919-39", *Studies in History and Philosophy and Biomedical Science*, No. 31, 2000, pp. 447-61.

Roemer, M.I., "Internationalism and Public Health", *Companion Encyclopaedia of the History of Medicine*, London, Routledge, 1993, p. 1417-35.

Roodhouse, M., "Popular Morality and the Black Market in Britain, 1939-1955", in Trentmann, F., Just, F. (eds.), *Food and Conflict in Europe in the Age of the Two World Wars*, New York, Palgrave, 2006, pp. 243-265.

Rose, N., *The politics of life itself: Biomedicine, Power, and Subjectivity in the Twenty- First Century*. Princeton, Princeton University Press, 2006.

Rosen, G., *A History of Public Health. Introduction by Elizabeth Fee: Biographical Essay and New Bibliography by Edward T. Morman*, Baltimore, Johns Hopkins University Press, 1993.

Rosenberg, E.S., *Financial Missionaries to the World: The Politics and Culture of Dollar Diplomacy, 1900-1930*, Cambridge MA, Harvard University Press, 1999.

Rossi, P., *I filosofi e le machine 1400-1700*, Milano, Feltrinelli, 2002.

Rotberg, R.I., Raab, T.K., *Hunger and History. The Impact of Changing Food Production and Consumption Patterns of Society*, Cambridge, Cambridge University Press, 1985.

Rouse, J., *Knowledge and Power. Towards a political philosophy of science*, Ithaca/London, Cornell Univ. Press, 1987.

Rumm-Kreuter, D., "Comparison of the eating and cooking habits of Northern Europe and the Mediterranean countries in the past, present and future", *International Journal for Vitamins and Nutrition Research*, No. 71, 2000, pp. 141-148.

Ruxin, J., "The United Nations Protein Advisory Group", in Smith, D.F., Phillips, J. (eds.), *Food, Science, Policy and Regulation in the Twentieth*

Century: International and Comparative Perspectives, London, Routledge, 2000, pp. 151-166.

Ryymin, T., "Tuberculosis-threatened Children. The Rise and Fall of a Medical Concept, *c.* 1900-60", in Andresen, A., Grønlie, T., Ryymin, T. (eds.), *Transferring Medico-Political Knowledge in Nineteenth- and Twentieth-Century Europe*, Bergen, Rokkan Centre for Social Studies, 2007.

Ryymin T., "Tuberculosis-threatened Children. The Rise and Fall of a Medical Concept in Norway, *c.* 1900-60", *Medical History*, Vol. 52, 2008, pp. 347-64.

Sabaté y Cañellas, F., "Las encuestas de alimentación y nutrición en España. Bibliografía 1939-1979", *Revista de Sanidad e Higiene Pública*, Vol. 58, 1984, pp. 117-1132.

Schneeman, B., "Evolution of dietary guidelines", *Journal of the American Dietetic Association*, No. 2, 2003 (supplement), pp. 5-9.

Scholliers, P. (ed.), *Food, drink and identity. Cooking, eatingand drinking in Europe since the Middle Ages*, Oxford/New York, Berg, 2001.

Scholliers, P., *Food culture in Belgium*, Westport/London, Greenwood Press, 2008.

Scholliers, P., Van den Eeckhout, P., "Hearing the Consumer? The Laboratory, the Public, and the Construction of Food Safety in Brussels (1840s - 1910s)", *Journal of Social History*, Summer 2011, pp. 1143 – 59.

Scott, J.C., *Seeing like a State: How Certain Schemes to Improve the Human Condition Have Failed*, New Haven, Yale University Press, 1998.

Scrimshaw, N., Gordon, J.E., *Malnutrition, learning, and behaviour.* Cambridge, Mass., The MIT Press, 1968.

Scrimshaw, N., "World Nutritional Problems", in Newman, L.F. (ed.), Crossgrove, W. *et al.* (ass.ed.), *Hunger in History: food shortage, poverty and deprivation*, Cambridge, Mass., B. Blackwell, 1990, pp. 353-373.

Secord, J.A., "Knowledge in transit", *Isis*, No. 95 (4), 2004, pp. 654-672.

Segers, Y., "Food Recommendations, Tradition and Change in a Flemish Cookbook: *Ons Kookboek*, 1920 – 2000", *Appetite*, No. 45 (1), pp. 4-14.

Sen, A.K., *Poverty and Famines. An Essay on Entitlement and Deprivation*, Oxford, Oxford University Press, 1982.

Sen, A.K., "Food Entitlement and Economic Chains", in Newman, L.F. (ed.), Crossgrove, W. *et al.* (ass.ed.), *Hunger in History: food shortage, poverty and deprivation*, Cambridge, Mass., B. Blackwell, 1990, pp. 374-386.

Shaw, J., *World Food Security. A History since 1945*, Hampshire, Palgrave Macmillan, 2007.

Simon, J., Herrán, N., Lanuza-Navarro, T., Ruiz-Castell, P., Guillem-Llobat, X. (eds.), *Beyond Borders: Fresh perspectivas in history of science*, Newcastle, Cambridge Scholars Publishing, 2008.

Simón Pérez, H., J. Escudero, A., "El bienestar en España: una perspectiva de largo plazo, 1850-1991", *Revista de Historia Económica*, Vol. 2, 2003, pp. 525-566.

Slater, D., *Consumer Culture and Modernity*, Cambridge, 1997.

Smith, D.F., (ed.), *Nutrition in Britain: Science, Scientists and Politics in the Twentieth Century*, London/New York, 1997.

Smith, D., "The Discourse of Scientific Knowledge of Nutrition and Dietary Change in the 20th Century", in Murcott, A. (ed.), *The Nation's Diet. The Social Science of Food Choice*, London/New York, Longman, 1998, pp. 311-31.

Smith, D.F., Phillips J. (eds.), *Food, Science, Policy and Regulation in the Twentieth Century. International and Comparative Perspectives*, London, Routledge, 2000.

Smith, D.F., "The rise and fall of the Scientific Food Committee during the Second World War", in Smith, D.F., Phillips, J. (eds.), *Food, Science, Policy and Regulation in the Twentieth Century. International and Comparative Perspectives*, London, Routledge, 2000. pp. 101-116.

Spiekermann, U., "Brown Bread for Victory: German amd British Wholemeal Politics in the Inter-War Period", in Trentmann, F., Just, F. (eds.), *Food and Conflict in Europe in the Age of the Two World Wars*, New York, Palgrave, 2006, pp.143-171.

Stanziani, A., *Histoire de la qualité alimentaire: XIXe-XXe siècle*, Paris, Editions du Seuil, 2005.

Stanziani, A., "Negotiating innovation in a market economy: foodstuffs and beverages adulteration in 19th century France", *Enterprise and society*, No. 8, 2007, pp. 375-412.

Staples, A.L.S., *The Birth of Development. How the World Bank, Food and Agriculture Organization, and World Health Organisation Changed the World, 1945-1965*, Kent, The Kent State University Press, 2006.

Stearns, P., *Fat History. Bodies and Beauty in the Modern West*, New York, New York University Press, 2002.

Steckel, R.H., "Stature and the standard of living", *Journal of Economic Literature*, No. 33, 1995, pp. 1903-1940.

Steckel, R.H., Rose J.C. (eds.), *The Backbone of History. Health and Nutrition in the Western Hemisphere*, Cambridge, Cambridge University Press, 2002.

Steckel, R.H., "Heights and human welfare: Recent developments and new directions", *Explorations in Economic History*, No. 46 (1), 2009, pp. 1-23.

Stüber, G., *Der Kamps gegen den Hunger, 1945-1950: die Ernëhrungslage in der britishen Zone Deutschland...*, Neumünster, K. Wachholtz, 1984.

Svedberg, P., *Poverty and undernutrition. Theory, measurement, and policy, With a foreword by Amartya Sen*, Oxford, Oxford University Press, 2000.

Szreter, S., Woolcock, M., "Health by association? Social capital, social theory, and the political economy of public health", *International Journal of Epidemiology*, No. 33, 2004, pp. 650-667.

Szreter, S., *Health and Wealth: Studies in History and Policy.* Rochester, Rochester University Press, 2005.

Taithe, B., *Defeated flesh. Welfare, warfare and the making of modern France*, Manchester, Manchester University Press, 1999.

Tanner, J.M., *A history of the study of human growth*, Cambridge, Cambridge University Press, 1981.

Tanner, J.M., "Growth as a mirror of conditions in society", in Lindgren, G. (ed.), *Growth as a mirror of conditions in society*, Stockholm, Stockholm Institute Education Press, 1990.

Tanner, J.M., "Growth as a measure of the nutritional and hygienic status of a population", *Hormone Research*, No. 38, 1992, pp. 106-115.

Tanner, J., *Fabrikmahlzeit: Ernährungswissenschaft, Industriearbeit und Volksernährung in der Schweiz, 1890 – 1950*, Zürich, Chronos, 1999.

Tauger, M., "Stalin, Soviet Agriculture, and Collectivisation", in Trentmann, F., Just, F. (eds.), *Food and Conflict in Europe in the Age of the Two World Wars*, New York, Palgrave, 2006, pp. 109-142.

Teuteberg, H.J., "The Discovery of Vitamins: Laboratory, Research, Reception and Industrial Production", in Fenton, A. (ed.), *Order and Disorder: the Health Impications of Eating and Drinking in the 19th and 20th Centuries*, East Linton, Tuckwell Press, 2000.

Thoms, U., "Industrial Canteens in Germany, 1850-1950", in Jacobs, M., Scholliers, P. (eds.), *Eating Out in Europe*, Oxford/New York, Berg, 2003, pp. 351-72.

Thoms, U., "From Cooking to Consultation: the Professionalization of Dietary Assistants in Germany, 1890 – 1980", in Oddy, D., Petranova, L. (eds.), *The Diffusion of Food Culture in Europe from the Late 18th Century to the Present Day*, Prague, Academia, 2005, pp. 107-18.

Thoms, U., *Anstaltskost im Rationalisierungsprozess. Die Ernährung in Krankenhäusern und Gefängnissen im 18. Und 19. Jahrhundert*, Stuttgart, F. Steiner Verlag, 2005.

Thoms, U., "Learning from America? The travels of German nutritional scientist to the USA in the Context of the technical Assistance Program of the Mutual Security Agencies and its consequences for West German Nutritional Policy", *Food and History*, 2004, Vol. 2, pp. 117-151.

Touraine, A., *Comment sortir du libéralisme*, Paris, Fayard, 1999.

Toussaint-Samat, M., *A history of food*, Chichester-Malden, Wiley-Blackwell, 2009.

Treitel, C., "Max Rübner and the Biopolitics of Rational Nutrition", *Central European History*, No. 41, 2008, pp. 1-25.

Trentmann F., Just, F. (eds.), *Food and Conflict in Europe in the Age of the Two World Wars*, New York, Palgrave, 2006.

Trentmann, F., "Coping with Shortage: The Problem of Food Security and Global Visions of Coordination, *c.* 1890s-1950", in Trentmann F., Just, F. (eds.), *Food and Conflict in Europe in the Age of the Two World Wars*, New York, Palgrave, 2006, pp. 13-48.

Trittel, G., *Hunger und Politik. Die Ernährungskrise in der Bizone (1945-1949)*, Frankfurt/New York, 1990.

Tucker, T., *The Great Starvation Experiment: Ancel Keys and the Men Who Starved for Science*, Minneapolis, University of Minnesota Press, 2007.

Van der Zee, H.A., *The Hunger Winter: occupied Holland 1944-5*, London, J. Norman & Hobhouse, 1982.

Van Otterloo, A., "Dutch Food Culture and its Cookery Teachers: the Rise, Diffusion and Decline of a Tradition (1880 – 1980)", Oddy, D., Petranova, L. (eds.), *The Diffusion of Food Culture in Europe from the Late 18th Century to the Present Day*, Prague, Academia, 2005, pp. 96-106.

Velasco, C., Rodergas, R., "Los productos alimenticios y la publicidad", *Como vivíamos: alimentos y alimentación en la España del siglo XX*, Madrid, Lunwerg, 2007, pp. 119-138.

Vereecken, C. *et al.*, "Food Consumption among Pre-schoolers. Does the School Make a Difference?" *Appetite*, No. 51, 2008, pp. 723-6.

Vernon J., "The Ethics of Hunger and the Assembly of Society: The Techno-Politics of the School Meal in Modern Britain", *American Historical Review*, Vol. 110, 2005, pp. 693-725.

Vernon, J., *Hunger. A Modern History*, Cambridge, Harvard University Press, 2007.

Viaje a las Hurdes. El manuscrito inédito de Gregorio Marañón y las fotografías de la visita de Alfonso XIII, Madrid, El País-Aguilar, 1993.

Villalbí, J.R., Maldonado, R., "La alimentación de la población en España desde la posguerra hasta los años ochenta: una revisión crítica de las encuestas de nutrición", *Med Clin Barc*, Vol. 90, No. 3, 1988, pp. 127-130.

Wanjek, Ch., *Food at work: workplace solutions for malnutrition, obesity and chronic diseases*, Geneva, International Labour Organization, 2005.

Warde, A., *Consumption, Food and Taste. Culinary Antinomies and Commodity Culture*, London, Sage, 1997.

Welshman, J., "School meals and milk in England and Wales, 1906 -1945", *Medical History*, 41: 1, 1997, pp. 6-29.

Weindling, P. "Public Health and Political Stabilisation: The Rockefeller Foundation in Central and Eastern Europe between the two World Wars", *Minerva*, No. 31, 1993, 253-67.

Weindling, P., "Social Medicine at the League of Nations Health Organisation and the International Labour Office Compared", in Weindling, P. (ed.), *International Health Organisations and Movements, 1918-1939*, Cambridge, Cambridge University Press, 1995, pp. 134-53.

Weindling, P., "The Role of International Organizations in Setting Nutritional Standards in the 1920s and 1930s", *Clio Médica*, Vol. 32, 1995, pp. 319-332.

Weindling, P. "Philantropy and World Health: The Rockefeller Foundation and the League of Nations Health Organisation", *Minerva*, No. 35, 1997, 13 p.

Weindling, P. "Health and Medicine in Interwar Europe", in Cooter, R., Pickstone, J. (eds.), *Companion to Medicine in the Twentieth Century*, London, 2003, pp.29-50.

Weindling, P., *Nazi Medicine and the Nuremberg Trials: From Medical War Crimes to Informed Consent*, New York, Palgrave Macmillan, 2005.

Wildt, M., "Promise of more. The rhetoric of (food) consumption in a society searching for itself: West Germany in the 1950s", in Scholliers P. (ed.),

Food, drink andidentity. Cooking, eating and drinking in Europe since the Middle Ages, Oxford/New York, Berg, 2005, pp. 63-80.

Wilt, A.F., *Food for War. Agriculture and Rearmament in Britain before the Second World War*, Oxford, Oxford University Press, 2001.

Wolf, J.H., *Don't Kill your Baby: Public Health and the Decline of Breastfeeding in the Nineteenth and Twentieth Centuries*, Columbus, Ohio University Press, 2001.

Worboys, M., "The Discovery of Colonial Malnutrition between the Wars", in Arnold D. (ed.), *Imperial Medicine and Indigenous Society*, Manchester, Manchester University Press, 1988, pp. 208-25.

Worboys, M., *Spreading Germs: Disease, Theories, and Medical Practice in Britain, 1865-1900*, New York, Cambridge University Press, 2000.

Zweiniger-Bargielowska, I., *Austerity in Britain: rationing, controls and consumption, 1939-1955*, Oxford, Oxford University Press, 2000.

European Food Issues

For several decades now, our attention has been drawn to expanding agricultural output and the proliferation of powerful food companies. At the same time, in the process of European integration, the adoption of the Codex Alimentarius (1963), the Food Law (2002), and the recognition of PGIs for many products have contributed to the creation of a common European "food space". Today, these systems of supply and distribution have between them given Europeans quite varied dietary possibilities. This situation stems from various developments, linking the economic to the technical and amounting to a long-term trend. Cultural issues bear upon this, whether culinary transmission from generation to generation or the increasingly diverse catering sector, and political decisions also contribute through the establishment of standards and regulations. Hence, traditions and ruptures, innovations and continuities are permanently unsettling the European diet. Using original sources, doctoral theses, conference papers, monographs and testimonies, this series examines historical developments at the national scale and also, more generally, in a transnational perspective. The series hopes to make a significant contribution to understanding the processes of food innovation, which are powerful factors of difference and identity in contemporary Europe.

Series editors:

Antonella CAMPANINI, Università degli Studi di Scienze Gastronomische, Pollenzo (Italia)

Peter SCHOLLIERS, Vrije Universiteit Brussel (België)

Jean-Pierre WILLIOT, Université François-Rabelais de Tours (France)

Editorial Board:

Virginie AMILIEN, SIFO, Oslo, (Norge)
Peter ATKINS, Durham University (UK)
Alberto CAPATTI, Università degli Studi di Scienze Gastronomiche, Pollenzo (Italia)
Jesús CONTRERAS, Universitat de Barcelona (España)
Jean-Pierre DEVROEY, Université Libre de Bruxelles (Belgique)
Henry NOTAKER, Bergen (Norge)
Massimo MONTANARI, Alma Mater Studiorum – Università di Bologna (Italia)
Jean-Robert PITTE, Université Paris-Sorbonne (France)

Series Titles

N° 1 – Antonella CAMPANINI, Peter SCHOLLIERS et Jean-Pierre WILLIOT (dir.), *Manger en Europe. Patrimoines, échanges, identités*, 2011.

N° 2 – Daniëlle DE VOOGHT, *The King Invites. Performing Power at a Courtly Dining Table*, 2012.

N° 3 – Josep L. BARONA, *From Hunger to Malnutrition. The Political Economy of Scientific Knowledge in Europe, 1918-1960*, 2012.

P.I.E. Peter Lang – The website

Discover the general website of the Peter Lang publishing group

www.peterlang.com

For the avoidance of doubt, input of the whole or any part of this publication into any generative artificial intelligence model, chatbot, program, software or technology is expressly prohibited without the prior written consent of the publisher.